Adventure and Extreme Sports Injuries

Omer Mei-Dan • Michael R. Carmont
Editors

Adventure and Extreme Sports Injuries

Epidemiology, Treatment, Rehabilitation and Prevention

Springer

Editors
Omer Mei-Dan
School of Medicine
Department of Orthopaedics
University of Colorado
Aurora
USA

CU Sports Medicine,
Boulder, Colorado
USA

Michael R. Carmont
The Department of Orthopaedic Surgery
Princess Royal Hospital
Shrewsbury and Telford NHS Trust
Telford
UK

The Department of Orthopaedic Surgery
The Northern General Hospital
Sheffield Teaching Hospitals NHS
Foundation Trust
Sheffield
UK

ISBN 978-1-4471-4362-8   ISBN 978-1-4471-4363-5 (eBook)
DOI 10.1007/978-1-4471-4363-5
Springer London Heidelberg New York Dordrecht

Library of Congress Control Number: 2012953003

© Springer-Verlag London 2013
This work is subject to copyright. All rights are reserved by the Publisher, whether the whole or part of the material is concerned, specifically the rights of translation, reprinting, reuse of illustrations, recitation, broadcasting, reproduction on microfilms or in any other physical way, and transmission or information storage and retrieval, electronic adaptation, computer software, or by similar or dissimilar methodology now known or hereafter developed. Exempted from this legal reservation are brief excerpts in connection with reviews or scholarly analysis or material supplied specifically for the purpose of being entered and executed on a computer system, for exclusive use by the purchaser of the work. Duplication of this publication or parts thereof is permitted only under the provisions of the Copyright Law of the Publisher's location, in its current version, and permission for use must always be obtained from Springer. Permissions for use may be obtained through RightsLink at the Copyright Clearance Center. Violations are liable to prosecution under the respective Copyright Law.
The use of general descriptive names, registered names, trademarks, service marks, etc. in this publication does not imply, even in the absence of a specific statement, that such names are exempt from the relevant protective laws and regulations and therefore free for general use.
While the advice and information in this book are believed to be true and accurate at the date of publication, neither the authors nor the editors nor the publisher can accept any legal responsibility for any errors or omissions that may be made. The publisher makes no warranty, express or implied, with respect to the material contained herein.

Printed on acid-free paper

Springer is part of Springer Science+Business Media (www.springer.com)

About the Authors

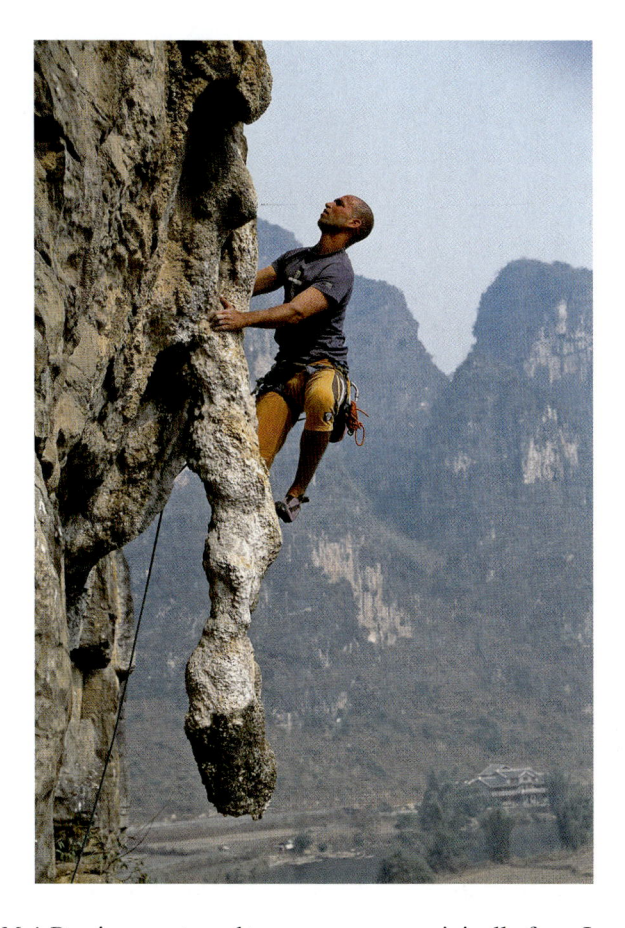

Dr. Omer Mei-Dan is a sports and trauma surgeon, originally from Israel, now practices in University of Colorado, located in Denver and Boulder, near the mountains he adores. Omer is a world renown extreme sports athlete himself who has been involved for more than 20 years in numerous disciplines within this area and was responsible for the establishment and production of many innovative events.

His achievements vary from mountaineering first ascents to be part of the evolvement of the sports of wing-suit flying and base jumping. In the past years Omer is involved in extreme sports research, mainly in the areas of climbing and base jumping injuries but also observing the mental characteristics and hormonal aspects of extreme sports athletes.

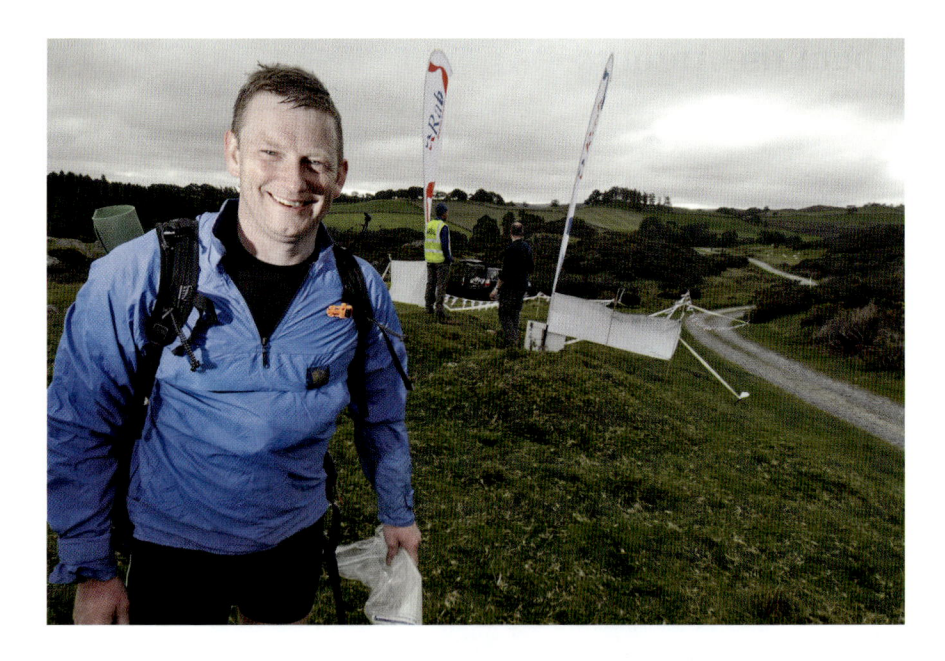

Mr. Mike Carmont is a knee and foot and ankle Orthopedic Surgeon from the north of England. He has competed at adventure sports for the last 20 years fell racing, orienteering, mountain bike orienteering and moutain marathon racing up to elite level and has completed the Devizes to Westminster Kayak marathon twice.

He has researched kayak and mountain bike injuries and has written many articles and scientific papers on this and other sports injuries. He is an instructor on several event side resuscitation courses.

Contents

1. **The Management of the Extreme Sports Athlete** 1
   Omer Mei-Dan and Michael R. Carmont

2. **Rock and Ice Climbing** 7
   Volker Schöffl

3. **Alpine Skiing and Snowboarding Injuries** 37
   Mike Langran

4. **Skydiving** 69
   Anton Westman

5. **BASE Jumping** 91
   Omer Mei-Dan

6. **Whitewater Canoeing and Rafting** 113
   Jonathan P. Folland and Kate Strachan

7. **Surfing Injuries** 143
   Andrew T. Nathanson

8. **Kite Surfing and Snow Kiting** 173
   Mark Tauber and Philipp Moroder

9. **Windsurfing** 189
   Daryl A. Rosenbaum and Bree Simmons

10. **Sailing and Yachting** 203
    Michael R. Carmont

11. **Mountain Biking Injuries** 225
    Michael R. Carmont

12. **Paragliding** 247
    Lior Laver and Omer Mei-Dan

13	**Mountain, Sky, and Endurance Running**	273
	Denise Park and Michael R. Carmont	
14	**Personality Characteristics in Extreme Sports Athletes: Morbidity and Mortality in Mountaineering and BASE Jumping**	303
	Erik Monasterio	
15	**Endocrine Aspects and Responses to Extreme Sports**	315
	Karen Tordjman, Naama Constantini, and Anthony C. Hackney	
16	**Preventing Injuries in Extreme Sports Athletes**	325
	John Nyland and Yee Han Dave Lee	
17	**Rehabilitation of Extreme Sports Injuries**.	339
	Peter Malliaras, Dylan Morrissey, and Nick Antoniou	
Index		363

Contributors

Nick Antoniou Melbourne Hand Therapy, Elgar Hill Medical Suites, Suite 7, 28 Arnold Street, Box Hill 3128, Melbourne, VIC, Australia

Michael R. Carmont, FRCS (Tr&Orth) The Department of Orthopaedic Surgery, Princess Royal Hospital, Shrewsbury and Telford NHS Trust, Telford, UK

The Department of Orthopaedic Surgery, The Northern General Hospital, Sheffield Teaching Hospitals NHS Foundation Trust, Sheffield, UK

Naama Constantini Department of Orthopedic Surgery, Sport Medicine Center, The Hadassah-Hebrew University Medical Center, Jerusalem, Israel

Lee Yee Han Dave, M.D. Division of Sports Medicine, Department of Orthopaedic Surgery, University of Louisville, Louisville, KY, USA

Jonathan P. Folland, Ph.D., FACSM School of Sport, Exercise and Health Sciences, Loughborough University, Sir John Beckwith Centre for Sport, Loughborough, Leics, UK

Anthony C. Hackney Endocrine Section-Applied Physiology Laboratory, Department of Exercise and Sport Science, University of North Carolina, Chapel Hill, NC, USA

Mike Langran Health Centre, Aviemore, Inverness-Shire, Scotland, UK

Lior Laver, M.D. Department of Orthopaedics and Sports Medicine Unit, "Meir" Medical Center, Kfar-Saba, Israel

Peter Malliaras Centre for Sports and Exercise, Queen Mary, University of London, Mile End Hospital, London, UK

Omer Mei-Dan, M.D. Division of Sports Medicine, Department of Orthopaedic Surgery, University of Colorado School of Medicine, Aurora, CO, USA

CU Sports Medicine, Boulder, Colorado, USA

Erik Monasterio Department of Psychological Medicnine,
University of Otago, Christchurch School of Medicine,
Christchurch, New Zealand

Philipp Moroder, M.D. Shoulder and Elbow Service, ATOS Clinic Munich,
Munich, Germany

Department of Traumatology and Sports Injuries,
Paracelsus Medical University Salzburg, Salzburg, Austria

Dylan Morrissey Centre for Sports and Exercise, Queen Mary,
University of London, Mile End Hospital, London, UK

Andrew T. Nathanson, M.D., FACEP Department of Emergency Medicine,
Alpert School of Medicine at Brown University, Injury Prevention Center,
Rhode Island Hospital, Providence, RI, USA

John Nyland, DPT, SCS, EdD, ATC, CSCS, FACSM Division of Sports
Medicine, Department of Orthopaedic Surgery, University of Louisville,
Louisville, KY, USA

Denise Park, M.Sc., MCSP, SRP Grad Dip Phys Denise Park Practice,
Clitheroe, UK

Daryl A. Rosenbaum, M.D. Department of Family and Community Medicine,
Wake Forest University School of Medicine, Winston, Salem, NC, USA

Volker Schöffl, Ph.D., M.D., MHBA Department of Sportsorthopedics
and Sportsmedicine, Orthopedic and Trauma Surgery, Klinikum Bamberg,
Sozialstiftung Bamberg, Bamberg, FRG, Germany

Bree Simmons, M.D. Wake Forest University School of Medicine,
Winston, Salem, NC, USA

Kate Strachan, MBChB, MRCGP, M.Sc., DRCOG FFSEM(UK) English
Institute of Sport – East Midlands, EIS/Loughborough Performance Centre,
Loughborough, Leics, UK

Mark Tauber, M.D., Ph.D. Shoulder and Elbow Service, ATOS Clinic Munich,
Munich, Germany

Karen Tordjman Institute of Endocrinology, Metabolism, and Hypertension,
Tel Aviv-Sourasky Medical Center, Tel Aviv, Israel

Sackler Faculty of Medicine, Tel Aviv University, Tel Aviv, Israel

Anton Westman, M.D., Ph.D. Department of Physiology and Pharmacology,
Karolinska Institutet, Stockholm, Sweden

Introduction

Adventure and extreme sports have developed significantly and gained enormous popularity over the past two decades, and are now performed by adventurous elite athletes as well as the recreational adventure sportsman. These sports, by definition, involve elements of increased risk, and are usually performed in beautiful, exciting and remote locations or in extreme environments, far away from medical assistance.

Mass media interest, lifestyle factors and a youth culture lead to an increased extreme sport's audience appeal. The impressive film footage of these sports, including breath-taking stunts, has attracted not only sports fans but also major television networks, their audiences and advertising, with it associated financial investment. The published footage frequently shows spectacular crashes and near misses but rarely shows injuries or fatalities.

The risks involved with these sports are often highlighted by the media, usually after a reported accident or fatality. These risks may vary according to the involvement of the participant. To the general public the challenge may seem unsurmountible and expose the participant to profound risk, and yet the event may be the culmination of hours of training and preparation. Every aspect of the activity may have been considered with safety being the paramount concern. Like everything else in life, it all depends on the eye of the beholder.

A wide variety of sports fall into the category of adventure and extreme sports and with an increasing number of disciplines, this field is ever expanding. Sports are performed in contact with the "ground", the air or in-on water. Some sports may be performed as a combination of few disciplines, e.g., kite surfing, and as so involve very unique mechanisms of injury. Sports events can also be merged to form a multi-sport race comprising many disciplines lasting from single to multi-day races. Sports may involve competition with others, against the environment or with oneself, frequently the most ferocious adversary.

These sports fields are becoming increasingly popular in the general public and a few elect to take it to the next extreme level, with the accompanying risks. Those that do, bring such time and dedication that they become professional in terms of training, preparation and finance, in parallel with their peers in "common professional sports."

As more and more people are enjoying adventure sports, unfortunately increased numbers are becoming injured as a result. Future research is progressing alongside the sport development, to allow the sport mechanisms, injury patterns and predisposing factors to be better understood. It is the hope of all researchers to make the sports safer without detracting from their adventurous nature.

Researching extreme sports requires thorough understanding of the activities, preferably from within, which also make it easier to approach the right population and get their will and approval to collect and analyze unique data. Being "part of it all" not only motivated us but helped us throughout this process.

Being extreme and endurance sports athletes, we wished to learn more about these adventure sports. We appreciate that there is currently little published literature in many of these sports available for reference. We have attempted to assemble a comprehensive text on extreme and adventure sports injuries. Each chapter is written or co-written by an experienced athlete, doctor or physiotherapist involved in the sport at an international level. In some cases new research is being presented, all chapters review the current literature and this is presented from an academic viewpoint and interpreted practically for all involved in adventure sports.

This book combines our love to the sports with our life as sports surgeons. The aim and scope of this text is to bring the "sports medicine" involved in each of these sports into one volume. Each sport and discipline is explained together with their subtle similarities and differences, the common injury mechanisms, patterns of injury and treatment options and, finally, the mental and physiological aspects of it all. In this book we hope that we were able to deliver useful valuable information to surgeons, physicians, physical therapists and whoever treats or interested in these amazing activities.

Omer and Mike

Introduction

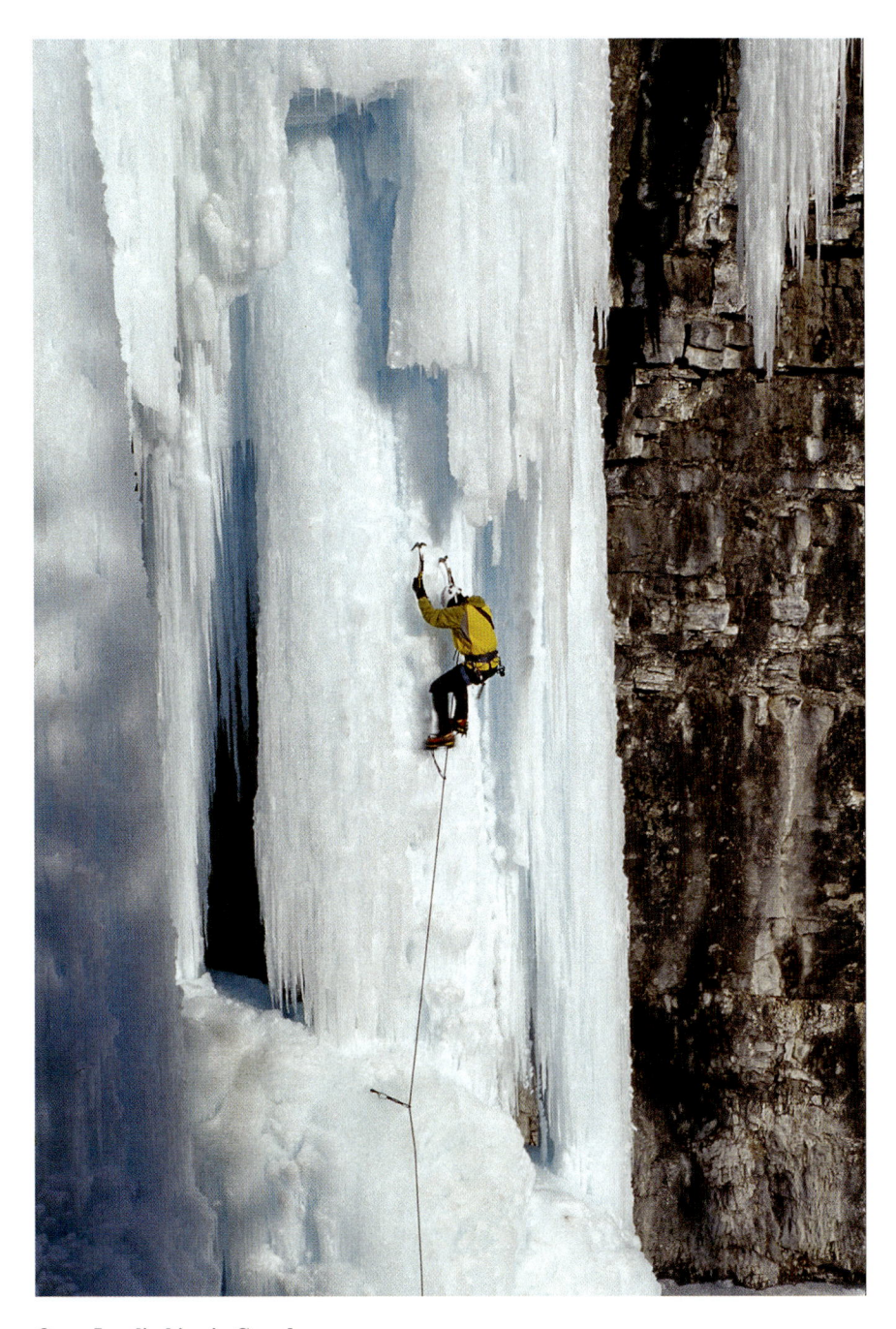

Omer Ice climbing in Canada
Photo: Barak Naggan

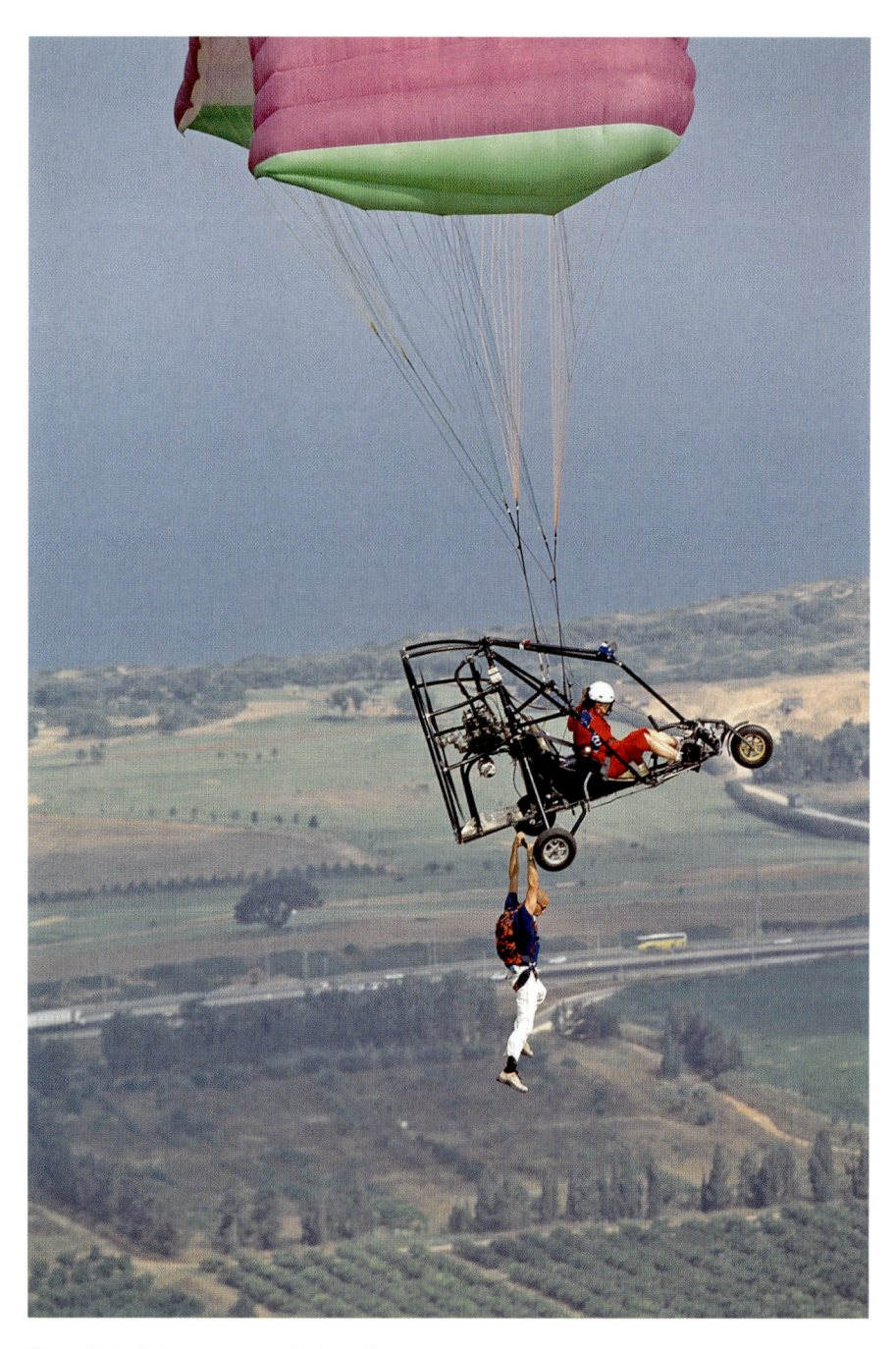

Omer test piloting new parachute system
Photo: Yaron Weinstein

Introduction xv

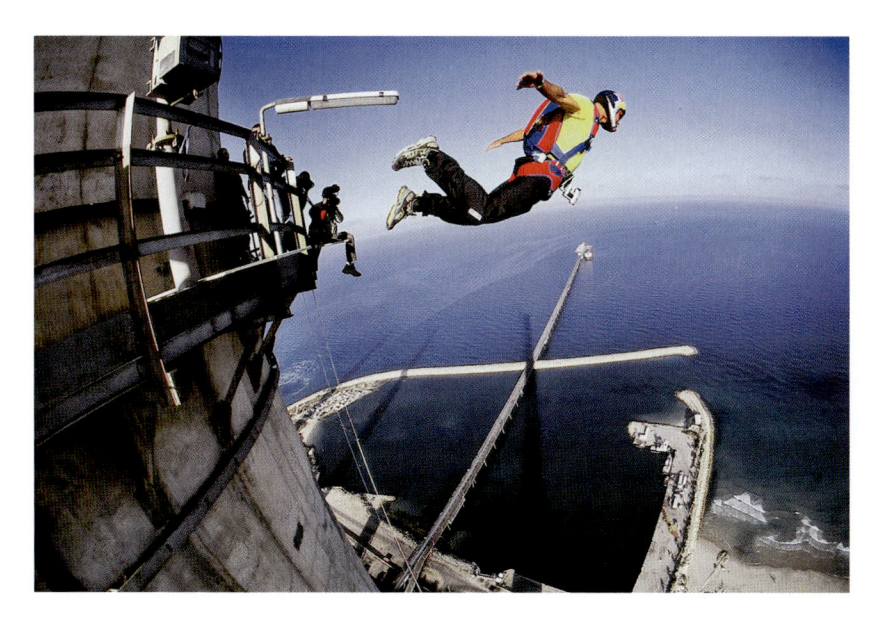

Omer Base jumping a smoke stuck in Israel
Photo: Ronen Topelberg

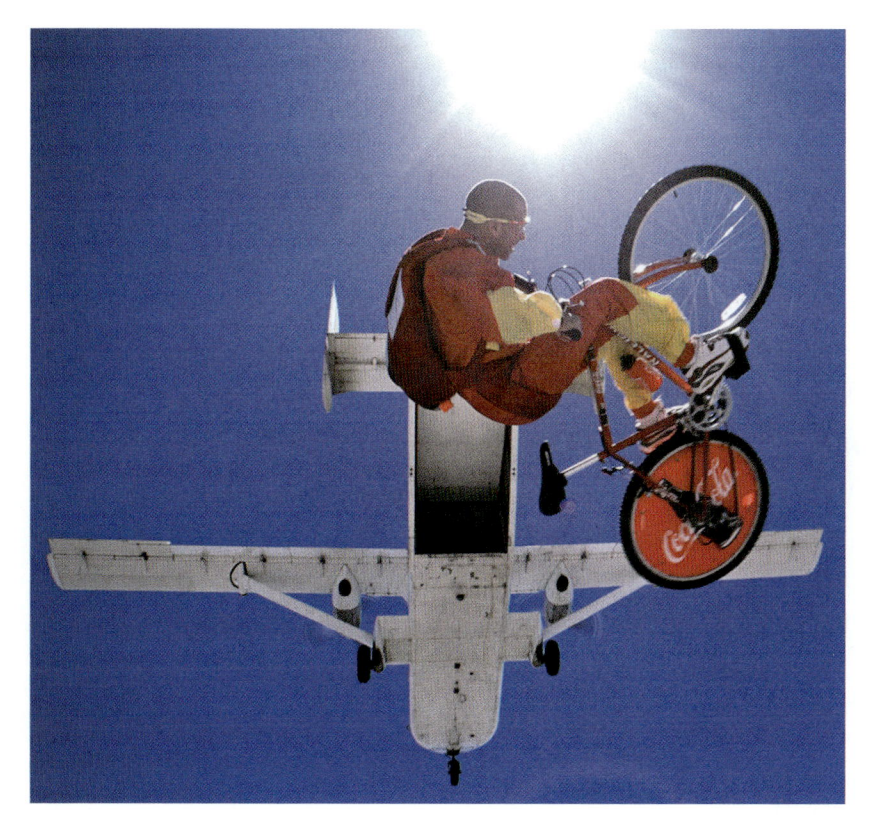

Omer during a commercial stunt, LA
Photo: Joe Jennings

xvi   Introduction

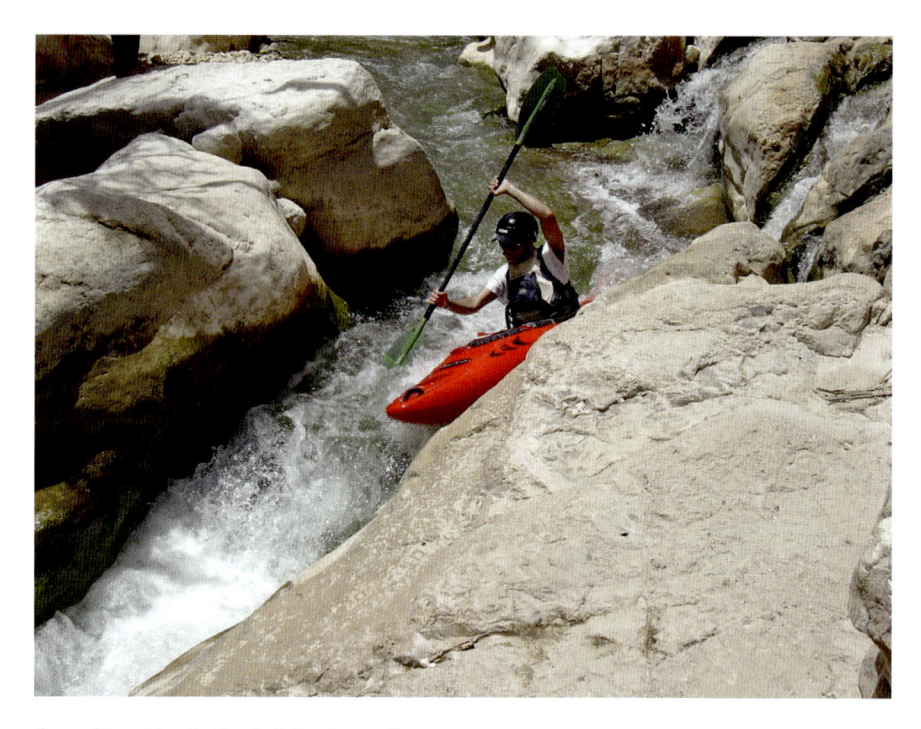

Omer Kayaking in the Judeha desert, Israel
Photo: Hagit Gal

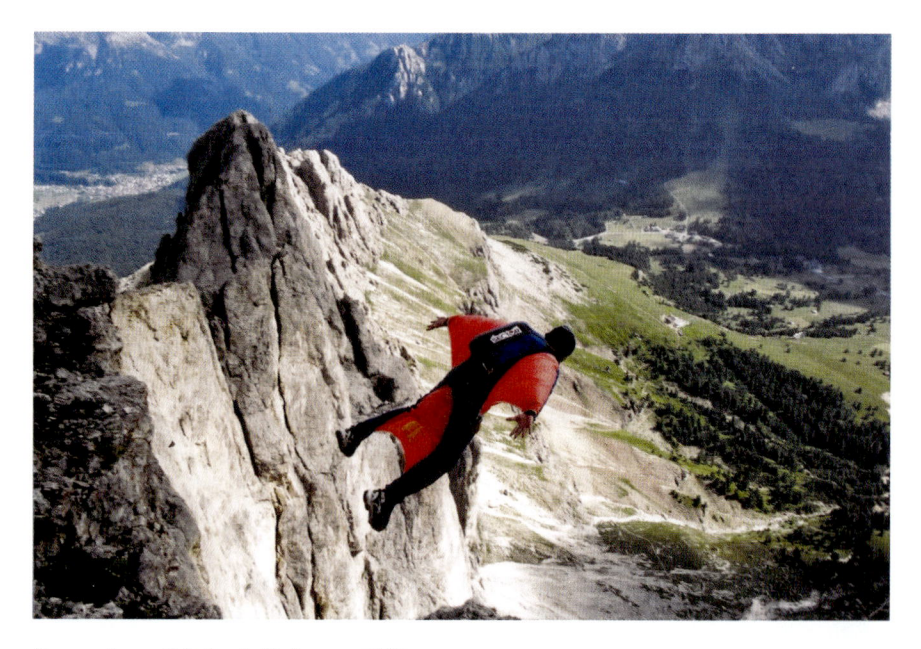

Omer wing suit flying in Italy, year 2000
Photo: DJ

Chapter 1
The Management of the Extreme Sports Athlete

Omer Mei-Dan and Michael R. Carmont

Contents

The Temperament of the Extreme Sports Athlete	2
Epidemiology	2
Resuscitation and Initial Management	3
Treatment Decisions	3
Rehabilitation	4
References	5

Extreme and adventure sports activities may be considered to be foolhardy by many but also exciting and applauded by others. The perception of the risk involved in these activities forms the opinion of the observer toward the participant. The majority of athletes performing these sports and challenges acknowledge that there is considerable risk involved but will have spent a great deal of time in preparation to minimize these risks. The rates of severe injury and death of inexperienced moun-

O. Mei-Dan, M.D. (✉)
Division of Sports Medicine, Department of Orthopaedic Surgery,
University of Colorado School of Medicine,
Aurora, CO 80045, USA

CU Sports Medicine,
Boulder, Colorado, USA
e-mail: omer@extremegate.com, omer.meidan@ucdenver.org

M.R. Carmont, FRCS (Tr&Orth)
The Department of Orthopaedic Surgery,
Princess Royal Hospital, Shrewsbury and Telford NHS Trust,
Telford, UK

The Department of Orthopaedic Surgery, The Northern General Hospital,
Sheffield Teaching Hospitals NHS Foundation Trust,
Sheffield, UK
e-mail: mcarmont@hotmail.com

taineers paying for supported trips up Everest or those participating in charity skydiving events are far higher, and yet these are frequently seen as laudable activities.

For many extreme sports, a considerable level of experience is required to make the sport safer or even to be able to engage with it in the first place; so frequently extreme sport athletes are experienced in many activities. BASE jumping may seem like a more exciting version of skydiving, but proficiency in the core skills of position control while falling through the air next to a cliff, canopy opening, and steering is vital to reduce the risk of ground or cliff strike. Most BASE jumpers would be expected to have completed several hundred skydives before undertaking their first BASE jump.

As medical personnel treating the extreme sports athlete, there are numerous differences we must appreciate between the common traditional sports and this newly developing era. These relate to the temperament of the athletes themselves, the particular epidemiology of injury, the initial management following injury, treatment decisions, and rehabilitation.

The Temperament of the Extreme Sports Athlete

Extreme sports athletes may self-select for their sport, in that they are more capable of responding appropriately in an adverse situation and thus do not perceive the situation as dangerous compared to the perception of the nonparticipating population. Most certainly, participants are aware of the risks and consequences of their actions including death or disablement. The ability to be able to respond immediately to an equipment malfunction or a "miss-hap" stands as a basic prerequisite for survival in the extreme sports world.

Studies of risk-taking sports people, such as mountaineers and BASE jumpers, indicated that their temperament traits scores differ significantly when compared to normative population [1, 2]. This data is presented with more detail in a following chapter dedicated to the topic. When BASE jumpers were assessed based on a temperament score of harm avoidance, they were actually found to have much lower scores than a non-jumping population. A subject which has scored low in this temperament trait of harm avoidance would be defined as carefree, relaxed, daring, courageous, outgoing, bold, optimistic even in situations which worry most people, and confident in the face of danger and uncertainty. As temperament traits are thought to be neurochemically regulated and moderately heritable, it is likely that to some extent engagement in these sports is genetically determined and "hardwired." However, no tightly defined personality profile among mountaineers and BASE jumpers was found [6].

Epidemiology

Injury epidemiology of traditional sports is being increasingly understood, with national surveillance and injury reporting programs. The mechanism of most of these injuries has been established, and when sustained, athletes tend to follow a management algorithm, featuring nonoperative care, surgical requirement, and rehabilitation, before return to play. By comparison, the injury mechanisms of extreme sports are less understood, particularly the pattern of injury in many sports. In addition, the athletes themselves, by their very nature, are keen to participate in new treatments or progress rapidly to the surgical option, even in the absence of established outcome studies. The highest rate of injuries in extreme sport justifiably belongs to two groups: new and inexperienced athletes who have just started engaging in extreme sports and experienced extremists.

Reported injury rates in extreme sports may be expected to increase during competition rather than training. This behavior is well known for common team sports [3, 4]. Similar observations are noted in head-to-head or judged competitions and are expected in extreme sports when athletes are trying to push their limits even further for prizes, audience, or fame. The published injury rate for various extreme sports series has been determined; however, in some disciplines, the fatality rate is hard to establish due to the lack of formal observed or recorded events. In many situations, the competition is against oneself or the forces of nature and the sport is practiced in relative isolation. Accordingly, some extreme sports fields, like BASE jumping, tend to eliminate official events where more fatalities could be expected.

Resuscitation and Initial Management

By their very nature, adventure sports involve high mountains, savage seas, tumbling rivers, and baking deserts. These are found in remote locations far away from habitation and settlements. The extraction of an injured recreational athlete relying on local and government assistance may take a considerable period of time, and an element of recovery may be required before surgical fixation can be achieved. Professional extreme sports athletes by comparison tend to have invested a considerable period of finance and planning for their sports and stunts. They usually have made arrangements for private extraction and transfer to private medical facilities so that their acts are not a burden on these frequently poorly supported local health-care resources.

When injury occurs, this typically results in multiple injuries with high Injury Severity Scores, and urgent rescue and transfer to high-level trauma center is required. Some geographical locations where extreme sports have evolved have become very popular, and local services have developed into designated rescue teams, usually air ones, to answer these needs. Examples for this are the Norwegian fjords and Swiss cliffs which attract many BASE jumpers year round, the Verdon or Chamonix rock faces considered as climbers' Meccas, or the establishment of many hyperbaric chambers in popular diving sites.

Treatment Decisions

Physicians must appreciate that extreme sports participants are likely to return to their sport irrespective of their functional outcome. In this respect, a poor outcome from nonoperative management is likely to increase the chances of reinjury or worse. It is understandable that some physicians may consider an adequate outcome as being acceptable and possibly act as a deterrent from future participation. They could be considered to be providing a good treatment option and from their point of view are looking after their patient's best overall interests. This, however, is simply not the case. Telling a climber that reports on finger pain only while climbing, "so stick to other sports," would just leave them upset and to seek other medical advice. This may be similar to surgeons treating obese patients with knee pain attributing all their problems to their obesity. If weight loss is mentioned early in the consultation, the rapport is frequently lost and the consultation breaks down. In our experience, extreme sports athletes tend not to modify their life patterns and sports participation as other athletes may do.

It is also unfortunate but understandable that some surgeons may also have the attitude of why should we go to all that trouble when these athletes are more likely to return to their sport with its possible consequences. It must be remembered that these patients undertake these sports as their passion, rather than merely a whim. By comparison, it can be argued that drink-driving leads to far more injuries and self-inflicted deaths than what occurs during extreme sports participation.

Professional or high-level competition in traditional sports tends to reduce in most high-profile sports with aging. Most top-level participants tend to retire in their 30s to 40s. The recreational aspect of many adventure sports encourages athletes to participate within the level of their physical ability for much longer and still with an element of competition, and possible danger. In some cases, the added experience and maturity (or courage) of the participant allows them to remain at the top level depending upon the sport and compensate for some age-related decline in physical performance, e.g., yacht racing or big wave surfing. These sports tend to feature a considerable aspect of endurance rather than focused strength or agility.

Similar to other sports participants, we recommend internal fixation should be removed following bone union due to the relatively high risk of traumatic reinjury. A periprosthetic fracture is complicated to manage in both young and old alike.

Rehabilitation

Published reports on extreme sports athletes, mentioned in the following chapters, suggest they return to active participation once rehabilitation is completed, even after life-threatening and disabling injuries [5]. Although half of injured whitewater kayakers sought medical care for their injury, and almost one third missed more than 1 month of kayaking because of their injury, almost all (96 %) reported a complete or good recovery with the best outcomes associated with impact injuries and the worst with overuse ones [6]. A recent report [6] by the editors has shown that of 68 studied BASE jumpers, 43 % have sustained at least one severe injury during their time in the sport, of which 52 % required acute surgical intervention. Also, 72 % of the jumpers had witnessed the death or serious injury of other participants in the sport, while 76 % had at least one "near miss" incident. Nevertheless, all of these jumpers maintained active participation in the sport. These reports, and others, imply that adventure sports athletes see injuries as integral part of the sport and are typically motivated to return to their sport. Specialized rehabilitation is frequently required as sports tend to feature one predominant key maneuver or action. A graduated return to extreme sports activity may not be possible as most require full commitment and an "all-or-nothing" level of performance is needed.

Simulation exercises can be performed in a reduced-risk environment prior to full return. Confirming that functional restoration has returned may be something that only the athlete themselves can determine. Resumption of their sport before body and mind are fully ready may be life-threatening injuries rather than "just" a reinjury for other traditional sports. A shoulder prone to dislocation for the skydiver or BASE jumper can result in inability to deploy the parachute on time or at all. Following a shoulder stabilization surgery, and rehabilitation program, the athlete would be better off testing his shoulder stability and function primarily in a wind tunnel environment rather than off the nearest 200-m cliff.

In summary, the management of the injured extreme sports athlete is a challenge to surgeons and sports physicians. The margins for error in these sports are small, and athletes as patients are more likely to return to their activities than the general sporting population following injury. We recommend that surgeons should plan their management with great care and attention to detail and pay particular attention to the requirements of this particular group of patients.

References

1. Monasterio E. Mental characteristics of extreme sports athletes. In: Mei-Dan O, Carmont MR, editors. Adventure and extreme sports injuries: epidemiology, treatment, rehabilitation and prevention. London, England: Springer; 2012 (in press).
2. Monasterio E, Mulder R, Frampton C et al. Personality variables in a population of BASE jumpers. J Appl Sport Psychol. 2012;24:391–400. doi: 10.1080/10413200.2012.666710.
3. Brooks JH, Fuller CW, Kemp SP, et al. Epidemiology of injuries in English professional Rugby Union. Part 1: match injuries. Br J Sports Med. 2005;39(10):757–66.
4. Brooks JH, Fuller CW, Kemp SP, et al. Epidemiology of injuries in English professional Rugby Union. Part 2: training injuries. Br J Sports Med. 2005;39(10):767–75.
5. Fiore DC, Houston JD. Injuries in whitewater kayaking. Br J Sports Med. 2001;35(4):235–41.
6. Mei-Dan O, Carmont MR, Monasterio E. The epidemiology of severe and catastrophic injuries in BASE jumping. Clin J Sports Med. 2012;22(3):262–7.

Chapter 2
Rock and Ice Climbing

Volker Schöffl

Contents

Introduction	7
Rock Climbing	8
Injury and Fatality Risk	12
Traditional Climbing, Sport Climbing, and Bouldering	12
Indoor Climbing	12
Ice Climbing	12
Mountaineering	13
Equipment	13
Training in Rock Climbing	14
Injuries and Overuse Syndromes	16
Clinical Examination and Diagnostics of Finger Injuries	16
Normal Musculoskeletal Adaptations in the Climber's Body	19
Main Climbing-Specific Injuries	19
Anorexia Athletica	29
Injury Prevention	30
Ice Climbing	31
Ice Climbing: Overuse Syndromes	32
Mountaineering	32
References	33

Introduction

Modern sport climbing, or its various versions, has developed from mountaineering which was a sport that started in the European Alps. By the mid-1980s, the popularity of this new-old sport has spread globally and diversified to include new

---

V. Schöffl, Ph.D., M.D., MHBA
Department of Sportsorthopedics and Sportsmedicine, Orthopedic and Trauma Surgery,
Klinikum Bamberg, Sozialstiftung Bamberg,
Bugerstr. 80, 96049, Bamberg, FRG, Germany
e-mail: volker.schoeffl@me.com; www.sportmedizin-bamberg.com

categories like ice climbing, bouldering, speed climbing, and aid climbing. The style in which a route is climbed and the difficulty involved now might be considered to be more important than reaching the summit itself. In style we refer to free climbing, which stands for a climb conducted using only the rock face formations, or aid climbing, when one can make his progress by using also various devices anchored into the wall, like a sling ladder. Simultaneously, in mountaineering, the routes to reach the summit became more and more difficult and started to fall into the definition of extreme climbing.

With increasing numbers of sport climbers, naturally the competition between individual climbers increased, progressing to actual formal sport climbing competitions. Since the inaugural World Championships in Frankfurt in 1991, the number of participants in the competition have gradually increased. The 2005 event included more than 500 athletes from 55 countries [1]. The International Federation of Sport Climbing (IFSC), the governing body for competition climbing, is currently seeking recognition as an Olympic sport [2].

The sport of climbing has also grown and diversified. It has also become more spectator-friendly with competitions attracting large audiences and being broadcast live on many sports television channels.

With any sporting participation, the enjoyment and benefits of this exercise must be balanced against the risk of injury or worse in the case of extreme sports.

The epidemiological analysis of sport-specific injuries helps form preventive measures to reduce the incidence and severity of injuries. Extensive injury-related studies in general rock climbing, indoor climbing, and competition climbing have been determined, and results are consistent. Most injuries in rock climbing involve the upper limbs, most commonly overuse finger injuries, rather than an acute injury mechanism [3].

Estimates as to the number of climbers worldwide vary greatly. The German Alpine Club estimates 300,000 rock climbers for Germany and two million for Europe. Nelson and McKenzie [4] report about nine million participants in rock climbing for the USA, based on the analysis of the Outdoor Industry Foundation (Boulder, CO, 2006). The numbers of mountaineers are even higher, but as the definitions in these analyses vary difficult to obtain.

Rock Climbing

Even the purest form of the sport now has several subdisciplines. The level of risk and difficulty tend to be determined by the subdiscipline practiced, the climber's experience and skills, difficulty grade of the route, equipment used, and environmental factors: the climbing surface, the remoteness of location climbed, the altitude, and the changing weather. It is common for climbers to regularly participate in more than one climbing subdiscipline, making the analysis and determination of risk difficult. This also increases the time involvement in the sport and, as a consequence, the risk of injury.

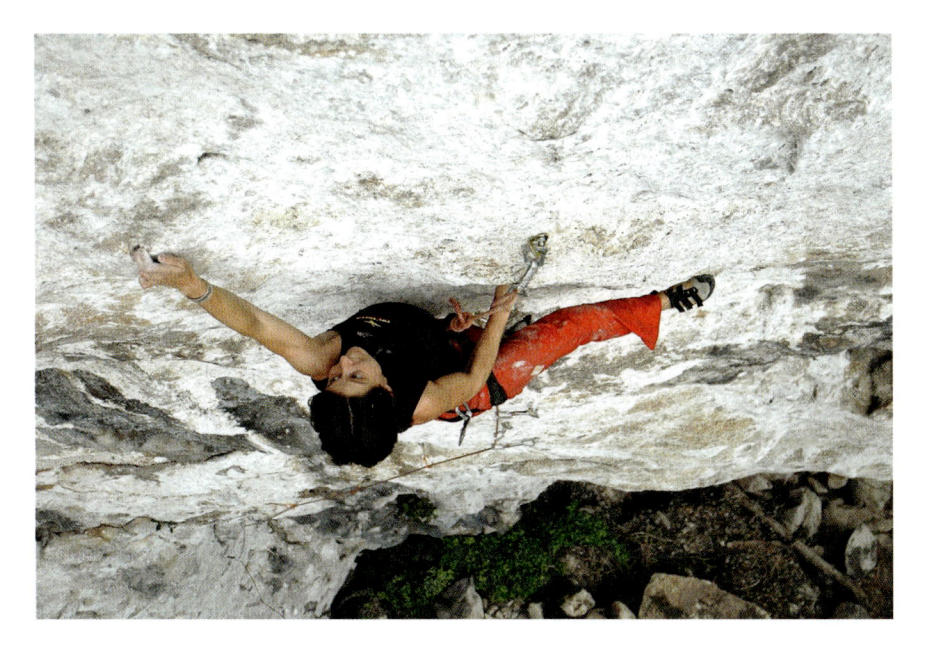

Fig. 2.1 Modern sport climbing, protected with bolts (Isabelle Schöffl in Dream Catcher, Laos 7b+)

Sport climbing or free climbing (Fig. 2.1) is similar to gymnastics in many ways. It requires flexibility, finger and overall limb strength, burst strength, and endurance used simultaneously and in a different manner dictated by the route climbed. The climbing is slightly prescriptive as the climber ascends toward mostly permanently fixed anchors, such as predrilled bolts, to clip the rope into for protection. The route length can range from 10 m to more than 100 m, with fixed anchors generally placed 2–5 m apart. Falls are frequent, trained for, mostly harmless, and considered common part of the discipline. Physical hazards (rock fall, weather changes, etc.) are small, and the neglect of wearing a climbing helmet is widely accepted.

Bouldering is defined as ropeless climbing involving a short sequence of powerful and technical moves to complete a graded route, or a sequence of few climbing moves, on large boulders, occasionally up to 10 m high.

Bouldering (Fig. 2.2) can be performed solo, without a partner, and with minimal equipment – climbing shoes and crash pad (a foam mattress designated to stop ones' fall). Falling onto one's feet or body is common in bouldering, whether a route is completed (defined as "topped") or not.

Traditional (alpine) climbing (or trad climbing) emphasizes the skills necessary for establishing routes in an exploratory outdoor environment. The lead climber typically ascends a section of rock while placing removable protective devices where possible and desirable along the climb. Falls can therefore be longer than those experienced when sport climbing. Unreliable fixed pitons may occasionally be found on older established routes. As physical hazards are likely, the use of a helmet is considered mandatory. If climbing is performed at an altitude of greater

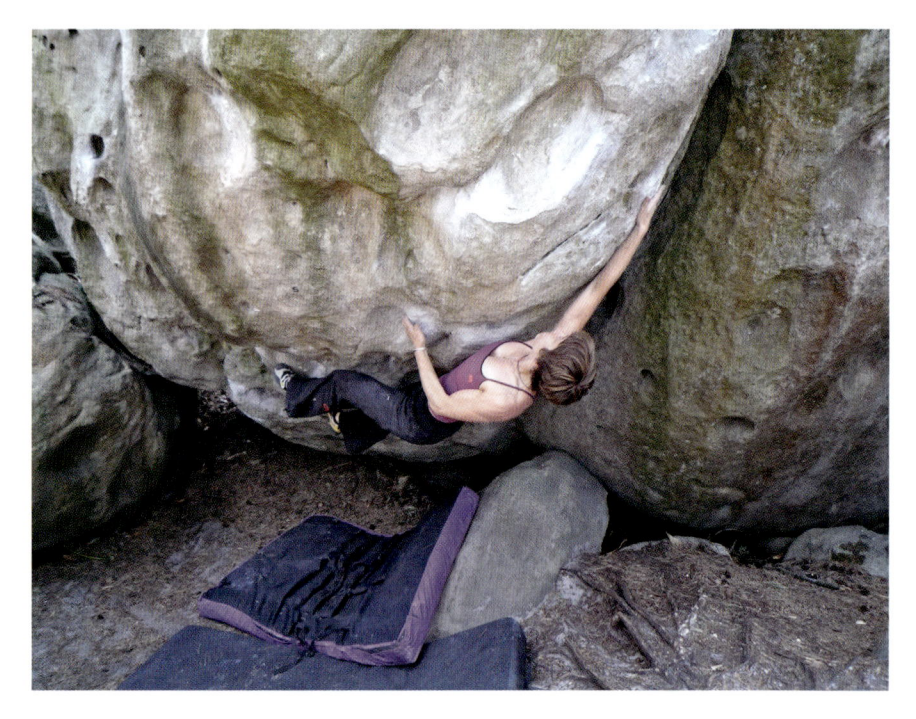

Fig. 2.2 Boulderer and protection (for protection, a bouldering mat (crash pad) is used)

than 2,500 m, physiological altitude-induced adaptations must also be factored into the climb.

Indoor climbing is performed on artificial structures that try to mimic climbing outdoors but in a more controlled environment. As physical hazards are almost totally eliminated, climbing became a popular extracurricular school sport in many countries. National and international competitions are held on such walls and involve three major disciplines – lead climbing (i.e., sport climbing), speed climbing, and bouldering. Indoor bouldering is performed above thick foam mat flooring.

Ice climbing (Fig. 2.3) normally refers to roped and protected climbing of features such as glaciers, frozen waterfalls, and cliffs or rock slabs covered with ice refrozen from flows of water. Equipment includes ice axes and crampons. Physical hazards such as avalanches and rock and icefalls or breaks are present [3].

Many different climbing grading systems exist, the most common of which are the Union Internationale des Associations d'Alpinisme (International Climbing Federation) UIAA, the French, and the Yosemite Decimal System scales. For scientific analysis, the decimal UIAA scale is recommended (Table 2.1) [5].

Lead climbing means that the leading climber attaches himself to a dynamic climbing rope and ascends the route while periodically placing protection consisting of metal wedges or bolts temporarily placed into cracks in the rock face or

2 Rock and Ice Climbing

Fig. 2.3 Ice climbing (Sam Lightner on The Pencil, Polar Circus, WI6, Alberta, Canada)

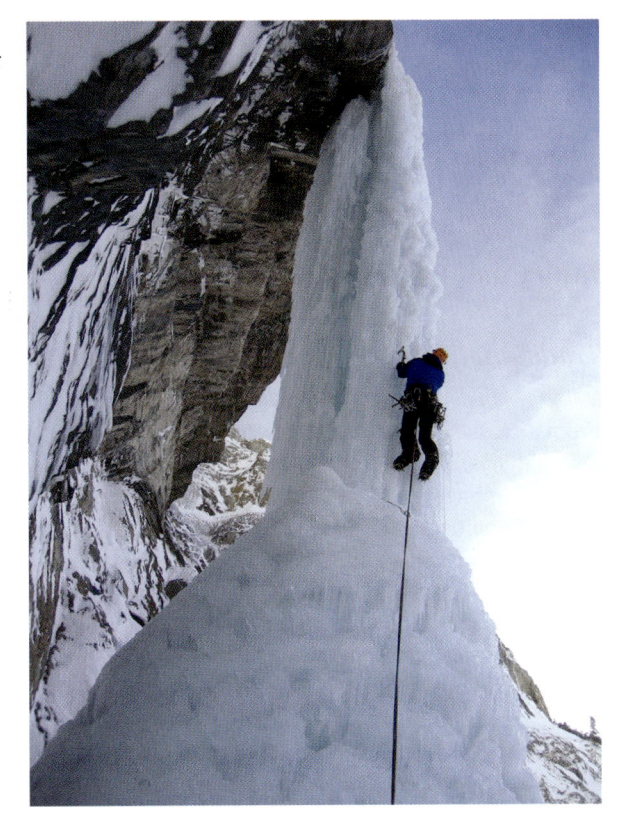

Table 2.1 The UIAA metric, the French, and the Yosemite Decimal System scales of climbing grades [5]

Metric scale	UIAA	French (Fr)	US-American (YDS)
5.66	6−	5b/c	5.8
6	6	5c/6a	5.9
6.33	6+	6a/6a+	5.10a
6.66	7−	6a+/b	5.10b/c
7	7	6b/b+	5.10d
7.33	7+	6b+/6c	5.11a/b
7.66	8−	6c+	5.11c
8	8	7a	5.11c/d
8.33	8+	7a+/7b	5.12a/b
8.66	9−	7b/7b+	5.12b/c
9	9	7c/7c+	5.12d
9.33	9+	7c+/8a	5.13a
9.66	10−	8a/8a+	5.13b/c
10	10	8b	5.13d
10.33	10+	8b+/8c	5.14a/b
10.66	11−	8c/8c+	5.14b/c
11	11	9a	5.14d
11.33	11+	9a+	5.15a
11.66	12−	9b	5.15b

"quickdraws" to bolts and attaching them to the climbing rope with carabiners. Top-rope climbing refers to climbing with a rope, used for the climber's safety and runs from a belayer at the foot of a route through one or more carabiners connected to an anchor at the top of the route and back down to the climber, usually attaching to the climber by means of a harness.

Injury and Fatality Risk

Traditional Climbing, Sport Climbing, and Bouldering

From a cross-sectional survey, Schussmann [6] concluded that rock climbing has a lower injury rate than football and horse riding; however, these sports rarely result in catastrophic events or fatalities. Climbing frequency and difficulty are associated with the incidence of overuse injuries in most studies [7, 8]. Most injuries are sustained by the lead climber, with falls being the most common source of acute injuries [9]. Repeatedly performing hard moves is the most common cause for overuse injuries [8]. In traditional climbing, falls resulting in wall or ground strike lead to most injuries, while in the safer discipline of sport climbing, performing strenuous moves tends to be the leading cause of injury. Overall, the majority of injuries described in climbing studies are of minor severity, with a fatality rate ranging from 0 to 28 % [3]. Given the range of mortality rates, it is understandable that differing methodology and data collection techniques exist, which makes direct comparison between series difficult.

Indoor Climbing

Of all climbing subdisciplines, indoor climbing reports 0.027–0.079 injuries per 1,000 h of participation and very few fatalities [3]. However, overuse injuries of minor severity predominantly involving the upper limbs, mainly the fingers, are commonly reported in rock climbing studies.

Ice Climbing

Ice climbing popularity is growing fast, while very little data on injuries and accidents exist for this subdiscipline. The overall injury rate published in the literature is comparable with other outdoor sports (2.87–4.07 injuries/1,000 h [3, 10]), with most injuries of minor severity. Nevertheless, objective danger is always present, and severe injuries and fatalities do occur [3, 10].

Mountaineering

Mountaineering also involves a wide range of activities, from hiking up to climbing peaks above 8,000 m. All these activities present different physiological demands and risks depending on climbing style, altitude, environmental conditions, climbing experience, and more [11]. Most studies on mountaineering fatalities and accidents are giving the fatality/accident number per 1,000 climbers or per 1,000 summits, which are therefore difficult to compare to the 1,000 h of sports performance used in other disciplines. For higher altitude, not only the accident and fatality rate is important but also the prevalence of altitude illness, which is between 28 and 34 % above 4,000 m [12, 13]. These illnesses can be a contributing factor to an injury, accident, or death. They are characterized by shifts of internal body fluid, being in places they should not be on exposure to altitude (i.e., brain, lungs). At "high altitude" (5,000+ m), there is a risk that these altitude-induced internal fluid shifts may accumulate in the brain (high-altitude cerebral edema – HACE) and/or in the lungs (high-altitude pulmonary edema – HAPE). Both HAPE and HACE are potentially fatal [12].

When assessing climbing risks, it is obvious that each climbing subdiscipline would determine different levels and types of risk, injury, and fatality. When climbing outdoors, there are objective dangers and physical hazards: variable rock and ice quality, extreme and changing weather conditions, weapon-like equipment (ice climbing), difficult approaches, and high mental and physical stress. In mountaineering, additional environmental factors (avalanches, crevasses, altitude-induced illnesses with neurological dysfunction, etc.) can sometimes directly influence injuries and fatalities [11]. Nevertheless, dangerous situations and predictable injury patterns or accident circumstances can still be avoided or successfully managed with adequate preparation, training, and experience. In contrast, in indoor and sport climbing, these objective and external dangers are greatly reduced, although the risk of a fatal injury is still present.

Equipment

In the early days of climbing, classic heavy mountaineering boots were worn for climbing in alpine regions as well as in rock faces. It was only in the early 1980s when the first real, or modern, climbing shoe with a friction sole was introduced. One common characteristic which all climbing shoes share is the tight, squeezed fit required to obtain optimal contact with the rock. This excessively tight footwear leads to foot problems, such as callosity, toenail infections, or, in a longer term perspective, a hallux valgus deformity [14]. The introduction of predrilled anchoring bolts was an important factor for the explosive development of the climbing grades scaled. Lead climber falls, relaying on the rope and anchoring bolts, are common for sport climbers now. The climbing harnesses used have improved.

While a combination of chest and sit harness has been used in traditional mountaineering, a pure sit harness design is now used in sport climbing. This allows maximum free movement while climbing and aims to reduce injury when falling [9, 15]. Bolts, ropes, harnesses, and other equipment used should carry the UIAA Safety Commission approval.

Ice climbing equipment also developed a long way from the tools used in classical mountaineering. Modern crampons with the prominent frontal spikes have initially become popular when Anderl Heckmaier and Wiggerl Vörg used them for the first ascent of the Eiger North Face. Nowadays, a single frontal spike or a heel spur is considered a state-of-the-art. Ice axes were already in use at the time of the first ascent of the Mont Blanc by Pascard and Balmat on 8 August 1786 and have evolved remarkably since. Recent technological advances have helped to transform these long-shafted tools into a short-shafted curved and surprisingly light crossbar that resembles a mythical medieval weapon. It is a topic of wide and hot discussion in the ice climbing community whether ice axes should be used with or without a leash. Leashes attach the ax to the climber's wrist, reduce stress onto the forearms, but increase the risk of injuring oneself from the ax during a fall where typically the ax bounces back into the climber's face. In parallel with the technological advancements in crampons and ice axes, Erich Friedli from Switzerland developed the first real ice screw [10]. This ice screw has played a pivotal role in increasing the safety of the sport. If placed correctly, in good ice and proper angle, it may guarantee a comparable pullout strength to bolts. All climbing disciplines use climbing ropes for protection. These ropes are dynamic ropes, in contrast to static ropes as used in sailing and caving. Dynamic ropes have a stretch of roughly 5 m per 50 m when stressed, which reduces the force onto the falling climber's body.

Training in Rock Climbing

The recent increase in levels of technical difficulty in rock climbing has intensified the impacts of the sport onto the musculoskeletal system. The age of the top athletes, especially in competition climbing, has steadily decreased. In 1986, the average competitive member of the German National Climbing Team spent about 10 h per week training and was 26 years old. By 1996, the competitive climber was spending 21 h a week training and his/her age had dropped to 22 years [2]. Today it is not uncommon for 50 % of World Cup finalists to be under 18 years old. In this age, the finger phalanges' growth plates have not fully closed yet in some of these young strong climbers, which frequently leads to unusual epiphyseal fatigue injuries [16]. While the majority of climbing activity and training is performed on rock or artificial climbing walls, certain climbing-specific training forms must also be considered. One of the most specific isolated and designated training forms is "to campus" (Fig. 2.4).

2 Rock and Ice Climbing

Fig. 2.4 Campus board training

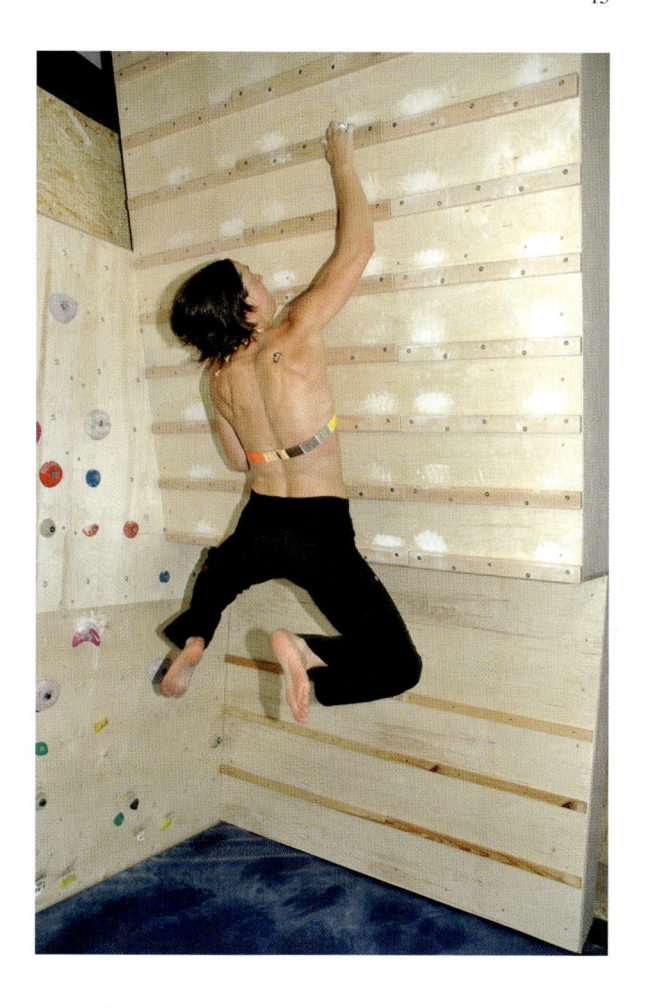

The legendary "campus board," built by Wolfgang Güllich and Kurt Albert at the Nuremberg "campus" gym, has become a household term among climbers. By training on the campus board, both in a positive and negative slope, Wolfgang developed his finger and forearm strength for the first ascent of "Action Directe" (the world's first UIAA 11/5.14d, in Frankenjura, Germany). The campus board is a slightly overhanging board with different-size rungs in a constant pattern screwed onto it. Basic exercises contain climbing up and down hand over hand without feet, increasing the distance between the rungs used. A special training technique is "double dynos." Based on the training principle of "plyometric training," the climber jumps up and down from small-sized rungs. This applies very high forces onto the fingers and, respectively, onto the ligaments, bones, and cartilage. While "campusing" is a good training exercise in the elite ranks, it should have no place in training of beginners, intermediates, and especially preadolescent climbers! According to the author's experience, two-thirds of junior climbers who trained regularly on the campus board sustained an injury! These injuries, commonly epiphyseal fatigue fractures, lead, if neglected, to a permanent damage of the affected finger. As a result, the main focus in the education of trainers, climbing instructors, parents, and young climbers should be focused on proper training methods and avoiding, as much as possible, techniques which may lead to these well-described injuries.

Injuries and Overuse Syndromes

While climbing relies on the synchronized and optimal function of the whole body, activity and performance are primarily limited by finger and forearm strength. The various gripping techniques (mostly crimp and hanging grip) (Figs. 2.5 and 2.6), which are used by the climber, led to the transmission of extremely high forces in the anatomical structures of the fingers. As a logical consequence, finger and hand injuries, predominantly overuse syndromes, are the most common complaints in rock climbers [7, 8, 17, 18]. A study evaluating 604 injured rock climbers found that 247 (41 % of injuries) sustained finger injuries (Table 2.2) [19, 20]. Some injuries, such as flexor tendon pulley ruptures or the lumbrical shift syndrome, are very unique and specific for the sport of climbing and are rarely seen in other patient populations [7]. As a result of this, it can be difficult to establish a diagnosis in uncommon and yet characteristic injuries for the general physician unfamiliar with climbing injury patterns (Table 2.3).

Clinical Examination and Diagnostics of Finger Injuries

A climber's injured finger, or a relevant complaint, requires a careful history, precise examination, and directed imaging. Both the active and passive range of motion of the proximal (PIP) and distal (DIP) interphalangeal joints should be measured. It is essential to examine the flexor tendons separately by isolating flexor digitorum profundus (FDP) and flexor digitorum superficialis (FDS) function. The collateral ligaments of the finger joints should be assessed through the application of lateral stress and the palmar plate through the translation test, which is analogous to Lachman test on the knee joint. For detection of a pulley rupture, an opposition of the injured finger against the thumb with forceful pressing in the crimp position may lead to a palpable or visual bowstring. Pressure tenderness on the palmar side of the base phalanx is present in both pulley rupture and tenosynovitis, while tenderness on the phalanges' side usually implies a lumbrical muscle injury.

High-energy acute injuries as well as any type of chronic problem require a radiograph in two planes. Further diagnosis may be provided by ultrasound, e.g., in

2 Rock and Ice Climbing

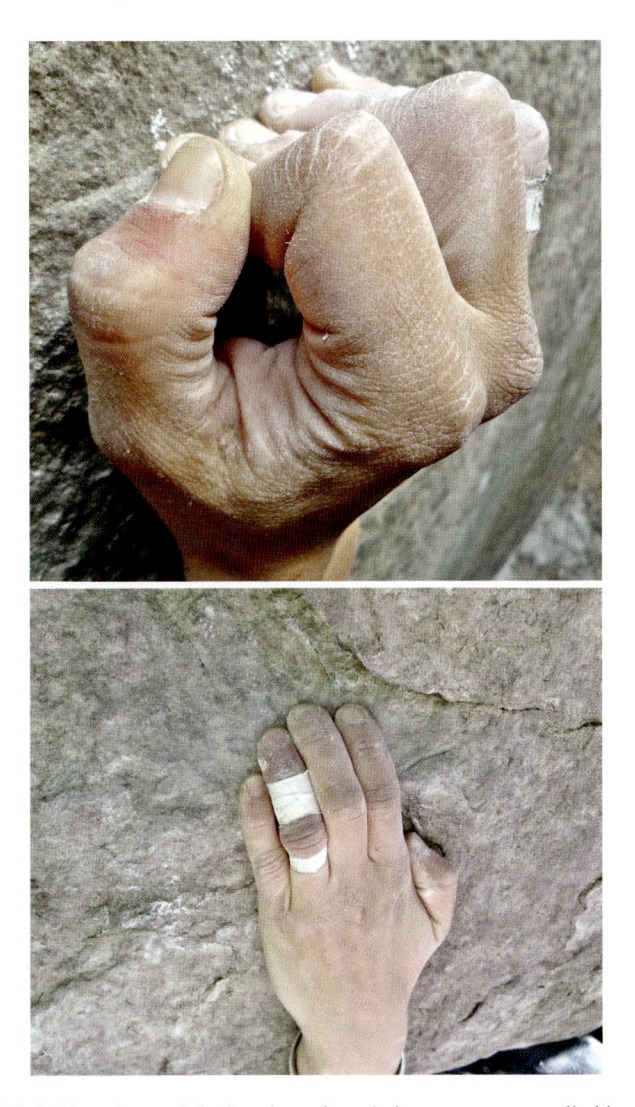

Figs. 2.5 and 2.6 The crimp and the hanging grip technique are common climbing finger holds involving very small rock face ledges or slopes which the climbers is holding to

detecting a pulley injury, ganglions or tenosynovitis of the fingers, biceps inflammations, or rotator cuff problems. The technique of finger ultrasound is easy to learn and is very accurate and cost-effective. A linear array transducer with 10–12 MHz in a prone position performing longitudinal and transversal planes is mostly used. For signal enhancement, a gel standoff pad or examination in a warm water basin is recommended. Only in rare cases an additional MRI (or CT) needs to

Table 2.2 The ten most frequent localization of climbing-specific diagnoses 1/98–12/01 ($n=604$) [20]

Fingers	247	(41.0 %)
Forearm/elbow	81	(13.4 %)
Foot	55	(9.1 %)
Hand	47	(7.8 %)
Spine/torso	43	(7.1 %)
Skin	42	(6.9 %)
Shoulder	30	(5.0 %)
Knee	22	(3.6 %)
Others	37	(6.1 %)
Polytraumatic	5	(0.8 %)

Table 2.3 Injuries and overuse syndromes in the fingers of rock climbers (types and onset) [7]

Diagnosis	N out of 271	Acute onset	Slow onset	Chronic onset
Pulley rupture	74	+	+	
Pulley strain	48	+	+	
Tenosynovitis	42	+	+	+
Joint capsular damage and ligamental injuries	37	+	+	
Arthritis (acute)	13	+	+	
Ganglion	11	+	+	+
Flexor tendon strain	7	+		
Fracture	7	+		
Arthritis (chronic)	7			+
Dupuytren contracture	5			+
Soft tissue injury, contusion	5	+		
Flexor tendon partial tear	4	+		
Collateral ligament injury	3	+	+	
Osseous tear fibrocartilago palmaris	2	+		
Epiphyseal fracture	2		+	+
Lumbrical shift syndrome	2	+	+	
Abscess/cellulitis	1	+		
Finger amputation	1	+		
Tendon nodules				+
Joint contracture[a]				+
Finger nerve irritation		+		
Extensor tendon irritation			+	+

Note: The numbers after certain injuries show their frequency in a group of 271 diagnoses in 247 analyzed finger injuries over a period of 4 years [7]; the other diagnoses are from recent years
[a]Joint contractures were not specified in the 271 diagnoses but classified as symptoms; nevertheless, climbers seek advice because of joint contractures even if no other complaints exist. An acute onset is defined as a single trauma, a slow onset as if the condition comes into being over an interval of up to 2 weeks

be performed in order to establish a clear diagnosis. In some cases, electromyography might be indicated when localized atrophy is suspected. That would be appropriate in nerve traction injury such as with suprascapular or long thoracic nerve for winging scapula.

Normal Musculoskeletal Adaptations in the Climber's Body

The high stresses involved in rock climbing, specifically at the fingers, lead to physiologic adaptations over the years, which need to be distinguished from pathologic changes. Through radiographic and MRI analysis, Hochholzer et al. [21] demonstrated the presence of these adaptations. They found an adaptive hypertrophy of the joint capsule, thickening of the collateral ligaments, cortical hypertrophy, and a hypertrophy of up to 50 % of the flexor tendons itself. The authors hypothesized that cortical hypertrophy could be adaptive signs to the high stress of the sport and not already pathological osteoarthrotic changes [22, 23]. Therefore, clinical and radiographic findings must be carefully interpreted. In an analysis of radiographs in young high-level climbers and 140 experienced climbers, Schöffl et al. [23] classified the following findings under the definition of a stress reaction: cortical hypertrophy, subchondral sclerosis/increased thickness of epiphysis, calcifications of the insertion of the flexor digitorum superficialis or the flexor digitorum profundus tendon, and broadened proximal and/or distal interphalangeal joint base (Table 2.4).

Main Climbing-Specific Injuries

Pulley Injuries

Injuries to the finger flexor pulley system are the most common finger injury in rock climbers. The pulley system of the index to little fingers consists of five annular (A1–A5) and three cross (C1–C3) ligaments (pulleys). Caused mainly through the crimping position (Figs. 2.5 and 2.6), the A2, A3, or A4 pulleys, which are considered the most important ones for this type of activity and which are prone to the highest stress level, can either be strained or ruptured. The most frequently injured pulley is the A2 pulley. Single pulley injuries would dictate a conservative therapy; multiple pulley injuries require surgical repair to preserve function (Table 2.5) [19].

The common presentation is a climber which reports of an acute onset of pain while "crimping" on a small finger hold. Occasionally, a "fatigue" rupture, with no adequate trauma, occurs after chronic tenosynovitis, which was treated with local cortisone injection. A pulley rupture may be accompanied by a loud "snapping" sound, similar to that associated with an Achilles tendon rupture. The climber would complain of palmar-sided pain at the level of the injured pulley, pressure tenderness, and swelling. Rarely, a hematoma would be present. The pain can extend into the palm or the forearm. If multiple pulleys are ruptured, a clinical "bowstring" becomes visible. With ultrasound, a larger than normal distance between the flexor tendon and the phalanx (Figs. 2.7 and 2.8) can be seen. If the ultrasound fails to establish an exact diagnosis, an MRI is the next most accurate investigation [25]. Based on a grading system and an algorithm proposed by Schöffl et al. [19], single

Table 2.4 Radiographic adaptations to rock climbing in the hand [22, 24]

Parameter	German Junior National Team 1999–2004	Recreational climbers (juniors)	Control group non-climbing juniors	Adults (2–5 climbing years)	Adults (<10 climbing years)	Adults (<15 climbing years)
Number	31	18	12	37	74	29
Stress adaption:	19 (61 %)	5 (28 %)	0	16 (43 %)	43 (58 %)	20 (69 %)
Cortical thickening	11 (36 %)	2 (11 %)	0	15 (40 %)	41 (51 %)	16 (55 %)
Subchondral sclerosis/epiphyseal concentration	11 (36 %)	1 (6 %)	0	5 (14 %)	11 (15 %)	4 (14 %)
Insertion calcification (FDP, FDS)	3 (9.7 %)	0	0	4 (11 %)	11 (15 %)	7 (24 %)
Broadened joint base PIP	13 (42 %)	5 (28 %)	0	11 (30 %)	39 (53 %)	16 (55 %)
Broadened joint base DIP	4 (13 %)	0	0	12 (32 %)	41 (55 %)	18 (62 %)
Osteoarthrotic changes	1 (3.2 %)	1 (6 %)	0	4 (11 %)	15 (20 %)	8 (28 %)
Bone spurs PIP	0	0	0	4 (11 %)	15 (20 %)	8 (28 %)
Bone spurs DIP	0	0	0	4 (11 %)	15 (20 %)	7 (24 %)
Narrowing joint space	0	0	0	0	1	6 (21 %)
Cysts, decalcification	0	0	0	1	1	4 (14 %)
Epiphyseal fracture	1 (3.2 %)	1 (6 %)	0			

FDP flexor digitorum profundus, FDS flexore digitorum superficialis, PIP proximal interphalangeal joint, DIP distal interphalangeal joint

Table 2.5 Therapy guidelines for annular pulley injuries [19]

	Grade I	Grade II	Grade III	Grade IV
Injury	Pulley strain	Complete rupture of A4 or partly rupture of A2 or A3	Complete rupture A2 or A3	Multiple ruptures, as A2/A3, A2/A3/A4, or single rupture (A2 or A3) combined with Mm.lumbricalis or ligamental trauma
Therapy	Conservative	Conservative	Conservative	Surgical repair
Immobilization	None	10 days	10–14 days	Postoperative 14 days
Functional therapy	2–4 weeks	2–4 weeks	4 weeks	4 weeks
Pulley protection	Tape	Tape	Thermoplastic or soft-cast ring	Thermoplastic or soft-cast ring
Easy sport-specific activities	After 4 weeks	After 4 weeks	After 6–8 weeks	4 months
Full sport-specific activities	6 weeks	6–8 weeks	3 months	6 months
Taping through climbing	3 months	3 months	6 months	>12 months

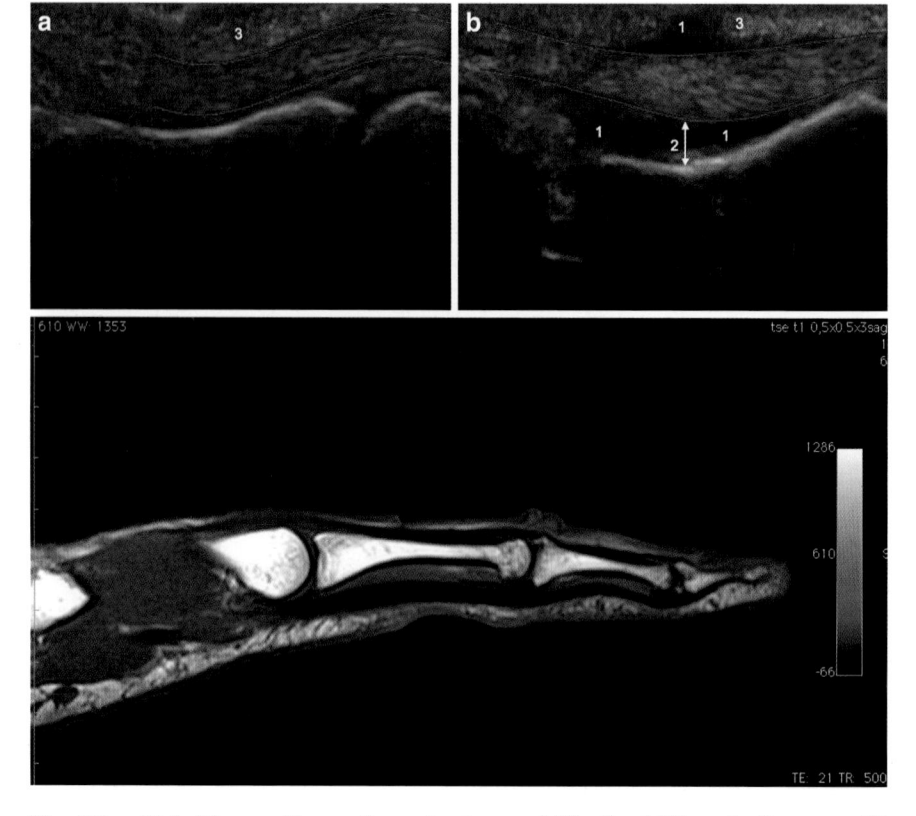

Figs. 2.7 and 2.8 Ultrasound image of normal and ruptured A2 pulley (**a**) Normal pulley system (**b**) A2 pulley rupture, note the increased distance of the flexor tendon to the bone (2) *1*: effusion and haematoma *2*: Tendon bone distance *3*: A2 pulley and tendon sheath, A2 pulley rupture in MRI image

ruptures would dictate a conservative treatment while multiple ruptures would require a surgical treatment (Fig. 2.9). Biomechanical analyses (Fig. 2.10) and strength measurements after conservative treatment for a single pulley rupture showed no strength deficit of the injured finger with the climbers returning to their original performance level after 1 year [26]. The outcome after surgical repair of multiple pulley injuries is also good, with >90 % of injured climbers reporting the resumption of previous climbing level after 1 year, in most cases. Nevertheless, a minor range of motion deficit is often present and may persist [26]. The main conservative recommended measure after a pulley injury is a protective taping with the biomechanically developed H-tape [27]. Therapy guidelines for annular pulley injuries are outlined in Table 2.5.

Tenosynovitis

Tenosynovitis (tendonitis, tendovaginitis) is the most important and common differential diagnosis with the pulley injury and the most frequent overuse syndrome in

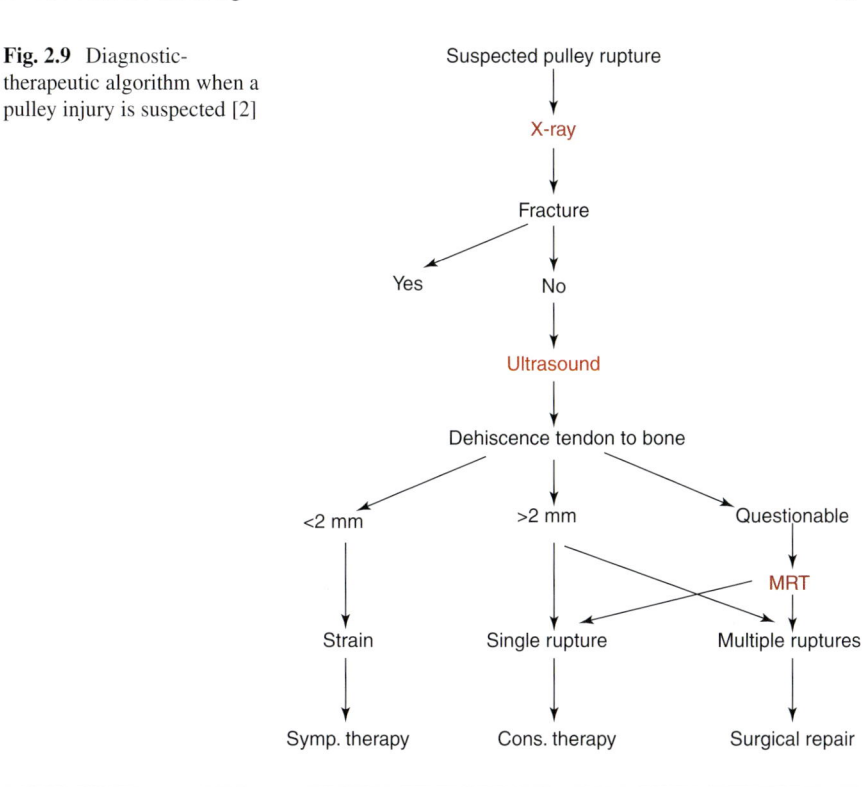

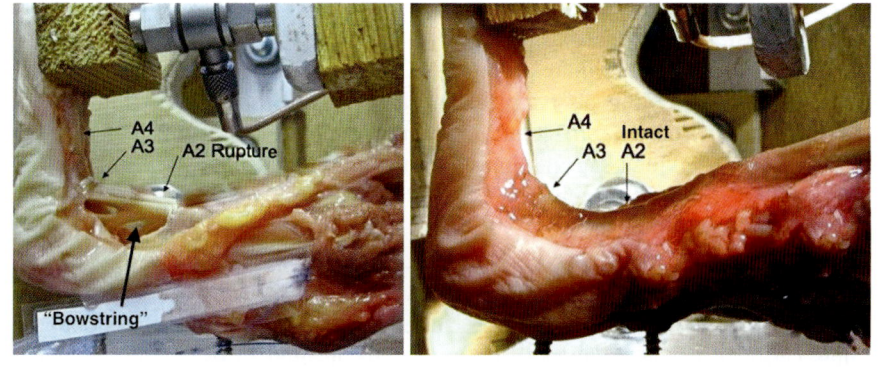

Fig. 2.9 Diagnostic-therapeutic algorithm when a pulley injury is suspected [2]

Fig. 2.10 Image of cadaver in biomechanic strength test with A2 pulley rupture: note the large distance between the flexor tendon and the bone (Picture courtesy of Schöffl I, Institute of Anatomy, FAU Erlangen-Nuremberg)

climber's fingers. An inflammatory response occurs after repetitive stress, and its onset can be acute, after one exceptional hard training or climbing session, or slow, which develop over days of continuous strenuous activity. The climber will present with pain and minor swelling along the palmar surface of the digit, similar to the anatomic location as in a pulley injury. The pain can also extend into the palm or the forearm. The diagnosis is best confirmed via ultrasound, which detects a "halo" phenomena around the tendon. This increased gathering of liquid around the tendon becomes most visible in the transverse plane. As climbers tend to have various ranges of increased fluid in their flexor tendon sheaths after high stress, no clear information can be given as for the normal range of this finding. It is best to compare the ultrasound findings of the injured finger to the contralateral one. The therapy consists initially of anti-inflammatory medication, rest using a splint for several days, brush massages, and ice therapy. In a persisting condition, local cortisone injection may be applied with the known risk involved. These injections, also being used as a last resort, are unavoidable in some instances, as the chronic tenosynovitis can be stubborn.

Joint Capsular Damage and Collateral Ligament Injury

Through directly pulling on "one-finger pocket" holds, a high stress is summoned upon the passive joint structures, the capsule, and the ligaments. By jamming the finger within the finger pocket hold (a hole in the rock), the climber is trying to divide the stress applied on the finger along its full length. This can strain or rupture both the joints capsule and the collateral ligaments. An injury to the palmar plate occurs typically when the finger is jammed in one- or two-finger pockets, and while the climber tries to continue with his next move advancing himself up, the finger gets stuck and as a result the joint is placed in a hyperextended position. This forced hyperextension can cause a palmar plate sprain, partial tear or complete tear, with or without displacement or entrapment. Radiographs will exclude a bony avulsion lesion. In the absence of detectable instability, the conservative therapy will be instigated consisting of immobilization in a cast, splint, brace, or buddy strapping to the adjacent digit. Only chronic instabilities or a complete rupture with joint entrapment of the palmar plate requires exploration and repair with or without reconstruction. Overextension of the palmar plate can cause an avulsion fracture. If neglected, this can result in a chronic stiff joint. Joint contractures are frequently the long-term results of untreated joint capsular injuries with chronic effusion and synovitis.

Arthritis and Osteoarthrosis

Acute arthritis (synovitis, capsulitis) is caused by the high-pressure peaks onto the joints cartilage in the crimp position potentially leading to osteoarthritis. Initial complains are of early morning stiffness and swelling of the finger joints, a reduced range of motion, and pain, which is improved after activity. An acute arthritis finger joint is swollen and feels warm but has no radiographic findings. The chronic condition, however, is characterized in the hand by massive bone spurs. The spurs can mechanically irritate the extensor tendon hood resulting in a local inflammation. The conservative therapy of these conditions consists of the common regimens with anti-inflammatories, ice, ointments, and massages. In the absence of improvement, an intra-articular injection of corticosteroids under image guidance is recommended. Alternatively, or in resilient cases, a radiosynoviorthesis is performed (RSO – a nuclear medicinal local therapy of chronically inflammatory affection of the joints through radioactive substances). Active movement therapy including compression therapy softballs, Thera-Band® Hand Exerciser, or Qigong balls is very important in both therapy and as a prophylaxis measure. The climber needs to be advised to perform these exercises not only as a warm up but also in order to cool down after a climbing session, to reduce intra-articular effusion.

The key question is whether long-term high-level climbing must lead to osteoarthrosis of the hands. The answer, as based upon current literature, concludes that climbing definitely increases the risk for osteoarthritis of affected joints, but this is not a direct consequence [28]. Schöffl et al. [22, 23] examined the German Junior National Team and a group of recreational young climbers and compared them to a group of non-climbers using clinical examination and radiographs' evaluation. They found no increase in osteoarthrosis rate in the climbers group; however, 47 % of the national team members showed bony stress reactions. These findings were evidenced in 28 % of the recreational climbers, while the non-climbers group had none. One member of the national team as well as one member of the recreational climbers had suffered from previous epiphyseal fracture, and one of them (recreational climber) showed early stages of osteoarthrosis. The 10-year controls are presently performed and will give further information.

Tendon Strains and Ruptures

Directly injured tendons are usually a result of the finger or hand being placed in a hanging position, which is then followed by a sudden additional stress. An example would be a loss of a foothold, resulting in a sudden full body weight load on the finger. The main presenting complaint is of pain running along the course of the flexor tendon. This pain increases in the hanging position, while it can disappear fully in the crimp position. Diagnosis can be rather difficult and the use of ultrasound and MRI is recommended. The anticipated recovery time can be rather lengthy, and the reoccurrence rate is high [2]. Treatment consists of early functional and manual therapy together with therapeutic ultrasound. In rare cases, a partial tear of the tendon is diagnosed, which can lead to the formation of tendon nodules and a trigger finger phenomena. Tendon avulsions or complete tears are rare, unless open traumatic injury is involved.

Fractures, Epiphyseal Fractures

Most fractures reported in climbing are caused by a direct trauma, such as rock fall or when striking the rock face, or the ground, during a fall. These trauma-related injury mechanisms can result in various fracture types, predominantly of the lower limbs. Another possible injury mechanism, which is more climbing activity related, involves a hand or a finger jammed in a crack or pocket hold which is prone to bending or an indirect trauma. The above fractures should be treated according to common orthopedic trauma conservative measures or by surgical fixation when indicated. Fixation should be considered in accordance with expected level of activity and the climber's goals regarding return to activity time frame. Note that some minor fractures can

Fig. 2.11 Epiphyseal fracture to the dorsal part of the epiphysis. (**a**) in the crimping position the dorsal part of the epiphysis gets most of the load, which can lead to a epiphyseal fracture (**b**) radiographic image of epiphyseal fracture

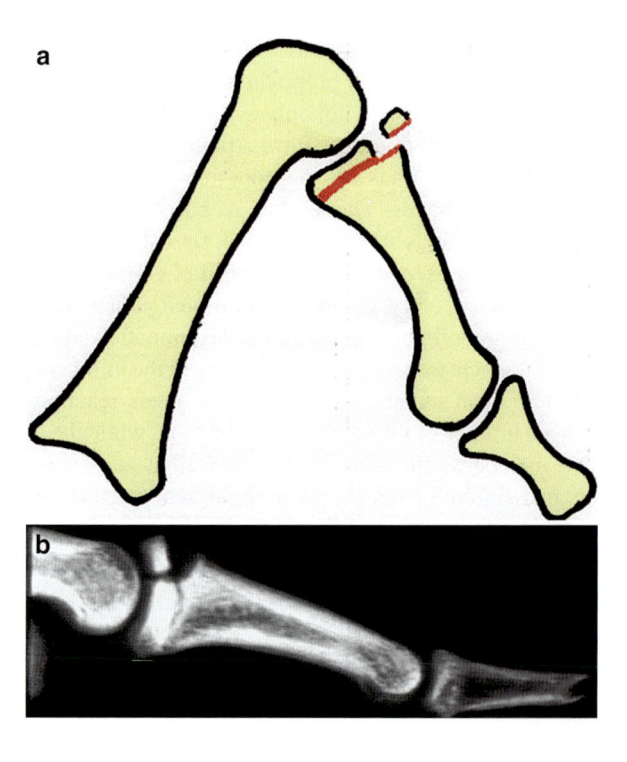

clinically mimic a pulley rupture, and as so, an x-ray should be performed, differentiating between the two. An alarming increase in the number of epiphysiolyses and epiphyseal fractures of young climbers without major trauma has been noted [16]. These injuries should be considered as fatigue fractures which can be related to the unique anatomy and histology characteristics of the immature bone [16]. The radiographs will commonly resemble a Salter-Harris type III fracture of the dorsal part of the PIP joint epiphysis (Fig. 2.11). This injury can be directly linked to the crimp position pathomechanism. Patients suffering from this injury report a slow onset of pain and a lack of a specific single event. They complained of pain and swelling at the interphalangeal joint. If a standard radiograph fails to show pathologic finding, an MRI is the most sensitive investigation. If left untreated, irreversible damage can occur. In non-displaced fractures and low-grade epiphysiolysis, conservative treatment with cast, splinting, and stress reduction is prescribed. In the presence of a fragment displacement, a surgical reduction, with or without fixation, must be performed. In addition to the applied treatment, information must be disseminated to parents, trainers, and the climbers themselves in order to prevent further injury.

Lumbrical Shift Syndrome

The lumbrical shift syndrome is another rare condition but very specific to climbing. It occurs when the climber pulls on a one-finger pocket, or isolated one-finger strength training, or when they extend one finger while pulling with the others in a

2 Rock and Ice Climbing

Fig. 2.12 Picture from A. Schweizer: lumbrical tears in rock climbers [29]. (**a**) lumbrical shift syndrome of the fourth finger (**b**) MRI image of lumbrical muscle tear (*arrow*)

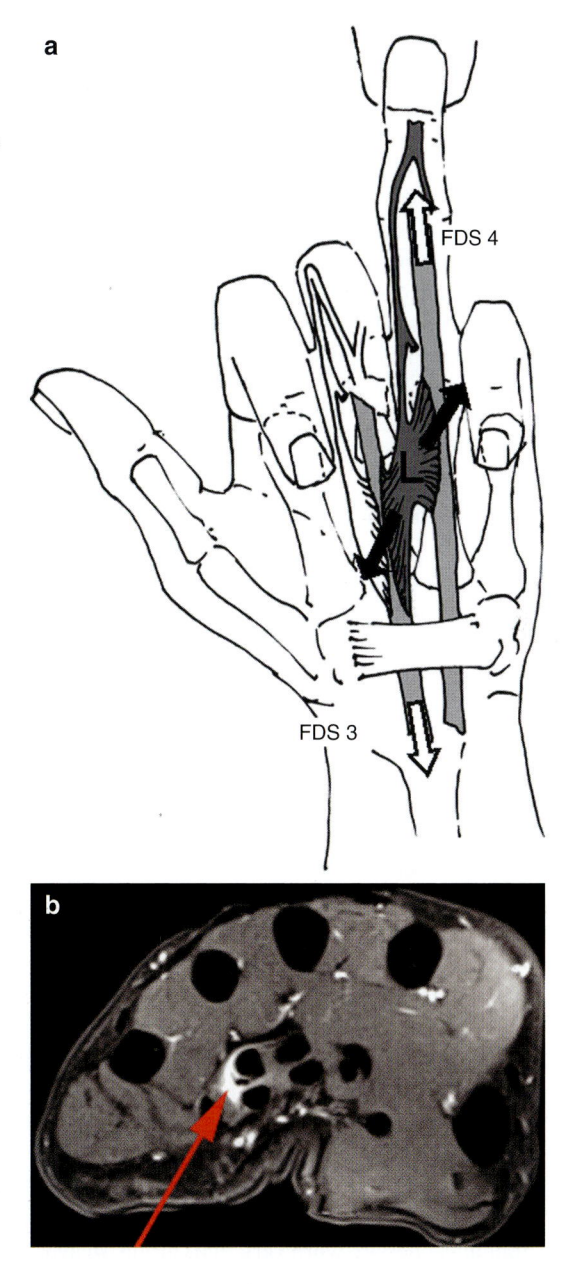

flexed position (Fig. 2.12). This maneuver is causing a shift of the FDP tendons and the lumbrical common muscle belly, of the various fingers, against each other, leading to muscle strains or partial tears. Pain only becomes apparent clinically if one finger is extended while the others are flexed. If the climber pulls with all his fingers in the extended position, no pain is evident. Treatment consists of symptomatic therapy, taping, and a careful stretching of the lumbrical muscles.

Dupuytren Contracture

This is a genetically predisposed pathology that tends to occur in people between the ages of 40 and 60 and is related to chronic microtraumas associated with hard labor or alcoholism. Nevertheless, Dupuytren contractures were recently correlated also with climbing [2, 30], where it tends to involve a less aggressive form. The pathomechanism is probably related to the constant stress and microtrauma of climbing placed upon the tendons and the connective tissue within the palm. This condition is rare in young people and understandably may resemble a malignant process. The authors have quite frequently diagnosed this condition within the younger climbers' population. The therapy is according to known disease stages with initial conservative strategy and in advanced stages by surgical revision.

Chronic Exertional Compartment Syndrome of the Forearms

Chronic exertional compartment syndrome is a well-described condition in sports medicine. Mostly affected is the tibialis anterior compartment in runners. A similar condition can also occur in rock climbers' population arising from the forearm compartments, predominantly the deep flexor compartment. This condition is also described in motorbike racers and piano players. The climber complaints are of a fast increasing "forearm-pump sensation," which is in no correlation to the stress endured. While pumped forearms are usual during long climbs, they normally resolve within a short time. In climbers with a chronic forearm compartment syndrome, the arms stay pumped for a long time period. Diagnosis is proven through intracompartmental pressure measurements, which can be up to over 40 mmHg in some cases (normal: basic <15, stress <30 mmHg) [31]. Schöffl et al. [31] defined an algorithm for the stress pressure and recovery. If an initial conservative therapy fails to improve symptoms, a surgical procedure may be considered.

Other frequently reported climbing-related injuries in the forearms are skin lacerations and bruises and elbow entities as epicondylitis or nerve entrapment syndromes.

Feet

Climbing shoes are worn very tight fitting, in average two to three sizes smaller than one's standard shoes. The reason is due to the need to press on the toes in an erect position, allowing a better strength transfer onto the tip of the shoe and the rock. This would be expected to lead to forefoot-related problems. Roughly, 90 % of climbers reported [14] suffering pain while using their climbing shoes and that they are happy to suffer this discomfort, for improved performance. Frequent problems are callosity, nail bed infections, pressure marks, and subungual hematomas. In the long term, using tight-fit climbing shoes can lead to the development of a hallux valgus deformity. The authors have evidenced 53 % incidence of hallux valgus deformity in long-term high-level climbers, in comparison to 7 % incidence in a similar matched age group of non-climbers [14]. The industry is currently trying to face and eliminate these "side affects" by modifying shoe designs and materials used.

Anorexia Athletica

Strength-to-weight ratio is one of the most important factors in climbing, perhaps more than in any other sport. A study conducted in the University of New Mexico in 1999 showed that climber's body fat below 6 % for males and 10 % for females does not significantly improve performance. Climbers frequently present to us with a body fat lower than the recommended 6 % limit. Their anthropometric data is very similar to gymnastics, and a similar development as in gymnastics can be evidenced in the top athletes' population. The top leading group of the high-level climbers show that they are getting smaller, younger, and thinner. Anorexia athletica, especially in top female climbers, is not an uncommon finding. Although many of the signs of anorexia athletica tend to mirror other eating disorders, some unique signs that pertain specifically to anorexia athletica are known, such as an exercising obsession. This obsession can lead to additional effects on the personal and social life of the climber which keeps on exercising instead of seeing friends and family.

Other signs, both unique to anorexia athletica and also shared with other forms of anorexia or bulimia, include the following:

- Exercising beyond the requirements for good health.
- Obsessive dieting: fear of certain foods and a total exclusion of fat in the diet.
- Obsessive-compulsive exercising: overtraining.
- Individual will not eat with teammates: tries to hide dieting.
- Amenorrhea
- Preference of wide clothes to hide the physical condition.
- Focusing on challenge and forgetting that climbing can be fun.
- Defining self-worth in terms of performance, climbing grades.
- Rarely or never being satisfied with climbing achievements.
- Mood swings: angry outbursts.

These issues need to be discussed openly and addressed properly. Some national federations demand a minimum BMI for entering a competition, although the Medical Commission of the International Federation of Sport Climbing (MedCom IFSC) has considered such a requirement currently unnecessary. Cooperation with the athletes and trainers and regular measures of body parameters, alongside a medical attention, are encouraged. World Cup climbers are currently monitored and regularly measured through the IFSC Medical Commission.

Injury Prevention

Injury prevention must be considered to reduce injury and health problems in climbing athletes. Injury preventive measures should be applied by all parties involved with the athlete's career and activity. Care should be taken by the climbers themselves and the organizers of competition and events, including the personnel in charge of route bolting.

The following points are of major importance although many were already largely improved:

Reducing the chance of an injury while climbing in an artificial indoor environment and while practicing sport climbing outdoors:

- Crash pad and spotting in bouldering
- Using mats in indoor climbing
- Closure of mat gaps
- Route setting outdoors
- Equipment with UIAA safety label
- Belay technique
- Fall technique

In bouldering, a "crash pad" and a spotter are recommended. A "crash pad" is a foldable matt, 10–15 cm thick, which is positioned underneath the climber's route. These mats are widely used and, together with spotting, are the reason bouldering does not result in higher injury rate than roped climbing. The obvious problem with the pads is that they need to be in the correct position beneath a moving climber; it is not uncommon to miss them after a fall. A spotter is usually a climber's partner, who helps position the falling climber in an erect position and onto the mat, when falling.

In indoor climbing, mats are now mandatory under bouldering walls where their thickness for competitions is defined strictly through MedCom IFSC. Also, the intersections in between the multimats used need to be sealed either by Velcro tarpaulin flaps or any similar accepted technique. Using the above recommendations helped to eliminate the "old" and common injury pattern of a climber foot being trapped in between the mats.

On bolted routes, common sense and experience are crucial when deciding where and how to place the bolts in a given route. The bolts should not be too far apart, especially the lower ones, so the possibility of a fall to the ground may be reduced. The bolts should be located at a point where they can be clipped into by all climbers, with consideration of those with a short reach. In addition, bolt planning should take into consideration rock face type (sandstone, granite, and limestone would require different types of bolts and fixation methods) and wall location (bolts adjunct to the ocean's salty air and rust corrode faster).

The UIAA Safety Commission (International Climbing Federation) gives safety labels or seals to approved safety equipment, and only such equipment should be used. There is an intensive ongoing research on injury mechanism and avoidance of technical failures, e.g., in belay devices. A good belay and fall technique must be trained and utilized so that the belayer does not stop his partner's fall too statically, leading to a sudden arrest of the climber's fall. This affects the climber both in the arrest of the fall and any recoil back into the rock surface. Similar consideration must be given to falls by the climber themselves by awareness of good falling techniques [9]. It is crucial for a climber to understand, plan, and train his body position and reaction to a fall, which is a common part of sport climbing. As in many other sports, awareness and preparation are essential.

General preventive measures such as warm up and cool down and stretching and training of the antagonists are important preventive measurements. Finger taping to further strengthen the pulleys, although very common among climbers, failed to prove a preventive effect in several studies. Junior and preadolescent climbers should avoid campus board to prevent epiphyseal fractures and early osteochondral damages. Posture training is important in junior climbers to minimize back problems (e.g., "climbers back", a hump back like postural adaptation [32]), and in general, highly active athletes as well as all junior athletes should be medically examined once per year. Guidelines for competing climbers' examinations are given by the IFSC Medical Commission (www.ifsc.org).

Ice Climbing

Much lesser numbers of studies have been performed reporting on ice climbing injuries and overuse syndromes. In our study [10], we found that most of the acute injuries (61.3 %) occurred while lead climbing, 23.8 % while climbing second, and the remainder were rare (6.3 % belaying, 3.8 % on return and 2.5 % on approach, other 2.5 %). Most of the acute injuries (73.4 %) happened in an icefall climbing, a smaller number on glacier ice walls (11.4 %), and the least on artificial ice walls (2.5 %). Climber fall-related acute injuries amounted to 10.5 %. Although over a quarter (27.3 %) of the injuries needed medical attention, only few (5.7 %) required hospitalization (Tables 2.6 and 2.7). Permanent damage however occurred in as much as 22.7 % of the injury cases. This was attributed to dysesthesia (2), cartilage damage (1), skin scars (6), and dental injuries (2). Injury type and anatomical distribution can be found in Tables 2.5 and 2.6. Surprisingly, most injuries were of minor severity.

Numbers for fatalities in ice climbing are difficult to obtain. According to the Canadian Alpine Club who document injuries and fatalities in the Canadian Rockies, there has been one fatality reported per year, for the last 30 years [3]. With the rising popularity of ice climbing, these numbers are likely to increase.

Table 2.6 Ice climbing injuries [10]

Ice climbing injuries		
Injury	n	%
Frostbite	9	8.8
Open wounds	53	52
Fractures	2	1.9
Hematoma	21	20.6
Other injuries	17	16.7
Total	102 (in 95 incidences)	100

Table 2.7 Location of ice climbing injuries [10]

Body part	n	%
Head	49	40.8
Finger	16	13.3
Leg	15	12.5
Foot	6	5
Arm	6	5
Shoulder	3	2.5
Chest	3	2.5
Back	2	1.7
Neck	1	0.8
Perianal	1	0.8
Others	18	15
Total	120	99.9

Ice Climbing: Overuse Syndromes

We investigated injuries in ice climbing in 2009, reporting a cross-sectional survey study of 88 ice climbers [10]. Seventeen (19.3 %) athletes reported a total of 35 different overuse syndromes related to ice climbing. Of these, 94.4 % involved the upper extremity. Interestingly, no persistent medical problems were reported by any climbers. In the majority (72.2 %) of cases, poor technique was perceived to be the predetermining factor for overuse problem. Overuse syndromes evidenced were muscle strains in the arm (28 %), in the shoulder (6 %), in the calf (6 %) and tendonitis in the arm (17 %), the fingers (22 %), and the shoulder (2 %). Training time correlated with the risk for development of an overuse problem ($p<0.01$). Conversely there was no correlation with body mass index.

In terms of risk perception and overuse problems, there was significant correlation between the risk of overuse problem reported and a climber's self-perception of risk (self-perception, scale from 1–4) ($p<0.01$). Icefall climbing also significantly correlated with overuse syndromes ($p<0.01$) [6].

Mountaineering

The term mountaineering encapsulates a wide field, and the specific medical problems and illness risks associated with high-altitude or expedition climbing is a very big topic by itself [11].

In high-altitude climbing, the risk of climbing at lower levels is complicated by the diminished oxygen concentration. Common altitude-related medical problems include acute mountain sickness (AMS), high-altitude pulmonary edema (HAPE), and high-altitude cerebral edema (HACE) [12]. Up to altitudes of about 5,000–6,000 m, symptoms of altitude illness are a direct result of poor acclimatization. Dependent on the ascent profile, up to 70 % of mountaineers suffer from some sort of altitude symptoms. Primary prevention is therefore considered the gold standard to avoid altitude illness. This includes a conservative ascent profile, adequate hydration and energy intake, and early recognition and management of potential medical problems, both before and during the trip [33].

For further details on high-altitude medicine, we refer to the specific literature. When comparing the injury profile of mountaineering, studies reveal a higher injury and fatality rate compared to rock and ice climbing [11]. Küpper [34] analyzed 2,730 rescue operations with 4,139 diagnoses recorded. The 72.8 % of trauma cases showed a significantly higher severity than those in sport climbing, especially more fractures, severe wounds, and polytraumatic patients. Firth et al. [35] calculated a mortality rate of 1.3 % when examining causes of mortality among those that climbed Mount Everest from 1921 to 2006 ($n = 192$ died from 28,276). Pollard and Clarke [36] similarly found that at extreme altitude, 70–80 % of mountaineering deaths were related to environmental factors. Salisbury [37] and Salisbury and Hawley [38] identified mortality rates between 0 and 0.126 deaths for every 100 mountaineers climbing above 6,000 m. In recent years, the mortality in mountaineering has appeared to decline [11]. On 8,000-m peaks, ascent success rates declined with summit height, but overall death rates, and death rates during descent from the summit, increased with summit height, while conversely overall death rates, and death rates during descent from the summits, increase with summit height [3, 11]. In mountaineering, additional environmental factors can directly influence injuries and fatalities (e.g., avalanches, crevasses, altitude-induced illnesses with neurological dysfunction), while these situations can still be avoided or successfully managed (e.g., using weather forecasts, training in alpine climbing/rescue skills, obtaining knowledge of local terrain, climbing permits, acclimatization and awareness of altitude-induced illnesses, access to helicopter mountain rescue). Also, coinciding existing medical conditions are more likely to cause injuries and fatalities in long mountaineering expeditions than in a single day rock climbing. Similar to many extreme sports, overuse injuries tend to predominate, typically involving the hands and arms in climbing sports. With the additional factors of cold and high altitude, there may be small misjudgments, which increase injury rates. Given the extreme environment, simple injuries may be significant consequences.

References

1. Schöffl V, Küpper T. Injuries at the 2005 world championships in rock climbing. Wilderness Environ Med. 2006;17:187–90.
2. Hochholzer T, Schöffl V. One move too many. 2nd ed. Ebenhausen: Lochner Verlag; 2006.
3. Schöffl V, Morrison AB, Schwarz U, Schöffl I, Küpper T. Evaluation of injury and fatality risk in rock and ice climbing. Sports Med. 2010;40:657–79.
4. Nelson NG, McKenzie LB. Rock climbing injuries treated in emergency departments in the U.S., 1990–2007. Am J Prev Med. 2009;37:195–200.
5. Schöffl V, Morrison AB, Hefti U, Schwarz U, Küpper T. The UIAA medical commission injury classification for mountaineering and climbing sports. Wilderness Environ Med. 2011; 22:46–51.

6. Schussmann LC, Lutz LJ, Shaw RR, Bohn CR. The epidemiology of mountaineering and rock climbing accidents. Wilderness Environ Med. 1990;1:235–48.
7. Schöffl VR, Schöffl I, Finger pain in rock climbers: reaching the right differential diagnosis and therapy. J Sports Med Phys Fitness. 2007;47:70–8.
8. Neuhof A, Hennig FF, Schöffl I, Schöffl V. Injury risk evaluation in sport climbing. Int J Sports Med. 2011;32:794–800.
9. Schöffl V, Küpper T. Rope tangling injuries – how should a climber fall? Wilderness Environ Med. 2008;19:146–9.
10. Schöffl V, Schöffl I, Schwarz U, Hennig F, Küpper T. Injury-risk evaluation in water ice climbing. Med Sport. 2009;2:32–8.
11. Schöffl V, Morrison A, Schöffl I, Küpper T. Epidemiology of injury in mountaineering, rock and iceclimbing. In: Caine D, Heggie T, editors. Medicine and sport science – epidemiology of injury in adventure and extreme sports. Basel: Karger; 2012.
12. Basnyat B, Murdoch DR. High-altitude illness. Lancet. 2003;361:1967–74.
13. Basnyat B, Lemaster J, Litch JA. Everest or bust: a cross sectional, epidemiological study of acute mountain sickness at 4243 meters in the Himalayas. Aviat Space Environ Med. 1999;70:867–73.
14. Schöffl V, Winkelmann HP. [Footdeformations in sportclimbers] Fußdeformitäten bei Sportkletterern. D Z Sportmed. 1999;50:73–6.
15. Hohlrieder M, Lutz M, Schubert H, Eschertzhuber S, Mair P. Pattern of injury after rock-climbing falls is not determined by harness type. Wilderness Environ Med. 2007;18:30–5.
16. Hochholzer T, Schöffl VR. Epiphyseal fractures of the finger middle joints in young sport climbers. Wilderness Environ Med. 2005;16:139–42.
17. Kubiak EN, Klugman JA, Bosco JA. Hand injuries in rock climbers. Bull NYU Hosp Jt Dis. 2006;64:172–7.
18. Logan AJ, Makwana N, Mason G, Dias J. Acute hand and wrist injuries in experienced rock climbers. Br J Sports Med. 2004;38:545–8.
19. Schöffl V, Hochholzer T, Winkelmann HP, Strecker W. Pulley injuries in rock climbers. Wilderness Environ Med. 2003;14:94–100.
20. Schöffl V, Hochholzer T, Winkelmann HP, Strecker W. [Differential diagnosis of finger pain in sport climbers] Differentialdiagnose von Fingerschmerzen bei Sportkletterern. D Z Sportmed. 2003;54:38–43.
21. Hochholzer T, Heuk A, Hawe W, Keinath C, Bernett P. Verletzungen und Überlastungssyndrome bei Sportkletterern im Fingerbereich. Prakt Sport Trauma Sportmed. 1993;2:57–67.
22. Schöffl VR, Hochholzer T, Imhoff AB, Schoffl I. Radiographic adaptations to the stress of high-level rock climbing in junior athletes: a 5-year longitudinal study of the German junior national team and a group of recreational climbers. Am J Sports Med. 2007;35:86–92.
23. Schöffl V, Hochholzer T, Imhoff A. Radiographic changes in the hands and fingers of young, high-level climbers. Am J Sports Med. 2004;32:1688–94.
24. Schöffl V. Rock climbing. In: Engelhardt M, editor. Sports injuries, vol. 1. Munich/Jena: Elsevier; 2011.
25. Schöffl V, Schöffl I. Injuries to the finger flexor pulley system in rock climbers – current concepts. J Hand Surg Am. 2006;31:647–54.
26. Schöffl V, Einwag F, Strecker W, Schöffl I. Strength measurement after conservatively treated pulley ruptures in climbers. Med Sci Sports Exerc. 2006;38:637–43.
27. Schöffl I, Einwag F, Strecker W, Hennig F, Schöffl V. Impact of taping after finger flexor tendon pulley ruptures in rock climbers. J Appl Biomech. 2007;23:52–62.
28. Hochholzer T, Schöffl V. [Osteoarthrosis in fingerjoints of rockclimbers] Degenerative Veränderungen der Fingergelenke bei Sportkletterern. D Z Sportmed. 2009;60:145–9.
29. Schweizer A. Lumbrical tears in rock climbers. J Hand Surg Br. 2003;28:187–9.
30. Logan AJ, Mason G, Dias J, Makwana N. Can rock climbing lead to Dupuytren's disease? Br J Sports Med. 2005;39:639–44.
31. Schöffl V, Klee S, Strecker W. Evaluation of physiological standard pressures of the forearm flexor muscles during sport specific ergometry in sport climbers. Br J Sports Med. 2004;38:422–5.

32. Förster R, Penka G, Bosl T, Schöffl VR. Climber's back – form and mobility of the thoracolumbar spine leading to postural adaptations in male high ability rock climbers. Int J Sports Med. 2009;30:53–9.
33. Küpper T, Gieseler U, Angelini D, Hillebrandt J, Milledge J. Emergency field management of acute mountain sickness, high altitude pulmonary oedema and high altitude cerebral oedema. In: Commission UM, editor. Consensus statement of the UIAA medical commission. 1st ed. Bern: UIAA; 2009.
34. Küpper T. [Workload and professional requirements for alpine rescue]. Professoral Thesis at RWTH Aachen Technical University/Germany, 2006 (English publication in preparation). Professoral Thesis (English publication in preparation). Aachen: Aachen Technical University; 2006.
35. Firth PG, Zheng H, Windsor JS, Sutherland AI, Imray CH, Moore GW, Semple JL, Roach RC, Salisbury RA. Mortality on Mount Everest, 1921–2006: descriptive study. BMJ. 2008;337:a2654.
36. Pollard A, Clarke C. Deaths during mountaineering at extreme altitude. Lancet. 1988;1:1277.
37. Salisbury R. The Himalayan database: the expedition archives of Elizabeth Hawley. Golden: American Alpine Club; 2004.
38. Salisbury R, Hawley E. The Himalayan by the numbers. 2007. www.himalayandatabase.com. Accessed on 11 Sep 2012.

Chapter 3
Alpine Skiing and Snowboarding Injuries

Mike Langran

Contents

The Origin of the Sports and Their Development to the Current Stage	37
The Equipment Used: Essential and Safety Requirements	39
Alpine Skiing	39
Snowboarding	41
Equipment Common to Both Sports	42
Off-Piste (Backcountry) Equipment	44
Injury and Fatality Rates and Specific Types of Injury Related to Each Sport	44
Overall Injury Risk	44
Risk of Death on the Slopes	46
Injuries from Alpine Skiing	47
Injuries from Snowboarding	47
Injuries by Anatomical Area	51
Common Treatments for Each Sport and Relevant Rehabilitation	58
Proposed Prevention Measures	58
General Advice on Preventing Snow Sport Injuries	58
Advising Alpine Skiers on Injury Prevention	62
Advising Snowboarders on Injury Prevention	64
References	64

The Origin of the Sports and Their Development to the Current Stage

Alpine skiing and snowboarding are regarded as the two main piste-based snow sports. Alpine skiing has its roots in Nordic (cross-country) skiing, which evolved as a method of transportation in Scandinavia many thousands of years ago. The first skiers are believed to be Sami tribes in Scandinavia. A Norwegian, Sondre

M. Langran
General Practitioner, Health Centre, Aviemore Medical Practice,
Inverness-Shire PH22 1SY, Scotland, UK
e-mail: mike@ski-injury.com

O. Mei-Dan, M.R. Carmont (eds.), *Adventure and Extreme Sports Injuries*,
DOI 10.1007/978-1-4471-4363-5_3, © Springer-Verlag London 2013

Norheim, is widely regarded as the father of modern skiing. His early designs have gradually evolved over time from a pure method of transportation into the recreational and competitive activities of the modern day. Downhill skiing per se began in the nineteenth century, and Alpine skiing became a winter Olympic sport in Garmisch in 1936. Since this time, many variations of Alpine skiing have come and gone. Currently Alpine skiing can be broadly divided into downhill and freestyle subspecialties. Noncompetitive Alpine skiing is generally known as recreational skiing. Competitive downhill disciplines include slalom, giant slalom (GS), supergiant slalom (super G), and downhill racing. Each discipline has its own technical specifications which largely relate to both speed and turning ability. These can be influenced by many factors including ski length and the turn radius of the ski. Freestyle skiing combines aerobatic and balance skills, and participants use a variety of natural and man-made features (such as terrain parks and rails) to perform aerial tricks and maneuvers. Freestyle skis have twin-tip designs which allow the user to land and travel backward as easily as forward. Freeride skiing involves performing similar tricks to freestyle skiing but in the natural environment using features such as cliffs, steep runs, and off piste to perform maneuvers.

Snowboarding developed from Sherman Popper's original "snurfer" concept in the 1960s. The sport really took off in the mid-1980s, enjoying a phenomenal subsequent rise in popularity as manufacturing pioneers like Jake Burton refined and diversified the appeal of their products. Snowboarding led to the initial development of terrain parks at ski areas offering features such as half- and quarter pipes, rails, and big air jumps. These allowed snowboarders to perform aerial tricks and maneuvers which initially were difficult to perform on traditional Alpine skis. It became an Olympic sport in 1998. As with Alpine skiing, there are several styles of snowboarding available, each with their own variations on equipment and technique. The most common are freeride, freestyle, and freecarve. Freeride is the most popular activity and involves riding down any terrain available, most commonly pisted runs. Freestyle snowboarding (as with skiing) involves aerial tricks and maneuvers using a variety of features to gain "air." Freecarving, which has become far less popular, involves high-speed slalom snowboarding using stiff and narrow boards.

Visually exciting side by side simultaneous racing by up to four competitors going over a series of obstacles is common to both sports and known as "skier cross" or "boarder cross."

Although absolute numbers vary from resort to resort, currently approximately 60 % of those on the slopes are Alpine skiers, 30–35 % snowboarders with the remainder participating in sports such as ski boarding (snowblading) and Telemark skiing. There are currently estimated to be around 200 million skiers and 70 million snowboarders active in the world today. Many enthusiasts participate in these sports both on and off piste (Fig. 3.1).

The Equipment Used: Essential and Safety Requirements

The fundamental difference between the two primary snow sports is that Alpine skiers have their legs attached to their skis such that one can move independent of the other. In snowboarding, both feet are attached to the same single-board axis (Fig. 3.1). This has important implications for balance and maneuverability particularly for beginners.

Alpine Skiing

Alpine skiers use two skis attached to plastic ski boots via releasable binding systems. Ski poles are used to aid balance. The boot and binding should really be regarded as a single interface that transmits forces in both directions between the skier and the ski. Many different types of ski binding are available, all with subtle differences. All modern ski bindings involve a safety system which can be adjusted so that the binding releases at different preset force levels depending on the individual characteristics of the skier and their specific preferences. The bindings are also fitted with a braking system such that if the ski detaches from the boot, brake

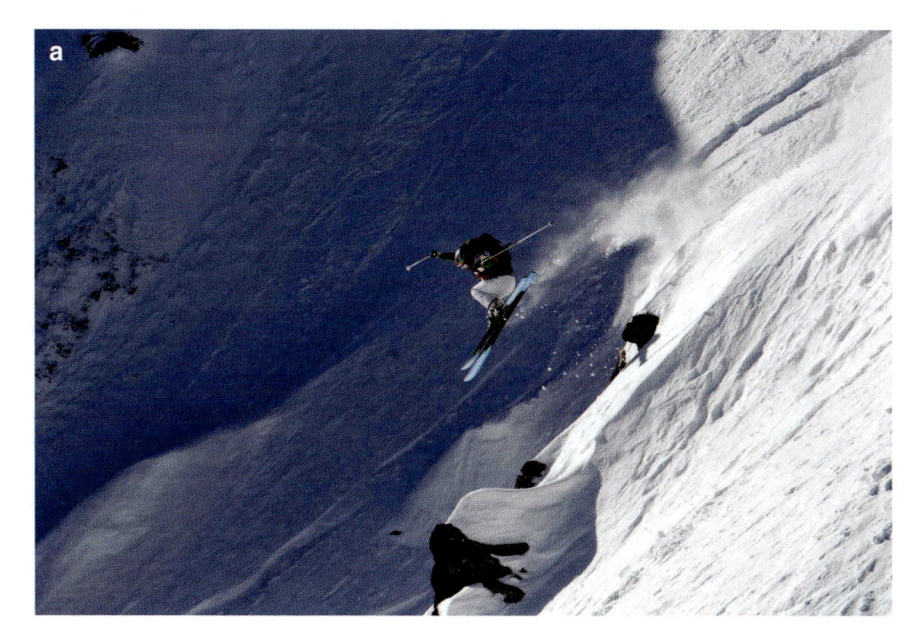

Fig. 3.1 Skier and snowboarder at the backcountry setup (By David Carlier)

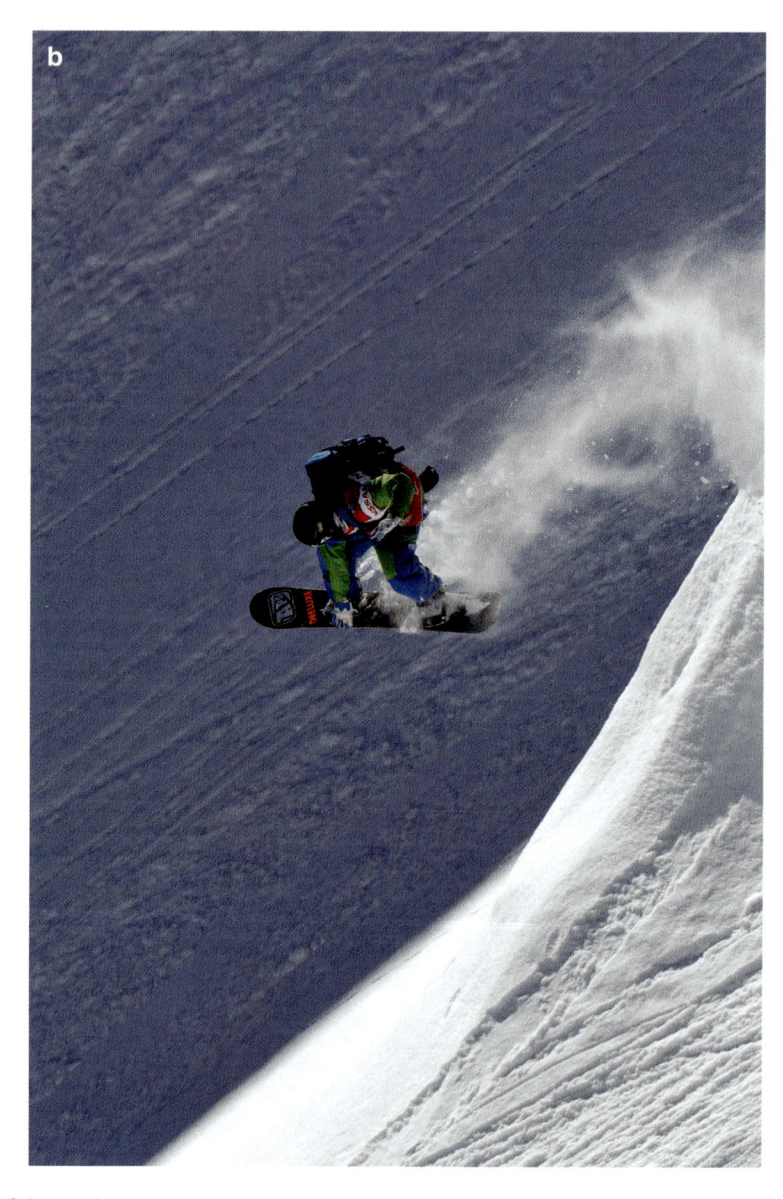

Fig. 3.1 (continued)

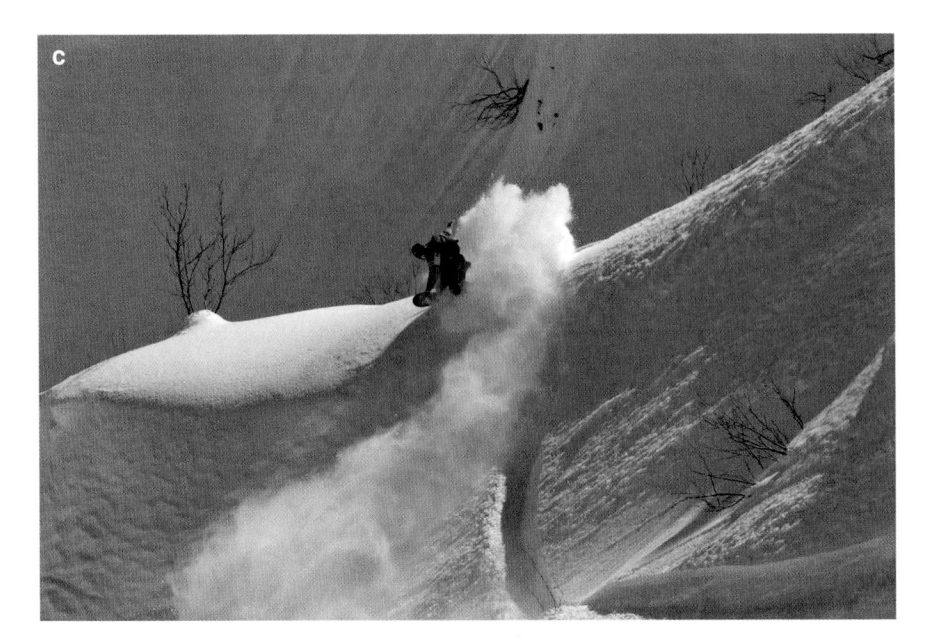

Fig. 3.1 (continued)

arms are activated. This function reduces the risk of a runaway ski sliding down the mountain causing injury. There is a huge variety of skis, boots, and bindings available depending on individual skiers' preferences on cost, performance, comfort, and appearance. In the early 1990s, a fundamental equipment change took place with the introduction of carving skis. Compared to older traditional skis which were long and relatively thin, carving skis have an hourglass shape with a wide tip and tail and a narrow waist. This improves the turning performance of the skis and in general makes them much easier to maneuver [1].

As a result, carving skis have helped to revive the popularity of skiing in the face of competition from snowboarding and have subsequently lead to the development of other ski designs such as twin tips which further broaden the performance spectrum.

Snowboarding

In contrast to Alpine skiers, snowboarders are attached to a single wide board by non-releasable bindings. The snowboard stance is angled relative to the board unlike Alpine skiers who face the same direction as their skis. About 95 % of snowboarders wear softer boots than Alpine skiers [2]. These aim to combine functionality with comfort. Harder plastic boots are used by a small minority (who prefer improved maneuverability at the cost of a small loss of comfort). Various binding systems are available including step-in plate bindings, strap, and flow designs. In general, snowboarders release one boot from its binding when using most lift systems. The majority of snowboard bindings have neither a release function nor an inbuilt braking system. Expert opinion has concluded that the biomechanics of snowboarding indicate that a releasable binding system is of no benefit to the majority of recreational snowboarders [3]. However, the potential exists for a runaway board if both boots are out of the bindings and the boarder loses control of their board. An extendable leash can be attached to the board in order to reduce this risk. The relatively recent advent of split snowboards (where the snowboard divides into two fat skis to which climbing skins can be attached) allows snowboarders the opportunity to explore the backcountry, previously the exclusive domain of skiers.

Equipment Common to Both Sports

In order to ski and snowboard in comfort in Alpine environments, skiers and snowboarders commonly wear layered outdoor clothing in order to be able to regulate their temperature according to their level of activity and the prevailing weather conditions. Outer clothing layers need to be both windproof and waterproof, and many different fabrics are available. Clothing layers near to the body should be able to wick moisture away from the body. Ambient temperatures can be extremely low which, combined with wind chill, can lead to a significant risk of hypothermia. Additional protection is needed in such circumstances including frostbite protection for the face, nose, and ears. Specific face masks are available for this purpose.

Helmets

The popularity of helmets among snow sport enthusiasts has increased considerably in recent years. The deaths of celebrities such as actress Natasha Richardson (after a seemingly innocuous fall while skiing in March 2009) inevitably lead to considerable media coverage and can significantly influence the use of helmets on the slopes [4]. Helmet design has improved considerably, and what was once viewed as a geeky piece of equipment has now attained a cool status. In America, currently about 60 % of all skiers and snowboarders now wear a helmet, and in Switzerland, the figure is almost 80 % [5]. Modern helmets provide superior comfort, ventilation, and attractive graphics (see www.skihelmets.com). They also allow the integration of an ever increasing number of modern devices such as helmet cams and portable music players/radios.

Not only should a helmet fit correctly, but it is imperative that it meets one of the three accepted manufacturing standards for snow sport helmets. These are CEN 1077, ASTM 2040, and Snell RS 98. All set minimum standards for impact protection from both blunt and sharp objects at prescribed speeds. To meet the standards for CEN 1077, for example, a helmet containing a simulated head must be able to withstand a drop from 1.5 m onto a flat anvil. The peak acceleration imparted to the "head" must not exceed 250 Gs. Helmets must also survive a drop from 0.75 m onto a conical metal punch, simulating the impact from a tree branch or ski pole.

There is now a large body of evidence supporting the view that wearing a helmet reduces the risk of sustaining a head injury by up to 60 % [6–9]. While the majority of this evidence to date concerns minor or moderate head injuries, recent American data has also shown a positive association between helmet use and a reduction in both skull fractures [10] and serious intracranial injuries [11].

Thankfully the actual risk of sustaining a potentially serious head injury is extremely low (approximately 24,000 mean days between injuries [11]). While helmet use is mandatory for competitive skiers and snowboarders, the consensus view of experts such as the International Society for Skiing Safety is that the overall risk of head injury is not high enough to make helmet use mandatory for all recreational users. Others disagree however [12], and this debate is certain to continue for some time [13, 14].

At present there is no evidence that wearing a helmet reduces the risk of traumatic death on the slopes, and those who wear a helmet must be aware that it does not make them invincible. It has been argued that helmet wearers may take more risks and ski/board faster than non-helmet wearers (the so-called risk compensation theory). The evidence to date on this is small but conflicting [15, 16].

Many of the arguments for not wearing a helmet have been questioned by recent research. For example, there is no evidence that helmets interfere significantly with vision or hearing, or that they place excessive force on the neck during an accident [8, 17–19]. Helmets that have been involved in a significant impact such that the physical integrity of the helmet has been damaged should be replaced.

Miscellaneous Equipment

Adequate eye protection is essential as Alpine areas have high levels of UV light. Sunglasses and goggles provide UV protection as well as enhancing the users' perception of physical terrain when traversing in bright or flat light. In general, sunglasses are preferred on calm sunny days, whereas goggles provide additional protection in more stormy weather. Goggles are however liable to fogging up, and adequate ventilation systems are required to prevent this.

Many skiers and snowboarders now routinely use portable digital music players to enhance their experience on the slopes. In addition, a variety of portable cameras have emerged specifically for the snow sport market. These can take a variety of still and video images along with audio recording and may be fitted to clothing, helmets, or even goggles. Indeed some modern goggles now offer integrated GPS systems. Care should be taken with all these items to ensure the user is not distracted by them from paying attention on the slopes.

Off-Piste (Backcountry) Equipment

Skiing or snowboarding out with the boundaries of recognized ski areas requires high levels of skill, knowledge of snow and mountain conditions, and the ability to navigate and survive independently. In addition to the standard equipment required for on-piste activities, backcountry skiers and boarders should carry supplementary equipment to assess and manage the risks and consequences of avalanche. This includes avalanche transceivers, probes, shovels, and airbag systems. Regular training in avalanche search techniques is recommended as time is a critical factor in avalanche survival [20]. Far too many potentially preventable avalanche deaths continue to occur every year [21]. Adequate communications, navigational equipment, and survival food/gear are required along with the skills to use them appropriately. While modern devices such as mobile phones and GPS units can greatly aid the backcountry enthusiast, overreliance on them should be avoided – GPS signals and batteries can both deteriorate unexpectedly. Participation in a specialist backcountry education program is highly recommended as is the use of a professional guide in unfamiliar areas. Those traveling abroad must read the small print of their insurance policy and ensure that it provides adequate cover should (potentially very expensive) rescue be required. Figure 3.2a, b shows a backcountry skier in a self-selected route and high jump. It is important to know how to land these high jumps to avoid major injuries. In Fig. 3.2b, a full-face helmet is almost mandatory in these types of stunts. A personal backpack would contain all the above-mentioned equipment.

Injury and Fatality Rates and Specific Types of Injury Related to Each Sport

Overall Injury Risk

Like most outdoor activities, skiing and snowboarding are associated with a risk of injury. The current risk of a snow-sport-related injury on recreational slopes is between 2 and 4 injuries per 1,000 participant days [22], much lower than most people imagine. Indeed, the risk is much lower than that seen in other popular sports such as football and rugby and has fallen steadily over recent years [23]. Improvements in equipment, ski area design and maintenance, and piste preparation have all contributed to this improvement [23].

There is some variation in the absolute injury rate seen between different studies. This usually relates to the individual design of the study. Those that rely on self-reported injuries not surprisingly tend to result in higher injury rates as individuals are likely to report every single minor injury that they sustain. In contrast, at the other end of the scale, hospital-based studies tend to see a smaller percentage of all injuries sustained and therefore report a lower rate [24]. The middle ground is occupied by studies that rely on ski patrol or mountain clinic data, and these generally give a more accurate reflection of overall injury rate. Nevertheless, some skiers and snowboarders do not seek medical attention near the slopes after their injuries, preferring to either self-treat or return home to seek help in a more familiar setting. This so-called bypass effect occurs to some degree in all injury studies, although its effect is generally believed to be less than 10 % [2, 25].

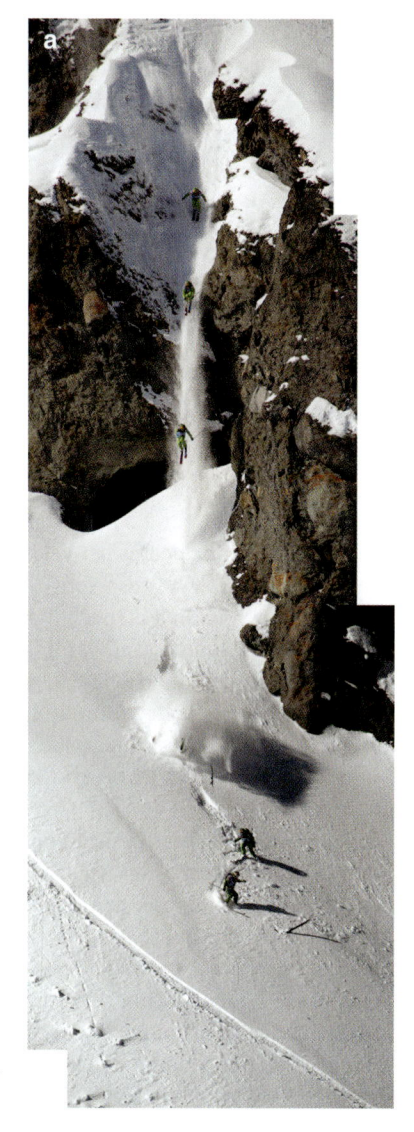

Fig. 3.2 (**a**) A skier lands badly, loose his skis but skis away from it… (**b**) Skier at the Freeride World Tour. Pay attention to full-face helmet, HD head-mounted camera. There is also full body armor underneath outfit (By David Carlier)

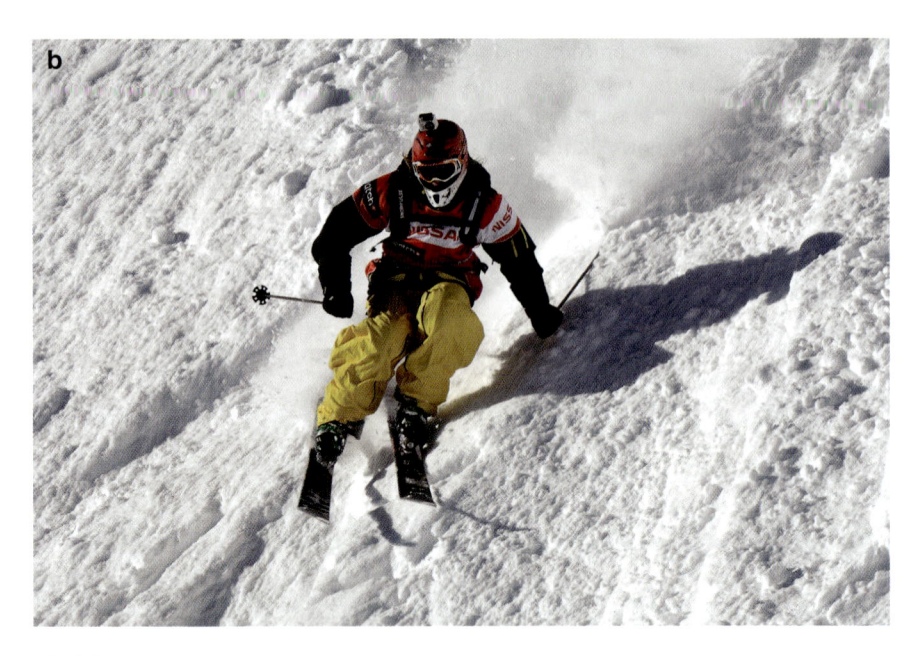

Fig. 3.2 (continued)

Risk of Death on the Slopes

The risk of sustaining a traumatic death from participating in snow sports is even lower at one death per 1.57 million participant days [26]. This equates to approximately 39 traumatic deaths per year in the USA out of a total of almost 60 m participant days (source: www.nsaa.org). As with the risk of injury, the risk of dying from skiing or snowboarding is much lower than that of other popular recreational activities such as swimming and cycling [26]. Nevertheless, snow-sport-related deaths usually attract disproportionate degree of media attention.

The commonest cause of a traumatic snow-sport-related death is a high-speed collision with a static object such as a tree, pylon, or another person [27, 28]. Many of these deaths involve injury to the head either in isolation or with other injuries [28].

Nontraumatic causes of death on the slopes include ischemic heart disease, hypothermia, and medical events such as acute severe asthma attacks [27]. A less frequent but nevertheless important mechanism of death is the so-called non-avalanche-related snow immersion death (NARSID), also known as a "tree well death" [28, 29]. In this scenario, skiers and snowboarders fall into a hidden pit underneath a tree. This is a particular risk when riding between trees either on the lifts or to the side of marked pistes. Unless the event is witnessed, self-extrication from the tree well is extremely difficult. The trapped individual tends to cause more snow to fall into the pit as they struggle to try to free themselves. Death usually results either from hypothermia or asphyxiation from snow falling in [30].

Injuries from Alpine Skiing

Overall Injury Risk

The risk of injury from recreational Alpine skiing is generally accepted to be between 1 and 2 injuries per 1,000 participant days [22, 31]. This rate has decreased considerably since the 1970s [23]. This is largely due to safety advances in equipment design such as the development of releasable ski bindings and ski brakes. Prior to release bindings, fractures of the lower leg in particular were common as twisting forces were regularly transmitted unmitigated from the ski up to the lower leg. Since their introduction, properly set and maintained bindings have been shown to significantly reduce the risk of lower leg fracture. Nevertheless, Alpine skiers are still more likely to injure their lower rather than their upper limb. The knee joint is the single commonest site of injury among skiers. Most of these injuries are soft tissue/ligamentous in nature.

Injury Classification

The breakdown of Alpine ski injuries by type is shown in Figs. 3.3 and 3.4. Muscle and ligament strains and sprains account for almost half of all injuries Fig. 3.5. The fracture rate from Alpine skiing is approximately 19 % [25]. Common sites of fracture include the clavicle, proximal humerus, and tibia. Lacerations may occur as a result of direct impact with objects such as rocks, pylons, and snow fences. Ski edges are also sharp and may inflict nasty wounds. Contusions of varying magnitude result from collisions either with the snow surface or other objects. Joint injuries usually affect either the thumb or the shoulder joint after falling onto an outstretched hand. As more and more skiers enter terrain parks seeking aerial thrills, there has been a slow but steady rise in the incidence of spinal injuries.

Injuries from Snowboarding

Overall Injury Risk

The risk of injury from snowboarding is generally regarded to be about twice that of Alpine skiing and currently stands at between 2 and 4 injuries per 1,000 participant days [31]. Snowboarders are more likely to injure their upper limb than their lower limb [25]. Learning to balance while fixed by both feet to a single board is a critical skill to develop. Unlike skiers, in the event of loss of balance, snowboarders cannot step out a leg to regain balance. As a result, falls due to loss of balance are frequent, and not surprisingly beginner snowboarders are at highest risk. Off-balance falls on

Injury breakdown by classification Alpine skiing

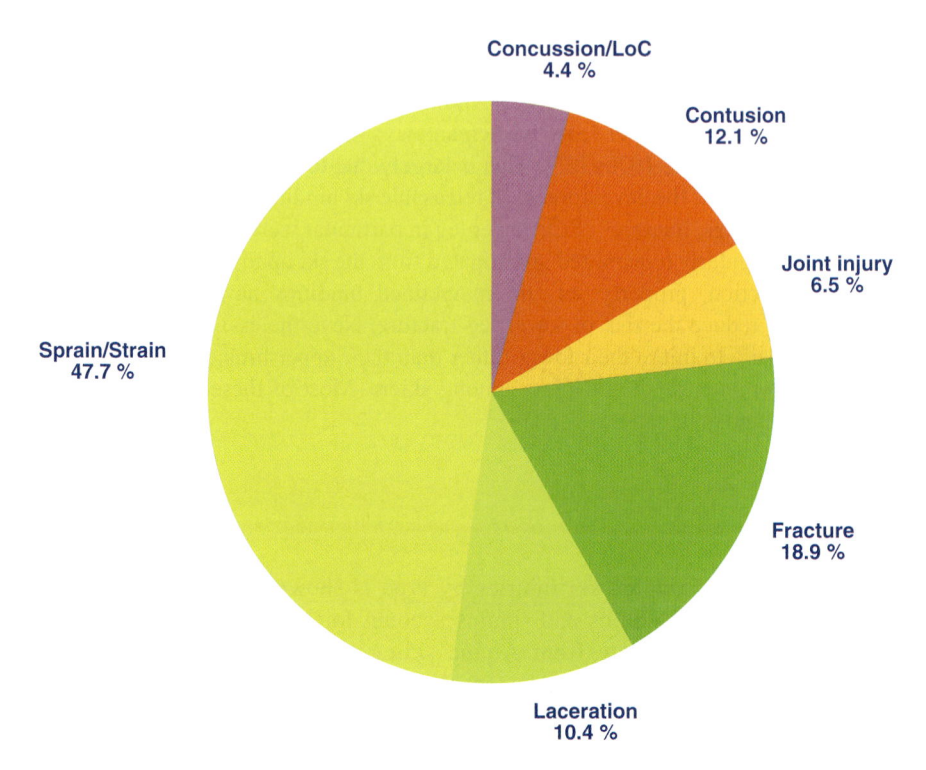

- Concussion/LoC 4.4 %
- Contusion 12.1 %
- Joint injury 6.5 %
- Fracture 18.9 %
- Laceration 10.4 %
- Sprain/Strain 47.7 %

Fig. 3.3 Alpine skiing – injury classification

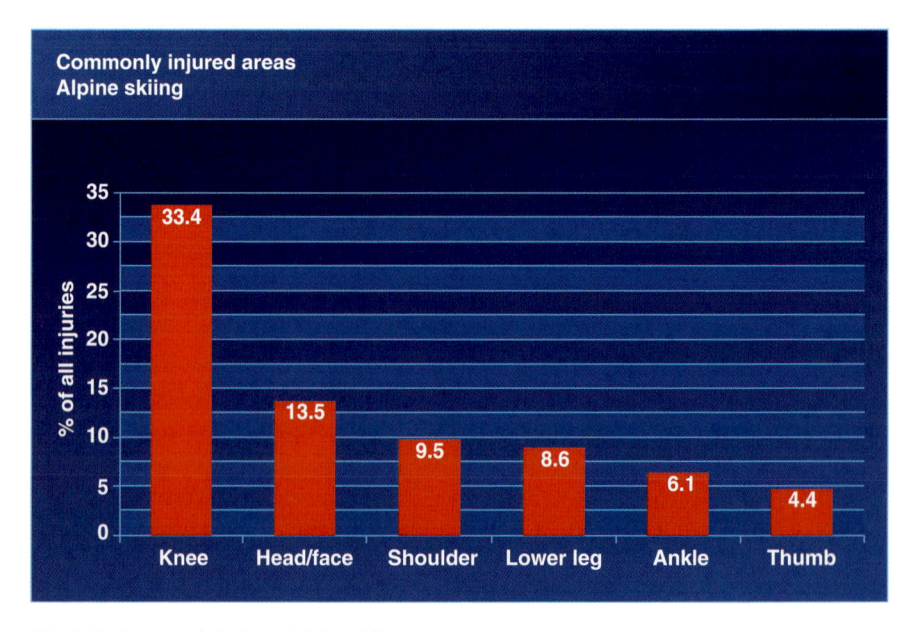

Commonly injured areas Alpine skiing

Area	% of all injuries
Knee	33.4
Head/face	13.5
Shoulder	9.5
Lower leg	8.6
Ankle	6.1
Thumb	4.4

Fig. 3.4 Common injuries – Alpine skiing

**Injury breakdown by classification
Snowboarding**

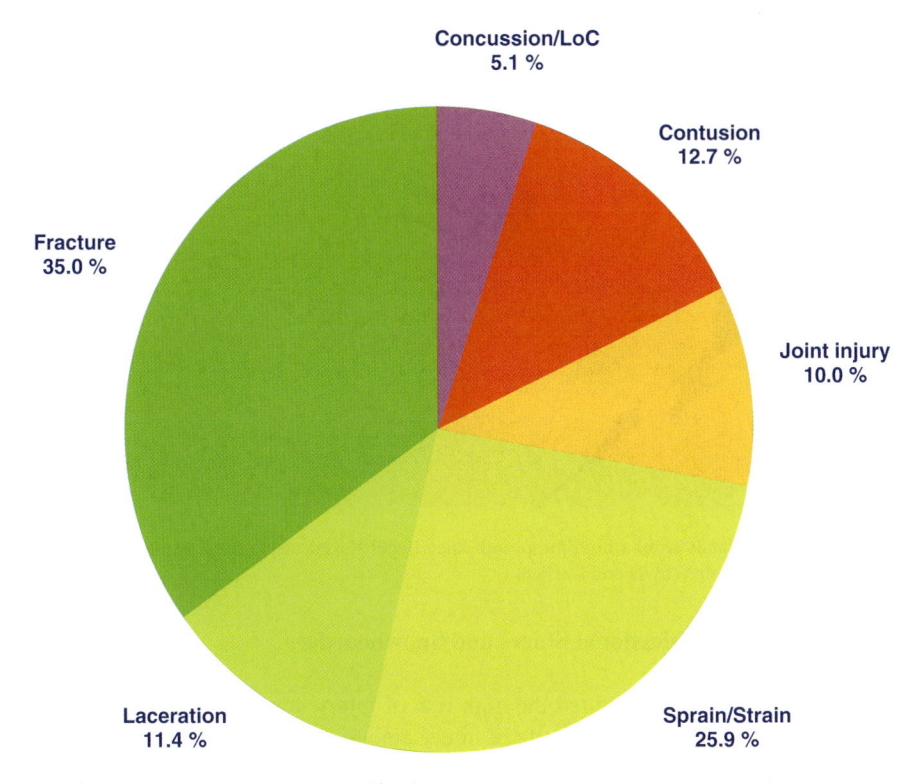

- Fracture 35.0 %
- Concussion/LoC 5.1 %
- Contusion 12.7 %
- Joint injury 10.0 %
- Sprain/Strain 25.9 %
- Laceration 11.4 %

Fig. 3.5 Snowboarding – injury classification

a snowboard generally lead to an instinctual reaction of outstretching the hand to break the fall. This places the upper limb, and the wrist joint in particular, at high risk of injury [32].

Injury Classification

The breakdown of snowboarding injuries by type is shown in Figs. 3.6 and 3.7. The fracture rate among snowboarders is twice that of Alpine skiers [25], and the high rate of wrist fractures (up to 33 % of all injuries [33]) largely accounts for this. Muscle and ligament strain/sprains are still common as are contusions from off-balance falls. Snowboarders suffer a higher rate of shoulder joint injuries due to an increased tendency to fall onto the upper limb [25]. Ever since its inception, snowboarding has been associated with jumps and other aerial maneuvers. These activities are associated with a relatively small but definite risk of injury to the spine [34–36].

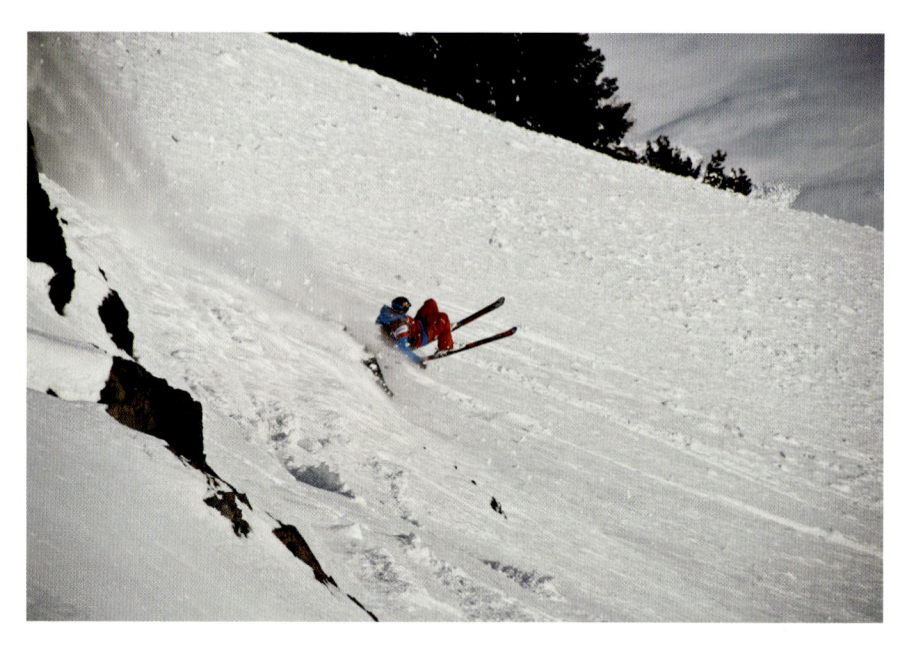

Fig. 3.6 A skier lands from a high jump with knee hyper-flexed which may result in injures to menisci/knee ligaments (by David Carlier)

Injuries Among Professional Skiers and Snowboarders

Recent research has highlighted the high risk of injury among professional skiers and snowboarders [37–40]. The rate of injury among professionals has been calculated to be as high as 17 injuries per 1,000 ski runs [38]. Extrapolation of this data indicates that the injury rate among professionals is approximately three times that of recreational participants [41]. While many of the injuries sustained are similar to those seen among recreational users, in general the incidence and severity of individual injuries is higher [39]. Almost one-third of all injuries among professional athletes were classified as severe, leading to an absence from participation of more than 28 days [39]. The knee is the commonest injury area among competitive Alpine skiers and snowboarders [38, 39, 41]. Having now identified the scale of the problem, the challenge for the FIS and national teams is to address this issue, balancing the potential conflict between performance and safety. Retrospective video analyses may help identify specific injury mechanisms among elite athletes [42].

Injuries Sustained in the Backcountry

There is no reliable data available specifically relating to the issue of backcountry injuries compared to on-slope injuries. Many backcountry users evacuate themselves to healthcare providers of their choice making study design challenging. Moreover, accurate assessment of the population at risk in the backcountry is extremely difficult to calculate. Those injuries that do come to the attention of ski

3   Alpine Skiing and Snowboarding Injuries

physicians indicate that backcountry users are susceptible to a similar range of injuries as other recreational users. In general, the injuries sustained tend to be less severe and less frequent, reflecting the higher ability levels in this group [2].

Injuries by Anatomical Area

Lower Limb Injuries

Knee Injuries

Injuries to the knee joint account for about one third of all skiing injuries. Most of these are minor soft tissue sprains. The medial collateral ligament (MCL) is commonly injured as a result of valgus twist to the knee as the ski unintentionally splays the lower leg outward, thus stressing the knee joint. Clinically, an MCL injury is suggested by the mechanism and description of the fall and is often associated with non-release of the binding. There is localized tenderness over the ligament, and stress testing may demonstrate some laxity in grade two and three injuries. The vast majority of grade one and two injuries will settle with conservative treatment. More aggressive treatment is often required for grade three injuries to permit return to sport.

The most serious soft tissue injury to the knee involves damage to the anterior cruciate ligament (ACL). This important ligament may be injured in isolation or in combination with other structures.

There are several documented mechanisms of ACL injury in skiing. Before the advent of carving skis, the commonest mechanism involved a backward twisting fall (Fig. 3.7). In this scenario (also known as the "phantom foot" mechanism), the large rear tail of the ski behind the binding acts as a twisting lever across the knee

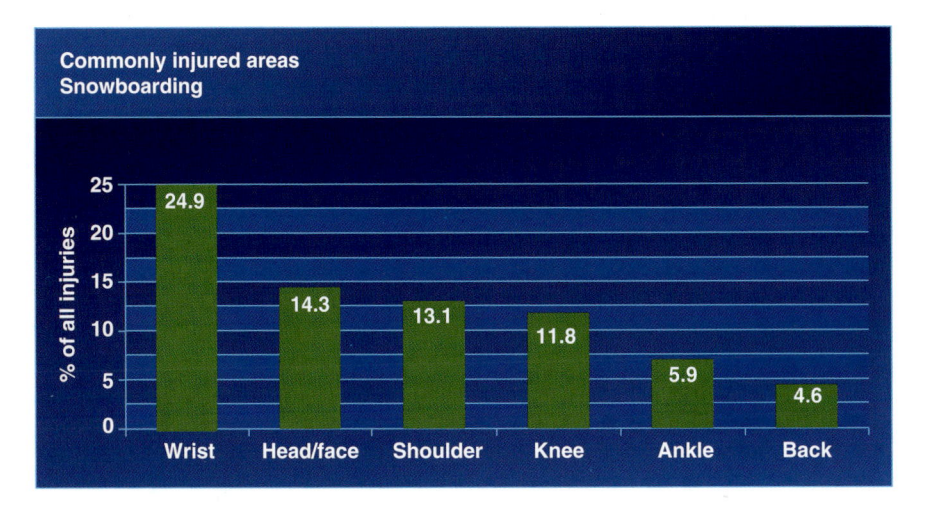

Fig. 3.7 Common injuries – snowboarding

joint, ultimately breaking the ACL [43]. Modern carving skis have a much smaller rear tail which reduces this risk. The commonest ACL injury mechanism currently is thought to be a forward twisting fall [44] with the knee flexed. The ACL can also be injured when a skier lands after a jump on the tail of the skis. The rear of the ski boot pushes the tibia forward relative to the femur causing ACL damage [45] with the knee hyperextended.

Clinically, skiers report hearing or feeling a "pop" or "snap" sensation, and the knee swells rapidly usually within the first 2 h of injury. Diagnosis may be made clinically although MRI is frequently used to ascertain the degree of damage to the ACL and associated structures.

While it is possible to ski without an ACL, this requires considerable effort and physiotherapy input to maintain stabilizing knee muscle bulk and proprioception. Most orthopedic surgeons recommend ACL reconstruction for those who wish to ski at or above an intermediate level.

No studies have yet shown that the wearing of a knee brace provides primary protection against ACL injury while skiing. There is some evidence that a custom knee brace can reduce the incidence of repeat injury after ACL surgery [46].

Knee injuries among snowboarders are much less common and usually result either from direct trauma to the anterior aspect of the knee during a fall or twisting injuries, most commonly when one foot is out of its respective binding. This most frequently happens when the snowboarder is using a surface or chairlift. If the board catches an edge at this time, significant twisting force can be applied to the leg still attached as the binding has no release function. Despite this, most experts agree that releasable snowboard bindings offer little protection to the average snowboarder and in fact inadvertent release may be more of a danger.

Lower Leg Injuries

Before the introduction of releasable ski bindings, fractures of the lower leg were the commonest injury to befall skiers. These injuries can still occur when the binding fails to release and can be subdivided into twist and forward bend injuries depending on the mechanism of fall (Fig. 3.8). The use of properly maintained and set bindings greatly reduces (although does not completely eliminate) this risk.

Direct trauma to the lower leg is the commonest cause of lower leg injury in snowboarders, and the leading leg is at highest risk. Significant twisting injury with one foot out of the binding (as described above) may lead to fractures of the tibia/fibula.

Ankle Injuries

Stiff modern Alpine ski boots in general provide the ankle joint with good protection. Nevertheless, ill-fitting or incorrectly sized boots that allow ankle movement

3 Alpine Skiing and Snowboarding Injuries 53

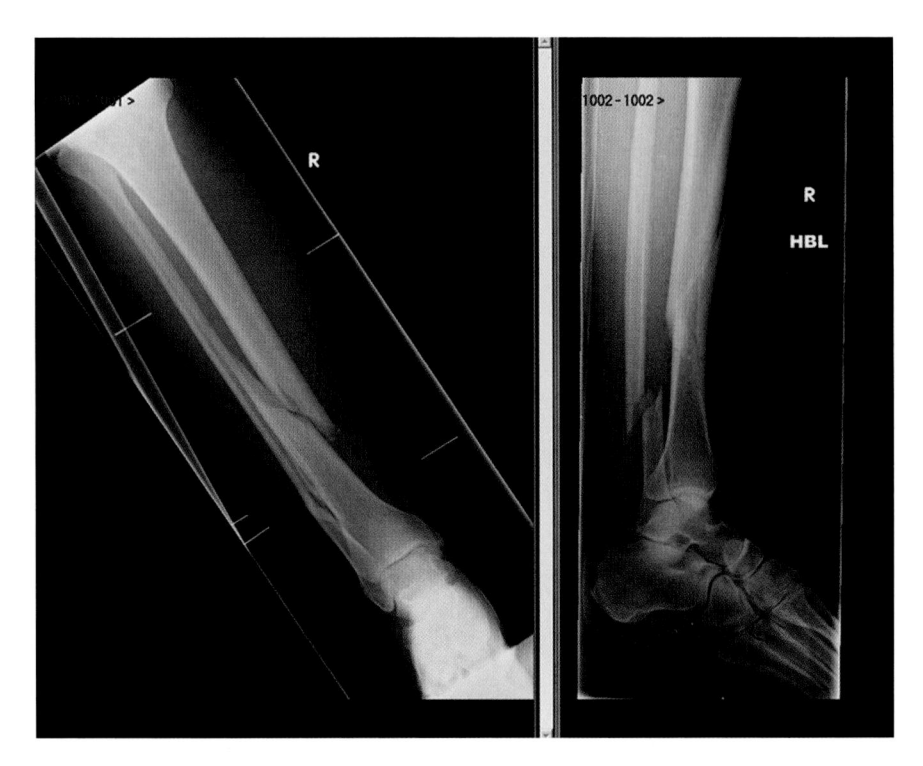

Fig. 3.8 Spiral lower leg fractures from Alpine skiing

can be associated with injury, usually soft tissue ligament sprains. Syndesmosis injuries have been reported in competitive slalom skiers, where excessive external rotation can cause injury to the tibiofibular syndesmosis [47].

Most snowboarders use soft boots as these provide a satisfactory compromise between performance and comfort. Unfortunately, soft boots offer less support to the ankle joint than stiffer ski boots, and, as a result, soft tissue ankle sprains are more common among boarders.

Snowboarders are susceptible to a specific ankle injury – namely, fracture of the lateral process of the talus bone [48]. This injury is rarely seen in other branches of medicine and has become known as "snowboarder's ankle" [49]. The injury mechanism involves compression and inversion often following aerial maneuvers. Clinically, the injury presents as a severe ankle sprain, and plain x-rays usually look normal. As a result, there is a tendency for these injuries to be missed by those not familiar with its occurrence. CT or MRI scanning is required to diagnose this condition which may require operative intervention to avoid early onset of osteoarthritis and long-term disability. Snowboarders who injure their ankles should be encouraged to seek specialist help if their ankle is not improving as would normally be expected.

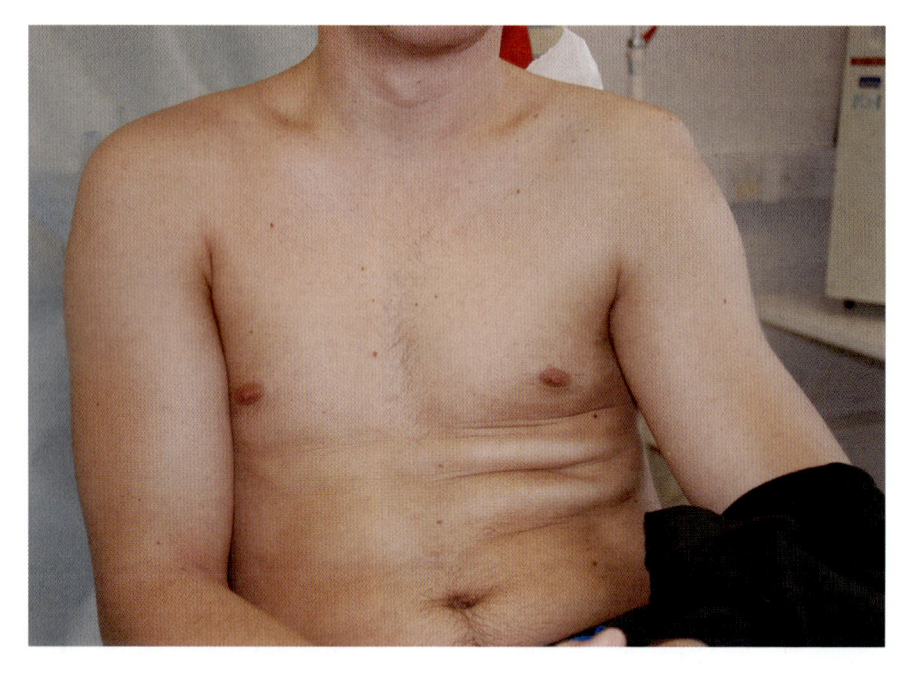

Fig. 3.9 Anterior dislocation of the left shoulder. Note the "squared off" appearance relative to the right shoulder

Femur Injuries

While relatively uncommon, bony injury to the femur requires substantial force and is associated with significant pain and potential concealed blood loss. Common mechanisms of injury include a fall from a height and collision with a static object. Localized severe pain and deformity are usually present.

Upper Limb Injuries

Shoulder Injuries

The four commonest shoulder injuries to affect skiers and snowboarders are anterior dislocation of the glenohumeral joint, acromioclavicular (AC) joint disruption, clavicle fracture, and fracture of the proximal humerus. The incidence of shoulder injuries is higher in snowboarders [50].

The mechanism of injury is the key to determining the injury sustained. Falls onto an outstretched hand can lead to either AC joint disruption or clavicle fracture depending on the level of force applied. If the body twists around the outstretched hand, then anterior dislocation may result. Falls resulting in direct impact of the upper arm onto a hard or icy snow surface may result in proximal humeral fracture.

Recognition of these injuries can be made clinically. Anterior dislocation (Fig. 3.9) is an extremely painful injury except when it has occurred recurrently.

Typically, the affected individual holds their arm to support it, and on examination the shoulder joint appears squared off compared to the uninjured side. Any movement is extremely tender. Clavicle fractures are locally tender, and there may be obvious deformity and palpable tenderness. Localized tenderness and swelling over the AC joint implies injury to this area, although distal clavicle fractures may present in a similar manner. If disruption of the AC joint is significant, then there may be associated deformity of the joint. X-ray may be required to differentiate between distal clavicle fracture and AC joint disruption.

Anterior dislocations should be reduced as soon as possible by clinicians familiar with the injury and methods of reduction. No one method of reduction has been shown to be superior to another. Axillary nerve dysfunction may be present and should be examined for prior to reduction. Many ski patrol physicians perform shoulder joint reductions on the mountainside or in ski patrol rooms. If associated bony injury is suspected, then a prereduction x-ray or CT scan in more complicated cases is ideal. After a first episode of dislocation, the risk of recurrence is high and surgical treatment may be indicated to reduce this risk [51].

The majority of AC joint disruptions (grades 1 and 2), clavicle fractures (with no major shortening or soft tissue compromise), and proximal humeral injuries may be treated conservatively with adequate analgesia and appropriate immobilization. Good functional recovery is the norm together with input from a skilled physiotherapist.

Wrist Injuries

Wrist injuries are relatively uncommon among skiers. The presence of the ski pole in the hand appears to provide a degree of protection against injury in this area. In contrast, the wrist is the commonest single site of injury among snowboarders [25, 50], largely due to falls on the outstretched hand after a loss of balance. Wrist injuries are more common among beginners and advanced snowboarders [25]. Beginners are at the highest risk of wrist injury due to their inherent instability on a board [33]. Advanced snowboarders tend to sustain wrist injuries due to high-velocity falls from aerial maneuvers gone wrong. Unfortunately, many of these injuries involve significant bony displacement, involvement of the growth plate, and/or bony comminution (Fig. 3.10). Consequently, many wrist injuries deter the individual from returning to snowboarding. The use of wrist guards has been shown to significantly reduce the risk of injury [52].

Thumb Injuries

In contrast to the wrist joint, thumb injuries almost exclusively affect Alpine skiers, so much so that the term "skier's thumb" is used to describe the commonest injury – an acute radial stress to the metacarpophalangeal (MCP) joint of the

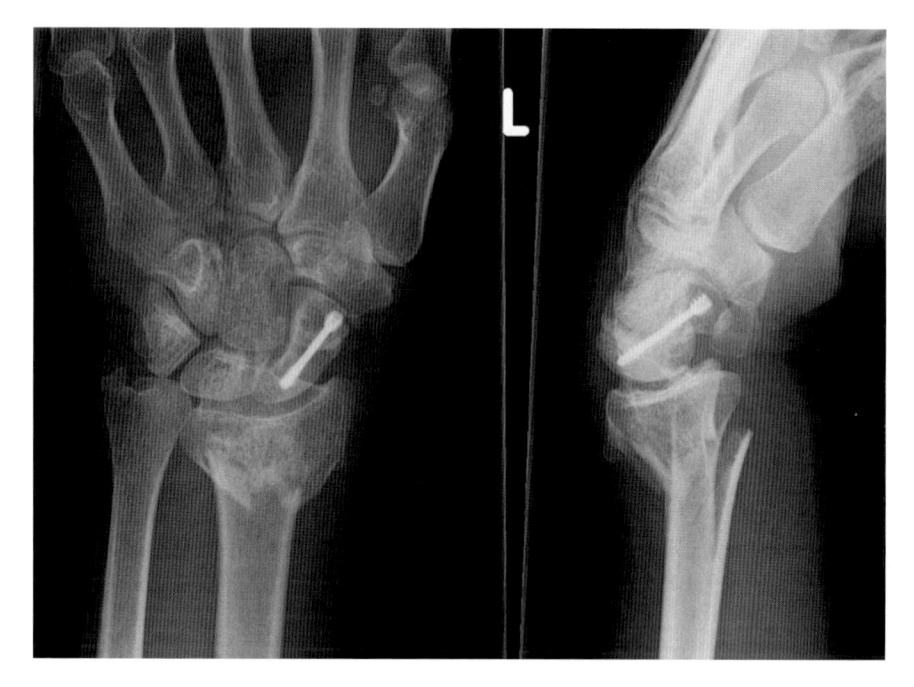

Fig. 3.10 Displaced wrist fracture in a snowboarder with a past history of a scaphoid fracture in the same wrist

thumb. In this injury, the handle of the ski pole acts as a fulcrum across the MCP joint leading to damage to the ulnar collateral ligament (UCL) [53]. If left untreated, this may lead to long-term functional disability. The stability of the UCL can be carefully tested once acute pain has settled, and ultrasound is a useful modality in this assessment. Grade one and two injuries may be treated conservatively, but if the ligament has been torn (grade three injury), then surgical repair is recommended [54]. Occasionally with grade three tears, the adductor aponeurosis interposes between the two torn ends of the UCL and prevents ligamentous healing. This is known as a Stener lesion and also requires surgical repair [55].

Elbow Injuries

In an off-balance backward fall, the elbow is at risk of hyperextension which can lead to either joint dislocation and/or bony injury to the distal humerus or proximal radius/ulnar. This mechanism is far commoner among snowboarders than skiers. Elbow dislocations in snowboarding are commonest on the same side as the sliding direction and tend to occur primarily due to backward falls [56].

Axial Injuries

Axial injury relates to any injury to the central axis of the body. It includes injury to the head, spine, chest, abdomen, or pelvis.

Head Injury

Injuries to the head account for up to 15 % of all skiing and snowboarding injuries [15]. Thankfully most of these are minor contusions and abrasions. Potentially serious head injuries (PHSI) include skull fractures and brain hemorrhage, and these injuries usually result from a collision at speed with a static object such as a tree, pylon, or other person.

Spinal Injury

Injuries to the spine are becoming more frequent among skiers and snowboarders as they attempt more and more daring aerial maneuvers [57, 58]. The majority of catastrophic injuries occur due to landing inverted, either directly onto the head or with forced flexion/extension of the neck. Unfortunately, the small bones of the cervical spine in particular are extremely vulnerable to relatively low forces, and, hence, even a bad landing from a relatively low jump may prove disastrous [59]. Much current research is focused on the design of terrain park features with specific emphasis on the landing area, in order to reduce the effective fall height (EFH) [60]. Nordic ski jumps, for example, use carefully controlled takeoff and landing areas which result in average EFHs of only 0.6 m despite jump lengths of over 100 m [61]. As a result, catastrophic injuries from Nordic jumping are rare events. It is argued that the same principles applied to terrain park design may make them safer [61]. In the meantime, skiers and snowboarders must exercise extreme care when performing jumps and tricks. If spinal injury is suspected, early intervention by ski patrol and careful application of full spinal immobilization are required with rapid transfer to an appropriate medical facility.

Other Axial Injuries

Depending on the mechanism of injury, skiers may sustain damage to their chest, abdomen, and/or pelvis. Such injuries usually involve high speeds and forces. While many injuries involve nothing more than contusions, significant visceral damage can result. In some instances of liver and splenic damage, it has been reported that individuals can continue skiing or snowboarding initially after injury before they become compromised. Careful assessment of such patients is required and treatment applied as appropriate.

Figure 3.11a–c A skier is airlifted after a major multitrauma injury. Most large alpine resorts now have a helicopter trauma service in place.

Common Treatments for Each Sport and Relevant Rehabilitation

Most of the injuries sustained by skiers and snowboarders are thankfully relatively minor in nature. Initial treatment should follow the standard guidelines for soft tissue injuries. Further treatment will depend on the specific individual injury and follows the normal pathways for trauma and orthopaedic care. Depending on the resources available, up to 70 % of all injuries may be dealt with on-site by the attending ski patrol staff. This includes the majority of lacerations, contusions, and other minor soft tissue injuries. In general, due to a lack of appropriate monitoring facilities, most ski patrols have a low threshold for transferring head-injured patients onto medical care. The majority of fractures are treated conservatively unless significant displacement, comminution, or ongoing functional disability is present.

Injury rehabilitation will depend on the specific circumstances of the injury and the individual involved. Early physical therapy is recommended, and emphasis should be placed on maintaining general cardiovascular fitness during the recovery phase. Some individuals face psychological barriers when planning a return to the slopes after a significant accident. Appropriate psychological intervention may be required to address this.

Proposed Prevention Measures

General Advice on Preventing Snow Sport Injuries

Skiing and snowboarding are exhilarating activities that nevertheless carry a degree of inherent risk. Accidents can happen for a variety of reasons, not all of which are under the control of the individual involved. Nevertheless, many simple preventative measures may reduce this risk considerably. All skiers and snowboarders should be aware of and adhere to the FIS code on piste safety (see Fig. 3.5). The majority of accidents occur when this code is broken.

The vast range of equipment options available can be confusing. Inexperienced skiers and snowboarders tend to hire their equipment initially and should be offered professional guidance on appropriate gear (in terms of both size and performance) for their needs. Hire facilities certified to ISO or TUV standards are recommended. Time must be taken to ensure that all equipment fits comfortably and is appropriate for the user's ability level. Carving skis should be standard issue for skiers. All slope users should be encouraged to wear a protective helmet that meets a recognized

3 Alpine Skiing and Snowboarding Injuries

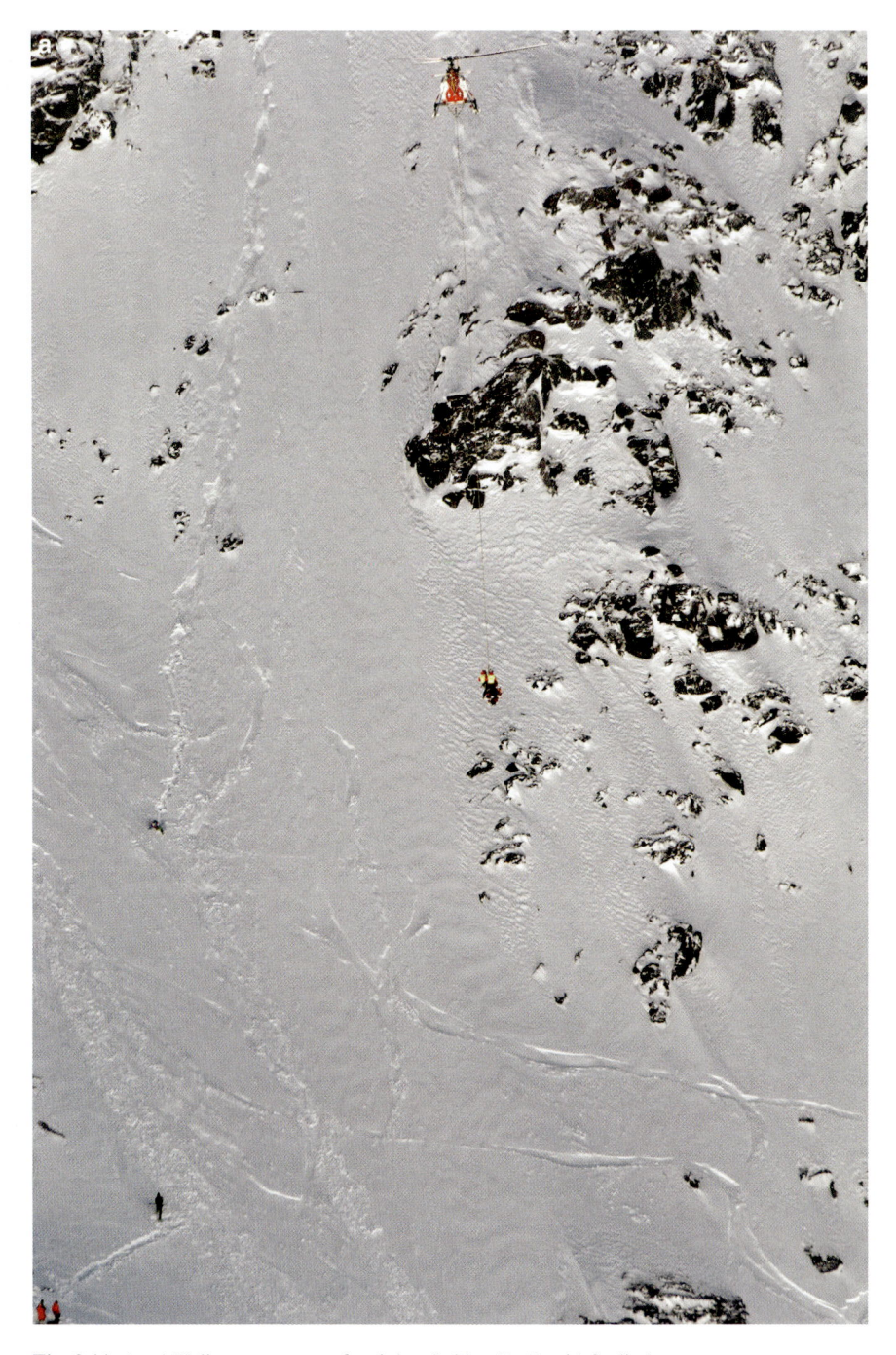

Fig. 3.11 (a–c) Helicopter rescue of an injured skier (By David Carlier).

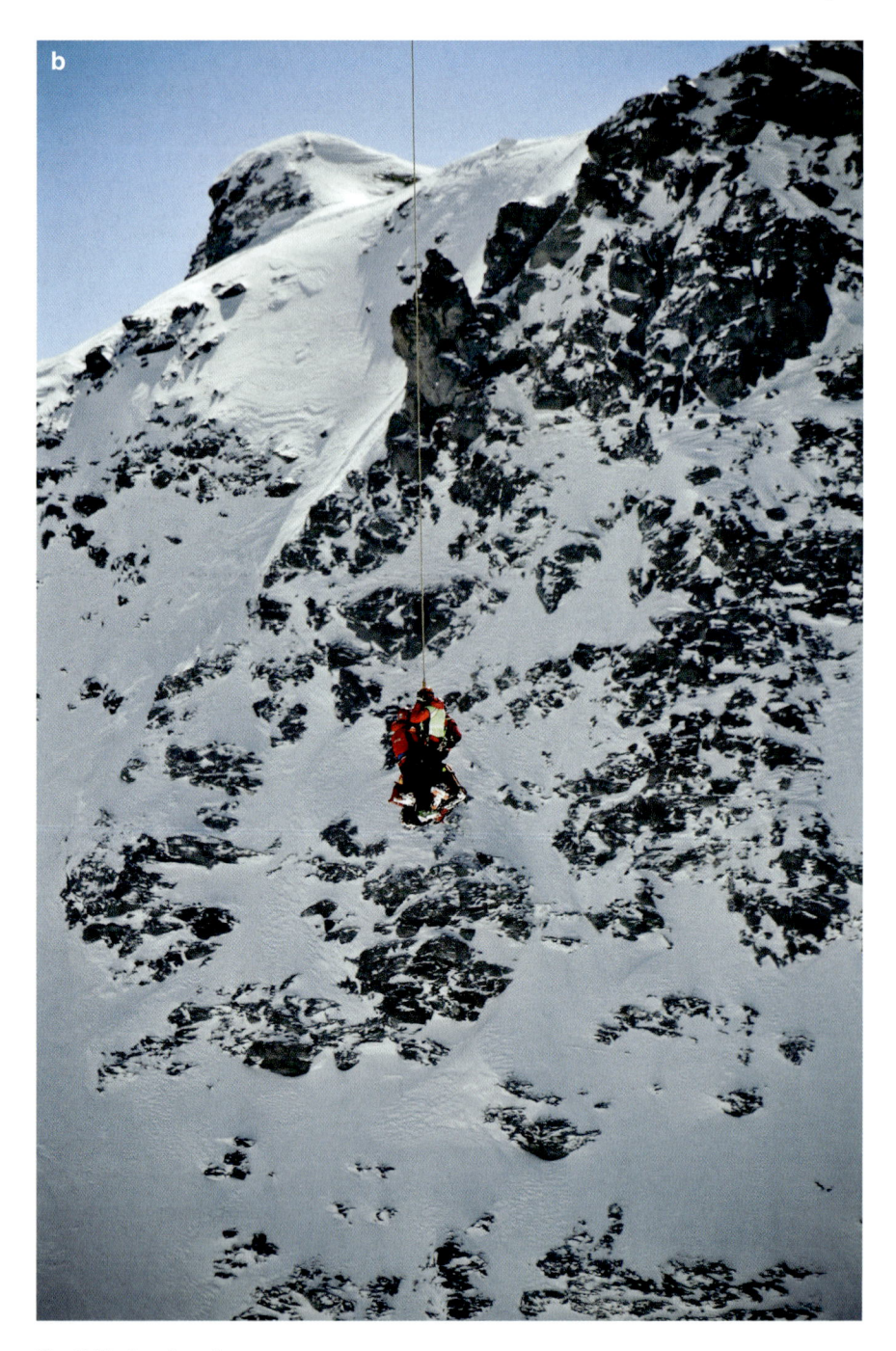

Fig. 3.11 (continued)

3 Alpine Skiing and Snowboarding Injuries 61

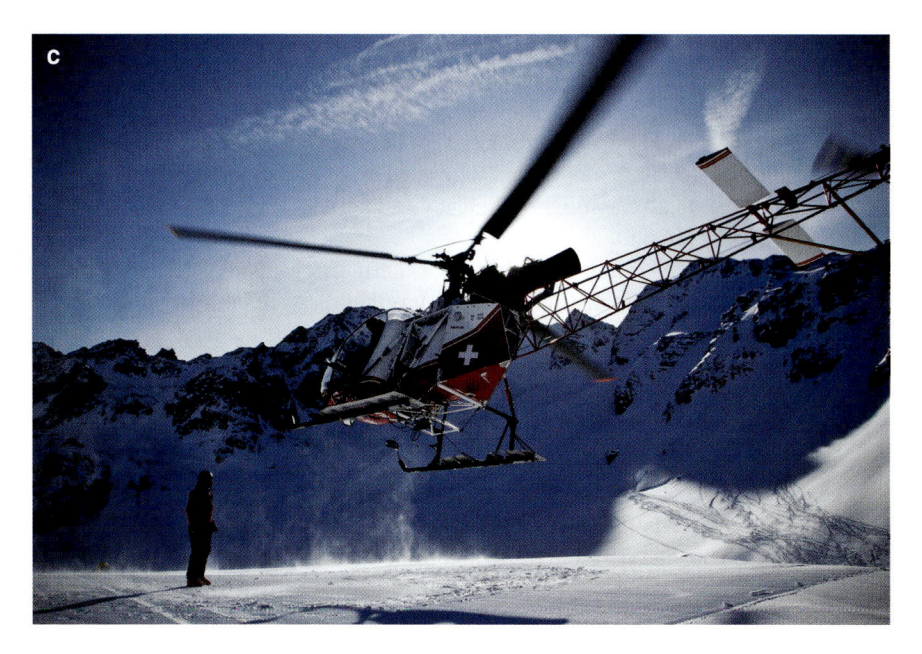

Fig. 3.11 (continued)

standard for snow sports. Helmets should fit correctly to provide adequate protection and must be replaced after a significant impact. Competitive athletes should augment their helmet with a face and/or chin guard. Helmets are now required by law for children skiing or boarding in Italy and some provinces in Austria.

Many skiers and snowboarders significantly underestimate the physical demands their sports place on them. Preseason snow-sport-specific exercises focusing on both cardiovascular fitness and muscle strength and flexibility are recommended. Before and after hitting the slopes, gentle stretches of the hamstrings, thigh muscles, hips, and calves may help to reduce the risk of muscular injury.

Ski patrols provide a multifaceted role that includes piste security, provision of first aid services and avalanche control. Ski patrol teams have intricate knowledge and experience of their own ski areas, and their advice on a range of topics including current snow conditions and off-piste safety should be treated with respect. Patrol instructions should be heeded at all times. In particular, signs indicating that a piste or area is closed should not be ignored. Those who transgress not only run the risk of serious injury or death to themselves but could be prosecuted and be held liable for the costs of any rescue. Pistes are only closed for good reason, even if those reasons are not immediately apparent.

Ski and snowboard instructors are extremely influential role models. They can ensure that those in their care are properly educated in all aspects of snow sport safety and etiquette. This is especially important for beginner skiers and snowboarders who often have little knowledge of equipment and general mountain safety. Taking professional lessons is recommended. Injuries are commoner in beginners and bad habits learned early on may be difficult to resolve later. It is important to emphasize that increasing ability usually results from a combination of instruction and experience, both best gained slowly over a period of time and in a variety of snow and weather conditions. Instructors should advise their students to avoid the temptation to try "too much too soon." Those who are proficient in one snow sport should not automatically assume proficiency in another. The techniques of skiing and snowboarding are quite different.

About 10 % of all injuries involve the ski lift mechanisms [62]. Individuals should receive appropriate instruction to ensure that they are competent to use the ski lifts safely.

Use of protective equipment by ski professionals sends out a strong message to others on the slope. It is important that patroller and instructor organizations keep abreast of the latest developments in snow sport safety so that these can be passed onto their members.

The potential hazards of off-piste skiing and snowboarding have already been highlighted. Individuals should never ski or board off-piste alone, must be aware of the prevailing avalanche risk, and, if in doubt, should consult a local guide or the ski patrol before setting out. All appropriate gear should be carried at all times.

Finally, an individual who falls near or into a tree well should try to tuck, roll, land upright, grab the tree trunk or a branch, and yell or blow a whistle to alert others. If buried upside down, the person should stay calm and try to create an air pocket in order to prolong the time available for rescue [63]. More information on tree wells can be found at www.treewelldeepsnowsafety.com.

Advising Alpine Skiers on Injury Prevention

Few skiers fully appreciate the critical role their boots and bindings play in providing functional performance while also safeguarding their lower legs from injury. Boots and bindings must be treated with care and respect and should be checked and serviced regularly by an appropriate ski technician. Skiers should minimize the amount of time they spend walking in their ski boots. The sole of the boot is designed to fit snugly into the binding plate so that it "transmits" accurate information between the ski, the binding, and the lower leg. Worn boot soles can significantly compromise the efficiency of the boot-binding interface which may lead to critical loss of performance. Releasable ski bindings and the reference charts used to set them are primarily designed to reduce the risk of lower leg fracture rather than knee sprains per se. As yet, no commercially available ski binding has been demonstrated conclusively to reduce the risk of ACL injury. Manufacturers continue to work on developments in this important area of injury prevention. All skiers should be made aware of the benefits of performing a self-test on their ski bindings every day. This simple procedure may help prevent many avoidable injuries to the knee. It is described in detail below.

Skiers are vulnerable to abduction injuries of the metacarpophalangeal joint of the thumb when they fall with their hands incorrectly positioned inside ski pole straps. The pole then acts as a lever across the MCP joint leading to injury. While no one device or piece of advice has any convincing evidence to support its use, using the pole straps correctly should help. Some researchers advocate skiing with the hands outside the pole straps (i.e., do not use the pole straps). Two exceptions to this rule would be when skiing in deep powder snow on piste though where the loss of a pole could be a major problem, or if skiing off-piste when poles may help skiers to "swim" in the event of an avalanche.

The Self-Test for Alpine Ski Bindings

This simple test ensures that at any given time, a pair of ski bindings is set correctly for an individual. It has been shown in a randomized intervention trial to reduce the risk of a knee injury by up to 30 % [64]. The test itself usually takes less than a minute or two to perform, especially if performed regularly. The basis of the test is the ability to self-release from the bindings at both the toepiece and heelpiece.

To test the toepiece
- With the ski angled so that the front inside edge is on the ground, the skier twists the boot inward. The toe should twist out and release from the front of the binding. Therefore, it should be applied gradually and progressively to avoid inadvertent injury.

To test the heelpiece
- With the ski flat on the ground, the skier slides their foot back until the leg is out straight. They then try and lift the heel of the boot out of the binding. Again, care should be taken to avoid applying too much force as this may strain the calf musculature or damage the Achilles tendon.
- If either the heel or the toe does not release from the binding, the binding setting should be reduced by 0.5 and the release procedure(s) repeated. Adjustments may be made using a variety of tools – many can be found at ski areas in self-help maintenance areas or else ask a ski patroller. The binding setting is reduced like this until the skier can release their boot themselves at both the heel and the toe. One might need more adjustment than the other. There is no evidence that the self-test – when applied correctly – makes bindings more liable to inadvertent release. At the end of each day, the skiers should reset the bindings back to their original settings ready for the next day and the next self-test.
- Some ski bindings released since 2010 are no longer easily amenable to adjustment by a lay person and require specialist tools in order to adjust the binding setting. On some bindings, the degree of movement needed to make an adjustment of 0.5 is so miniscule that it is only within the realm of a ski technician to do it accurately. In these circumstances, it is advisable to perform the self-test near to a facility where the adjustments may be made.

Advising Snowboarders on Injury Prevention

- Wrist guards are recommended for all snowboarders, especially beginners who are at highest risk of wrist injury. While in general any guard is better than no guard, there is evidence to suggest that longer, semirigid, and flexible guards provide a superior degree of protection [32]. Examples include the Flexmeter and Biomex guards. Short rigid guards (designed for in-line skating but used by many snowboarders) have been associated with a risk of severe "underguard" injury [32].
- As snowboard bindings do not incorporate a braking system, a leash, secured before getting into the bindings, may help to prevent a "runaway" board which can cause injury to others. Snowboarders usually ascend lifts with one foot detached from the bindings. In effect this leaves them with a "fat ski" on one leg which may twist unexpectedly causing knee injuries. The risk has been shown to be highest when using a surface lift like a T-bar or when dismounting from a chairlift [62].
- If using terrain parks, snowboarders should not attempt aerial maneuvers beyond their level of ability. If jumping, someone else should always act as a "spotter" near the landing area to reduce the risk of inadvertent collisions. Snowboarders should also be aware of the risk from falling into tree wells inadvertently.

In conclusion, snow sports offer exhilarating exercise to a wide spectrum of the population in beautiful mountain environments. They are associated with a risk of injury although this is much lower than commonly perceived. Specific injury patterns are recognized for each sport, and knowledge of and adherence to a few simple facts may help to minimize the risk of injury.

References

1. Senner V, Schaff P. Carving – the new dimension in skiing from the viewpoint of experts. Sportverletz Sportschaden. 1997;11(4):117.
2. Langran M, Jachacy GB, MacNeill A. Ski injuries in Scotland. A review of statistics from Cairngorm ski area winter 1993/94. Scott Med J. 1996;41(6):169–72.
3. Shealy J, Johnson R, Ettlinger C. Review of research literature on snowboarding injuries as might relate to an adjustable/releasable snowboard binding. Skiing Trauma and Safety 17th volume. ASTM STP. 2009;1510:111–25.
4. Jung CS, Zweckberger K, Schick U, Unterberg AW. Helmet use in winter sport activities-attitude and opinion of neurosurgeons and non-traumatic-brain-injury-educated persons. Acta Neurochir (Wien). 2011;153(1):101–6.
5. The Swiss Council for Accident Prevention (bfu). Statistics on non-occupational accidents and the level of safety in Switzerland – 2010 report. 2010. www.bfu.ch/PDFLib/1418_75.pdf.
6. Ruedl G, Sommersacher R, Woldrich T, Pocecco E, Hotter B, Nachbauer W, et al. Who is wearing a ski helmet? Helmet use on Austrian ski slopes depending on various factors. Sportverletz Sportschaden. 2010;24(1):27–30.

7. Ruedl G, Kopp M, Burtscher M. The protective effects of helmets in skiers and snowboarders. BMJ. 2011;342:d857.
8. Russell K, Christie J, Hagel BE. The effect of helmets on the risk of head and neck injuries among skiers and snowboarders: a meta-analysis. CMAJ. 2010;182(4):333–40.
9. Sulheim S, Holme I, Ekeland A, Bahr R. Helmet use and risk of head injuries in alpine skiers and snowboarders. JAMA. 2006;295(8):919–24.
10. Rughani AI, Lin CT, Ares WJ, Cushing DA, Horgan MA, Tranmer BI, et al. Helmet use and reduction in skull fractures in skiers and snowboarders admitted to the hospital. J Neurosurg Pediatr. 2011;7(3):268–71.
11. Shealy JE. The role of helmets in mitigation of head injuries: a case control study. Presented at 19th congress of The International Society for Skiing Safety 2011. Keystone, Colorado; May 2011.
12. Josefson D. US call for mandatory skiing helmets. BMJ. 1998;316(7126):172.
13. Ruedl G, Kopp M, Burtscher M. Mandatory ski helmets? CMAJ. 2010;182(9):942.
14. Ruedl G, Brunner F, Kopp M, Burtscher M. Impact of a ski helmet mandatory on helmet use on Austrian ski slopes. J Trauma. 2011;71(4):1085–7.
15. Bianchi G, Brugger O, Niemann S, Cavegn C. Helmet use and self-reported risk taking in skiing and snowboarding. J ASTM Int. 2011;1525:32–43.
16. Scott MD, Buller DB, Andersen PA, Walkosz BJ, Voeks JH, Dignan MB, et al. Testing the risk compensation hypothesis for safety helmets in alpine skiing and snowboarding. Inj Prev. 2007;13(3):173–7.
17. Macnab AJ, Smith T, Gagnon FA, Macnab M. Effect of helmet wear on the incidence of head/face and cervical spine injuries in young skiers and snowboarders. Inj Prev. 2002;8(4):324–7.
18. Mueller BA, Cummings P, Rivara FP, Brooks MA, Terasaki RD. Injuries of the head, face, and neck in relation to ski helmet use. Epidemiology. 2008;19(2):270–6.
19. Hagel BE, Russell K, Goulet C, Nettel-Aguirre A, Pless IB. Helmet use and risk of neck injury in skiers and snowboarders. Am J Epidemiol. 2010;171(10):1134–43.
20. Brugger H, Paal P, Boyd J. Prehospital resuscitation of the buried avalanche victim. High Alt Med Biol. 2011;12(3):199–205.
21. Boyd J, Haegeli P, Abu-Laban RB, Shuster M, Butt JC, Boyd J, et al. Patterns of death among avalanche fatalities: a 21-year review (see comment). CMAJ. 2009;180(5):507–12.
22. Ekeland A, Rodven A. Skiing and boarding injuries on Norwegian slopes during the two winter seasons 2006/07 and 2007/08. Skiing Trauma and Safety 18th volume. ASTM STP. 2011;1525:139–49.
23. Johnson R, Ettlinger C, Shealy J. Update on injury trends in alpine skiing. Skiing trauma and safety 17th volume. J ASTM Int. 2011;1510:11–22.
24. McBeth PB, Ball CG, Mulloy RH, Kirkpatrick AW. Alpine ski and snowboarding traumatic injuries: incidence, injury patterns, and risk factors for 10 years. Am J Surg. 2009;197(5):560–3.
25. Langran M, Selvaraj S. Snow sports injuries in Scotland: a case–control study. Br J Sports Med. 2002;36(2):135–40.
26. National Ski Areas Association. Facts about skiing/snowboarding safety. NSAA Online publications 2010. Available at: http://www.nsaa.org/nsaa/press/facts-ski-snbd-safety.asp Accessed 16th Sep 2012.
27. Sherry E, Clout L. Deaths associated with skiing in Australia: a 32-year study of cases from the Snowy Mountains. Med J Aust. 1988;149(11–12):615–8.
28. Shealy J, Johnson R, Ettlinger C. On piste fatalities in recreational snow sports in the US. Skiing trauma and safety 16th volume. ASTM STP. 2006;1474:27–34.
29. Cadman R. Eight nonavalanche snow-immersion deaths. A 6-year series from British Columbia ski areas. Physician Sportsmed. 1999;27(13):1–7.
30. Cadman R. How to stay alive in deep powder snow. Physician Sportsmed. 1999;27(13):18–9.
31. Ekeland A, Sulheim S, Rodven A. Injury rates and injury types in alpine skiing, telemarking and snowboarding. Skiing trauma and safety 15th volume. ASTM STP. 2005;1464:31–39.

32. Binet M. French prospective study evaluating the protective role of all kinds of wrist protectors for snowboarding. Presented at the 17th congress of The International Society for Skiing Safety 2007. Aviemore, Scotland; 2007;31–39.
33. Langran M, Selvaraj S. Increased injury risk among first-day skiers, snowboarders, and skiboarders. Am J Sports Med. 2004;32(1):96–103.
34. Yamakawa H, Murase S, Sakai H, Iwama T, Katada M, Niikawa S, et al. Spinal injuries in snowboarders: risk of jumping as an integral part of snowboarding. J Trauma. 2001;50(6):1101–5.
35. Wakahara K, Matsumoto K, Sumi H, Sumi Y, Shimizu K. Traumatic spinal cord injuries from snowboarding. Am J Sports Med. 2006;34(10):1670–4.
36. Koo DW, Fish WW. Spinal cord injury and snowboarding – the British Columbia experience. J Spinal Cord Med. 1999;22(4):246–51.
37. Florenes TW, Nordsletten L, Heir S, Bahr R. Recording injuries among World Cup skiers and snowboarders: a methodological study. Scand J Med Sci Sports. 2011;21(2):196–205.
38. Florenes TW, Bere T, Nordsletten L, Heir S, Bahr R. Injuries among male and female World Cup alpine skiers. Br J Sports Med. 2009;43(13):973–8.
39. Florenes TW, Nordsletten L, Heir S, Bahr R. Injuries among World Cup ski and snowboard athletes. Scand J Med Sci Sports. 2012;22(1):58–66.
40. Florenes TW, Heir S, Nordsletten L, Bahr R. Injuries among World Cup freestyle skiers. Scand J Med Sci Sports. 2012 Feb;22(1):58–66.
41. Florenes TW. Injury surveillance in World Cup skiing and snowboarding. MD Thesis. Faculty of Medicine, University of Oslo; 2010.
42. Bere T, Florenes TW, Krosshaug T, Koga H, Nordsletten L, Irving C, et al. Mechanisms of anterior cruciate ligament injury in World Cup alpine skiing: a systematic video analysis of 20 cases. Am J Sports Med. 2011;39(7):1421–9.
43. Ettlinger CF, Johnson RJ, Shealy JE. A method to help reduce the risk of serious knee sprains incurred in alpine skiing. Am J Sports Med. 1995;23(5):531–7.
44. Ruedl G, Nachbauer W, Burtscher M. Mechanism of ACL injury in skiers. Am J Sports Med. 2011;39(10):NP5–6.
45. McConkey JP. Anterior cruciate ligament rupture in skiing. A new mechanism of injury. Am J Sports Med. 1986;14(2):160–4.
46. Sterett WI, Briggs KK, Farley T, Steadman JR. Effect of functional bracing on knee injury in skiers with anterior cruciate ligament reconstruction: a prospective cohort study. Am J Sports Med. 2006;34(10):1581–5.
47. Fritschy D. A rare injury of the ankle in competition skiiers. Schweiz Z Med Traumatol. 1994;1:13–6.
48. Nicholas R, Hadley J, Paul C, James P. "Snowboarder's fracture": fracture of the lateral process of the talus. J Am Board Fam Pract. 1994;7(2):130–3.
49. McCrory P, Bladin C. Fractures of the lateral process of the talus: a clinical review. "Snowboarder's ankle". Clin J Sport Med. 1996;6(2):124–8.
50. Hedges K. Snowboarding injuries: an analysis and comparison with alpine skiing injuries. CMAJ. 1992;146(7):1146–8.
51. Owens BD, DeBerardino TM, Nelson BJ, Thurman J, Cameron KL, Taylor DC, et al. Long-term follow-up of acute arthroscopic Bankart repair for initial anterior shoulder dislocations in young athletes. Am J Sports Med. 2009;37(4):669–73.
52. Russell K, Hagel B, Francescutti LH. The effect of wrist guards on wrist and arm injuries among snowboarders: a systematic review. Clin J Sport Med. 2007;17(2):145–50.
53. Demirel M, Turhan E, Dereboy F, Akgun R, Ozturk A. Surgical treatment of skier's thumb injuries: case report and review of the literature. Mt Sinai J Med. 2006;73(5):818–21.
54. Ritting AW, Baldwin PC, Rodner CM. Ulnar collateral ligament injury of the thumb metacarpophalangeal joint. Clin J Sport Med. 2010;20(2):106–12.
55. Anderson D. Skier's thumb. Aust Fam Physician. 2010;39(8):575–7.

56. Yamauchi K, Wakahara K, Fukuta M, Matsumoto K, Sumi H, Shimizu K, et al. Characteristics of upper extremity injuries sustained by falling during snowboarding: a study of 1918 cases. Am J Sports Med. 2010;38(7):1468–74.
57. Harris JB. Spinal injuries in skiers and snowboarders. Am J Sports Med. 1999;27(4):546.
58. Tarazi F, Dvorak MF, Wing PC. Spinal injuries in skiers and snowboarders. Am J Sports Med. 1999;27(2):177–80.
59. Richards D, et al. Neck force and injury potential during head first impacts on snow. Presented at 19th congress of The International Society for Skiing Safety 2011. Keystone; May 2011.
60. Swedberg A, Hubbard M. Terrain park table-top jumps do not limit equivalent fall height. Presented at 19th congress of The International Society for Skiing Safety 2011. Keystone; May 2011.
61. Hubbard M, Swedberg A. Safer terrain park jump design based on equivalent fall height is robust to uncontrollable factors. Presented at 19th congress of The International Society for Skiing Safety 2011. Keystone; May 2011.
62. Langran M. Injuries associated with the use of ski lifts in Scotland. Presented at the 19th congress of The International Society for Skiing Safety 2011. Keystone; May 2011.
63. Van TC. Non-avalanche-related snow immersion deaths: tree well and deep snow immersion asphyxiation. Wilderness Environ Med. 2010;21(3):257–61.
64. Jlrgensen U, Fredensborg T, Haraszuk JP, Crone KL. Reduction of injuries in downhill skiing by use of an instructional ski-video: a prospective randomised intervention study. Knee Surg Sports Traumatol Arthrosc. 1998;6(3):194–200.

Chapter 4
Skydiving

Anton Westman

Contents

The Origins of the Sport and Its Development to the Current Stage	70
History	70
Sporting Events	71
The Equipment Used: Essential and Safety Requirements	73
The Parachute	73
The Reserve Parachute	73
Automatic Reserve Activation Devices	75
Wing Loading	75
Supplemental Oxygen	76
Injury and Fatality Rates and Specific Types of Injury	77
Fatalities	77
Injuries	79
Common Treatments and Relevant Rehabilitation	80
Local Emergency Services	80
"The Golden Hour"	83
Immediate Care	83
Initial Hospital Care	84
Rehabilitation	84
Proposed Prevention Measures	85
Aviation School Considerations	85
Parachute Flight and Landing	85
Medical Fitness	86
Hypoxia	86
Skydiving After Subaquatic Diving	87
Water Landings	87
Impact Energy	87
The Human Factor	88
References	88

A. Westman, M.D., Ph.D.
Department of Physiology and Pharmacology, Karolinska Institutet,
Stockholm, Sweden
e-mail: anton.westman@ki.se; anton@worldwidewestman.com

The Origins of the Sport and Its Development to the Current Stage

History

If the reader, bored by extreme sports injuries, throws this book out the window, it will tumble and turn, catching air while descending down through earth's relatively thick lower atmosphere. Medical textbooks or their readers do not really fall through air; they sink. Their sink rates can be lowered with extra drag, such as can be provided by a *parachute* (Greek/French: "against fall"). This principle was suggested in Chinese literature two millennia ago as a means to safely jump from a high object and possibly put to practical use in that country during the 1100s. Leonardo da Vinci designed a rigid-frame parachute in the 1480s, and reports of parachuting activities in Siam (Thailand) during the 1600s may have served as inspiration for European parachute designers in the 1700s [1–4]. The invention of the hot air balloon provided a high, mobile exit point from which a number of daredevil exhibition jumpers made parachuting known to a wider audience. Among early parachutists were Elisa Garnerin, who made 39 jumps from balloons in the early 1800s, and Käthe Paulus, who made 147 jumps at the end of the same century. In 1912, Albert Berry jumped from an airplane using a pack on the aircraft parachute system, and in 1914, Georgia Thompson performed a manual free fall activation of a parachute [1, 5].

The military use of parachutes was implemented in the First World War with safety parachutes for aviators and with the use of airborne soldiers, or paratroopers, in the Second World War [1, 5–7].

After the Second World War, civilian parachute organizations were formed in several countries. The World Air Sports Federation, Fédération Aéronautique Internationale (FAI), was proposed to include parachuting in 1948. The first world championships in sport parachuting were held in 1951, and by the end of that decade, athlete skills in aerial free fall flight had increased significantly and the prevailing English term for sport parachuting from aircraft came into use: *skydiving* [5, 7].

Until the 1960s, most parachutes in practical use were round drag parachutes, creating air resistance in opposition to the pull of gravity. In 1964, Domina Jalbert filed for a patent for a wing parachute, in essence a flyable textile wing, creating aerodynamic lift [8]. This landmark invention came to change the sport profoundly.

The 1970s saw further developments in free fall flying techniques, equipment improvements, and an increasing amount of fixed object parachute jumps, or BASE jumping, covered in a separate chapter. During the 1980s, tandem skydiving, in which a tandem passenger (typically, a first-time jumper) is connected via a harness to a tandem instructor operating the equipment, grew into both an introductory experience and a student training method. In some countries, such as the United Kingdom, tandem skydiving also came to be used for charity events. In the 1990s, faster and smaller wing parachutes were introduced, as were ram-air wingsuits.

The 2000s brought an increased availability of vertical wind tunnels allowing training for free fall flight techniques, raising athlete skills to unimaginable levels compared to those who first learned to fly the human body 50 years previously.

Today, skydiving is a major air sport. In 2009, approximately 5.5 million jumps, made by almost one million jumpers in 40 countries, were reported to the International Parachuting Commission (IPC) of the FAI. Most of those jumpers were tandem passengers – the reported number of jumpers operating their equipment by themselves added up to some 220,000 skydivers doing some 4.7 million skydives [9].

Sporting Events

The sport of skydiving now encompasses several disciplines and individual events (Fig. 4.1). In formation skydiving and vertical formation skydiving, teams of skydivers build predetermined sequences of free fall formations (drawn from an international pool) as fast as possible with each correctly completed formation scoring one point.

Freeflying, freestyle skydiving, and skysurfing are artistic events in which free fall moves performed by two or more skydivers are scored by judges in a manner somewhat similar to figure skating, but with the peculiar feature that one of the team members wears a video camera and records the video to be judged, encompassing both free fall flying skills in all three dimensions and cinematography into the artistry. Judging criteria are separated in technical and presentation items. In free fall style, an athlete performs a predetermined sequence of free fall maneuvers in the least amount of time possible.

During speed skydiving (claiming the title of "fastest nonmotorized sport on earth"), an athlete strives to achieve and maintain as high free fall vertical velocity as possible, typically by diving head down. The current speed skydiving world record is 527 km/h [10]. This is to be compared with the more typical terminal vertical velocity of a skydiver falling straight down, belly-to-earth, of around 200 km/h, or circa 55 m/s.

Canopy formation is similar to formation skydiving but with opened wing parachutes – teams of skydivers build sequences of parachute formations as fast as possible. In canopy piloting, also called swooping, an athlete performs a high-speed landing of a wing parachute judged by speed, distance, or accuracy. Accuracy landing is a separate landing event using larger and slower wing parachutes for centimeter accuracy. Para-ski combines accuracy landing with giant slalom skiing, the landing pad being located on a snowy slope of between 25 and 35°. Free fall style and accuracy landings are the two oldest competitive events in skydiving.

Other events include large formation jumps ("big ways"), night jumps, and high-altitude jumps. The latter require supplemental oxygen and are sometimes referred to as HALO jumps, acronym for high-altitude low opening, and HAHO jumps, acronym for high-altitude high opening. The highest parachute jump to date was made on August 16, 1960, when Joseph Kittinger in the US Air Force jumped from

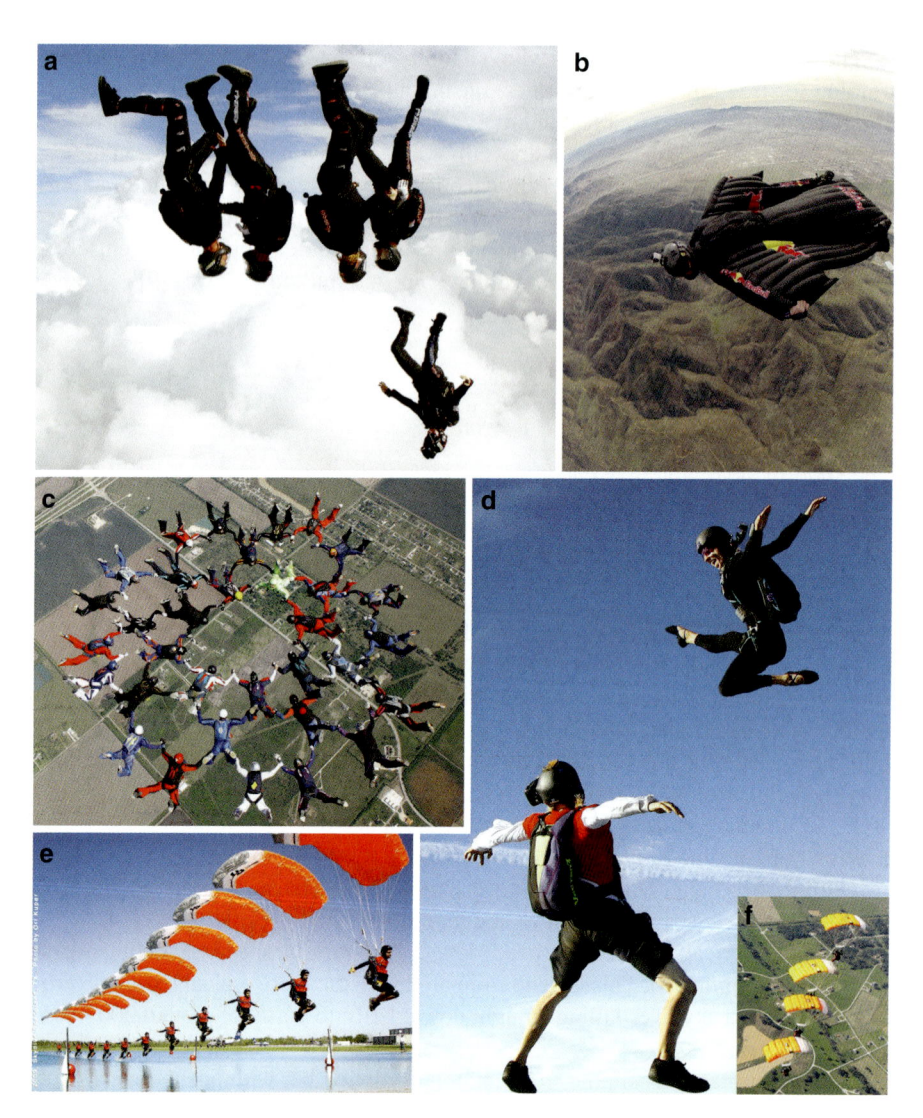

Fig. 4.1 Among the diverse disciplines and events that the sport of skydiving encompasses are formation skydiving and vertical formation skydiving (**a**), in which teams of skydivers build predetermined sequences of free fall formations as fast as possible. Wingsuit flying (**b**) utilizes garments that enhance the free fall glide ratio, and in large formation jumps (**c**), skydivers strive to build large free fall formations, sometimes in predetermined sequences. Freeflying and freestyle skydiving (**d**) are artistic events in which free fall moves are scored by judges in a manner somewhat similar to figure skating. In canopy piloting (**e**), also called swooping, an athlete performs a high-speed landing of a wing parachute judged by speed, distance, or accuracy. In canopy formation (**f**), teams of skydivers build sequences of formations with opened wing parachutes as fast as possible (Photos courtesy of Ori Kuper and Craig O'Brien)

31-km (102,800 ft) altitude above New Mexico [1, 11]. Attempts to break this record are underway.

The Equipment Used: Essential and Safety Requirements

The Parachute

The technical term for a parachute is *aerodynamic decelerator*, meaning that it slows down motion against air. The wing parachute is commonly referred to as a *ram-air parachute*, in reference to it being pressurized into its wing (air-foil) shape by ram-air intake of air in the front. This was the invention of Domina Jalbert: a wing that self-inflates by ramming air. To reduce opening shock, skydiving ram-air parachutes are fitted with a reefing device, typically a rectangular piece of fabric called a "slider" that slides down the lines on grommets during the parachute opening sequence. Parachute deployment is initiated by releasing a small round parachute, called a pilot chute, that anchors into the airstream and pulls out the wing parachute. An overview of modern, state-of-the-art skydiving equipment is given in Fig. 4.2.

Today, high-performance skydiving main parachutes are regularly flown and landed at speeds exceeding 100 km/h and require a bit of a runway to land safely, that is, a large open level field. During extreme high-speed landing approaches, they can achieve sink rates nearing a skydiver in free fall terminal vertical velocity. In skydiving vernacular, both round drag parachutes and rectangular ram-air wing parachutes are called "canopies," hence the names for the events canopy piloting and canopy formation.

The Reserve Parachute

Skydivers leave the aircraft carrying two packed separate parachutes, a main parachute and a reserve parachute. These are almost independent of each other, meaning that the risk of a double malfunction, that both should fail on the same jump, is very small. The philosophy of the skydiving reserve parachute is built upon two heights: one being the lowest required altitude for the reserve parachute to deploy and the other being the lowest required altitude for the main to deploy. Added, these two form the lowest required altitude for main parachute activation. Current Swedish regulations set this imaginary glass floor at 700 m (higher for several specific types of jumps) [12]. At a sink rate of 55 m/s, typical for a skydiver falling straight down, belly-to-earth, this equals to 13 s before impact. If the used reserve parachute model and configuration has a lowest required altitude to deploy of circa 300 m, the altitude margin from the lowest required altitude for main parachute activation is 700–300 = 400 m, equal to 7 s. Visual altimeters are usually worn on the wrist or chest strap and audible altimeters inside the helmet.

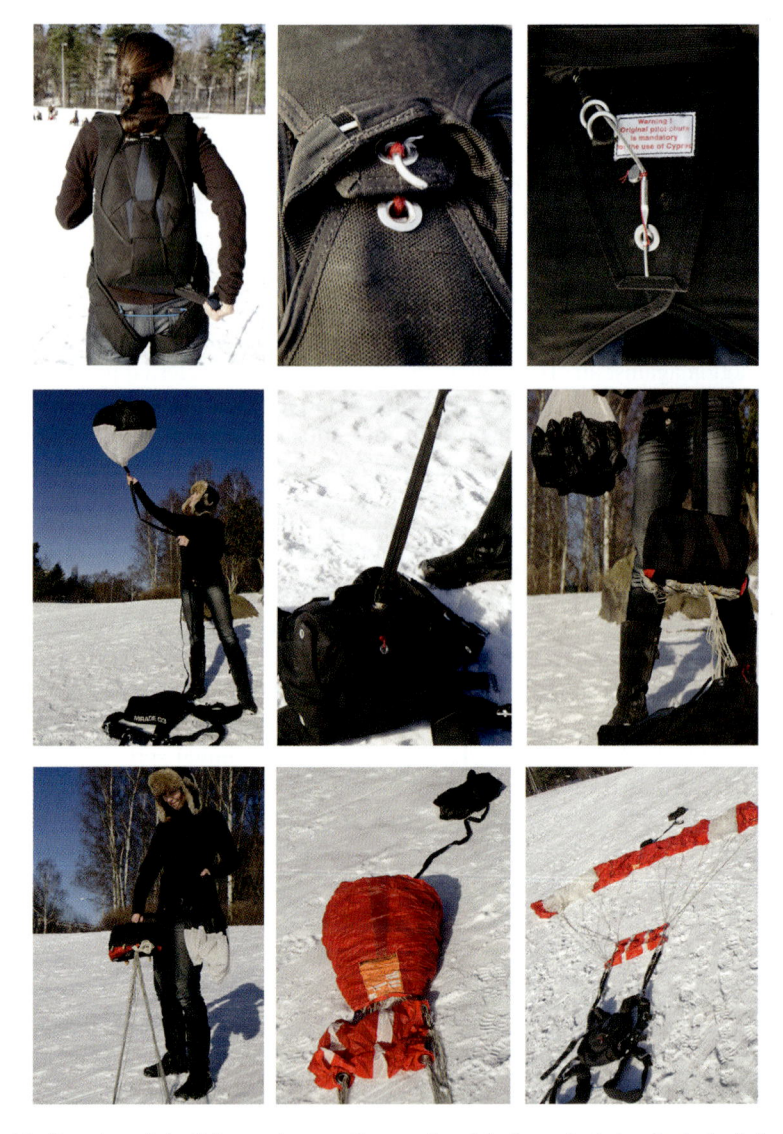

Fig. 4.2 Overview of skydiving equipment. *Top row from left*: A standard piggyback skydiving harness. It contains a main and a reserve parachute, packed in separate containers closed by metal closing pins. Should the main parachute malfunction, it is manually disconnected with a "cutaway" handle, and the reserve deployed by means of the reserve rip cord. This equipment is fitted with an automatic activation device, installed inside the reserve container, which activates the reserve at a preset altitude and vertical velocity, if the skydiver has lost altitude awareness or become incapacitated. In a pouch at the bottom of the main container is a small round parachute, called a pilot chute. *Middle row from left*: Main parachute deployment is initiated by manually releasing the pilot chute into the airstream, where it acts like an anchor and pulls out the deployment bag with the main parachute from its container. The lines are stowed with rubber bands on the deployment bag. *Bottom row from left*: The lines are stretched and the wing parachute emerges from the deployment bag. To reduce the opening shock, skydiving ram-air parachutes are fitted with a device that slows down the inflation. Typically, this is a rectangular piece of fabric called a "slider" that catches air like a small sail and slides down the lines on grommets during the parachute opening sequence (Photos courtesy of Linda Persson)

Since independence of the two parachute systems is paramount, activating the reserve in response to a main malfunction entails pulling two handles: First, the skydiver disconnects ("cuts away" in skydiving vernacular, though there is no cutting involved) the failed primary system and then activates the secondary. If this is performed in reversed order, the reserve canopy may entangle with the malfunctioned main canopy. A very dangerous situation arises if fabric or lines become tangled around the athlete. A few years ago in Sweden, a student skydiver practicing free fall flight techniques on his own, in accordance with the training program (it was his second free fall jump from 1,500 m), flipped over on his back when he pulled the main parachute, and it entangled with his foot. He disconnected the main parachute from the harness but it was still wrapped around his foot, and when he pulled the reserve parachute, it entangled with the entangled main parachute. He died on impact some seconds later.

Automatic Reserve Activation Devices

Responding to a persistent problem of no-pull (no parachute activation) and low-pull (too low parachute activation) fatalities, the industry developed a new generation of automatic reserve activation devices (AAD) that came out on the market in the 1990s [13]. The reliability of these led to widespread acceptance and use, reducing the number of no-/low-pull fatalities markedly. For the year 2009, at least 38 lives saved by AADs were reported to the IPC, and 10 of the reported 2009 fatalities (16 % of 62) might have been avoided by the use of an AAD [9].

Wing Loading

Various types of garments that enhance the jumper's free fall glide ratio (ratio of the horizontal to vertical distance traveled), such as the wingsuit (Fig. 4.3), are widely used today in sport parachuting. The wingsuit follows the same concept of the wing parachute, using layers of fabric between arms and body and between legs. During the fall, the air is pressurized into the ram-air wing shape cells. Some wingsuit designs give the parachutist a maximum glide ratio of >3:1 [14], similar to a high-performance skydiving main parachute. The most important factor to determine the glide ratio is the athlete himself, with his ability to control and navigate the wingsuit. A wingsuit, a very small skydiving main parachute, a large skydiving main parachute, a skydiving reserve parachute, and a BASE parachute can all be considered a continuum of variations of Domina Jalbert's ram-air fabric wing. What differs between them is the ratio of total suspended weight to wing platform area of the wing. This measure, called wing loading, is an important determinant of airspeed. Wingsuits have high wing loadings and consequently fly at high airspeeds and are as yet not intended for landing. BASE parachutes have low wing loadings and consequently fly at low airspeeds and are very soft to land. Highly loaded skydiving main parachutes can be flown at speeds approaching wingsuits.

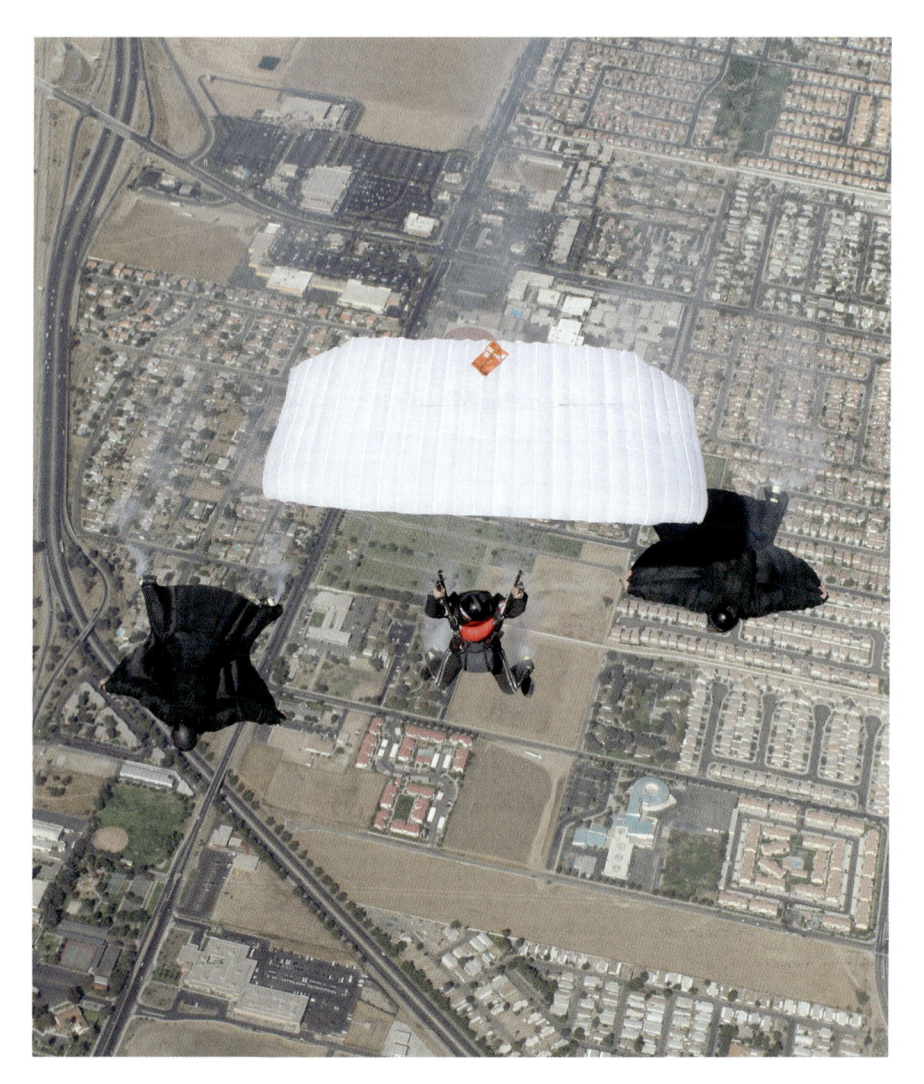

Fig. 4.3 A skydiver flying a wing parachute flanked by two skydivers flying wingsuits. The wing parachute and wingsuits alike are pressurized into their wing shapes by ram-air intake of air (Photo courtesy of Craig O'Brien)

Supplemental Oxygen

The regular exit altitude in skydiving, routinely using unpressurized aircraft without supplemental oxygen, is 4,000 m (13,000 ft). This is higher than the 3,000-m (10,000 ft) altitude at which hypobaric hypoxia (oxygen deficiency caused by low air pressure) is believed to be of physiologic importance. The rationale for this practice is an assumption that the relatively brief durations (usually less than half an hour) of hypobaric exposure do not cause hypoxic incapacitation to a significant degree [11].

4 Skydiving

Table 4.1 The international fatality rate reported to the International Parachuting Commission of the Fédération Aéronautique Internationale 1989–2009 [9]

Year and number of countries	Number Jumpers	Number Jumps	Number Fatalities	Jumps Per jumpers	Per fatality	Jumpers per fatality
1989 – 34 countries	340,715	5,564,137	97	16	57,362	3,513
1990 – 32 countries	316,994	5,189,991	70	16	74,143	4,528
1991 – 35 countries	245,162	4,848,025	74	20	65,514	3,313
1992 – 35 countries	300,586	4,591,980	59	15	77,830	5,095
1993 – 38 countries	370,679	5,267,754	101	14	52,156	3,670
1994 – 40 countries	285,253	5,064,125	70	18	72,345	4,075
1995 – 38 countries	322,322	5,562,691	64	17	86,917	5,036
1996 – 40 countries	323,300	6,013,691	76	19	79,128	4,254
1997 – 37 countries	404,198	6,843,299	78	17	87,735	5,182
1998 – 33 countries	332,603	5,596,753	72	17	77,733	4,619
1999 – 26 countries	335,867	5,594,191	60	17	93,237	5,598
2000 – 27 countries	355,405	5,750,464	63	16	91,277	5,641
2001 – 31 countries	417,202	6,872,438	92	16	74,700	4,535
2002 – 33 countries	357,155	5,769,010	73	16	79,028	4,893
2003 – 39 countries	402,513	6,335,624	82	16	77,264	4,909
2004 – 39 countries	493,250	5,332,756	53	11	100,618	9,307
2005 – 36 countries	806,515	6,147,351	64	8	96,052	12,602
2006 – 39 countries	832,683	5,958,194	51	7	116,827	16,327
2007 – 41 countries	837,831	6,222,629	68	7	91,509	12,321
2008 – 44 countries	918,436	5,770,169	70	6	82,431	13,121
2009 – 40 countries	955,558	5,452,521	62	6	87,944	15,412

In-aircraft supplemental oxygen is used when the exit is at higher altitudes. During the large formation world record jumps over Thailand in 2004 and 2006, over 400 skydivers jumped out of multiple C-130 Hercules aircraft at >7,300 m (>24,000 ft). The in-aircraft oxygen system used for these jumps were individual oxygen hoses fed into the skydiving helmets, without oxygen breathing masks (H. Berggren, 2011, Thailand 2004 big way hog hojd, Personal Communication; J. Hansson, 2011, Skydiving_Chapter_of_Adventure_and_Extreme_Sports_Injuries2 Kommentar LUL5, Personal Communication; S.Mörtberg, 2011, world team 2006, Personal Communication) [15, 16].

Injury and Fatality Rates and Specific Types of Injury

Fatalities

International fatality statistics are collected by the IPC and published as an annual report (Table 4.1). The 2009 number was one fatality per 88,000 jumps [9]. Skydiving in Sweden during the years 1994–2003 suffered nine fatalities in 1.1

million jumps, or one fatality per 125,000 jumps [17], a risk slightly less than maternal deaths per live birth in Sweden during the same period (Mödradödlighet (dnr 32346/2011), 2011, Personal Communication) [18]. A review of postmortem autopsy records in 22 fatalities in Swedish skydiving 1964–2003 showed massive injuries to the central nervous, cardiovascular, respiratory, musculoskeletal, and urinary systems and to the liver, spleen, pancreas, and skin. In many cases, more severe injuries were found in body parts having hit the ground first. One skydiver in this group who fell into a lake with no parachute inflated died with severe lacerations of the central nervous system [17]. Main causes of fatal skydiving incidents reported to the IPC for 2009 (40 countries, 62 fatalities) were "fast canopies" (e.g., fast wing parachutes) – 12 (19 %), "landing errors" – 11 (18 %), "no/low main pull" – 7 (11 %), tandem – 7 (11 %), and "canopy collisions" (e.g., midair wing parachute collisions) – 6 (10 %). The IPC concluded that 44 (71 %) of the 62 fatalities in 2009 happened with the jumper having at least one good parachute on his or her back, and that 49 (79 %) of the 62 fatalities may have been caused by human error [9]. The introduction of high-performance wing parachutes in the 1990s has rendered it the epithet "A Decade of Landing Deaths" [19]. Between 1986 and 2001, 507 people in the United States died from injuries sustained in skydiving, with an increase in landing fatalities with open parachute and fully functional gear, but without change of overall fatality rate [20]. Thus, perhaps counterintuitive to a non-skydiver, it may be concluded that the fatality risk in a skydive is not exclusively related to whether the parachute will open or not but also to the parachutist's piloting skills of a perfectly functioning parachute. When flying and landing a highly loaded skydiving main parachute, the margin of error is small.

Off Drop Zone Landings

A designated area for skydiving activities including landing is called a drop zone. Off drop zone landings into trees, buildings, power lines, etc. are prone to injury and fatality. Landing unintentionally by parachute in deep water may not seem overly risky, but equipment entanglement with the lines and the fabric can contribute to the difficulty of the situation, and the environmental factors of cold, waves, or currents provide additional hazards. As a result, there have been a number of drownings in skydiving. Further, some licensed skydivers use weight vests to match free fall rates, which after unintentional landing in deep water may worsen the situation considerably.

Jump Plane Crashes

Airplane crashes have caused a substantial number of skydiving fatalities. A recent example is the crash of a Pilatus PC-6 "Turbo-Porter," in which a skydiver had elected not to jump and descended with the aircraft. The parachute equipment of the skydiver was fitted with an AAD configured for student use, having a lower preset activation sink rate than models for licensed skydiver use. Against the recommendation of the manufacturer [21], the AAD was not switched off during the aircraft descent, and it activated the reserve parachute during the landing approach. The reserve parachute slipped out into the air current, pulling the skydiver out of the copilot's seat, and got caught at the horizontal tail. The skydiver was instantly killed by internal decapitation, and because of the low altitude, the pilot had no time to leave the plane and use his rescue parachute before the fatal impact [22].

Injuries

Specific types of nonfatal injuries sustained in skydiving incidents in Sweden in 1999–2003 are noted (Fig. 4.4), and their causative mechanisms of injury have been determined (Fig. 4.5). The chain of events that led to the most severe incident (pelvic fracture, bilateral femur, and tibia fractures) was initiated by one skydiver "hookturning" (performing a steeply diving high-speed landing approach) into another before landing. It appears in this material that the risk of an injury is higher for students than for licensed skydivers, but that among those most severely injured, there has been a shift toward higher experience level. Non-minor injuries occur at a rate of almost double that of Swedish road traffic. Most injuries are caused by wing parachute pilot errors, both high-speed landing approaches as well as standard and straight-approach landings. Figure 4.6 shows the exposure of extremities and spine to impact energy during wing parachute landing.

Barrows et al. pointed out that comparative analysis of skydiving injury studies is confounded by discrepancies in methods. They themselves defined a skydiving injury as something treated at first aid stations at the World Freefall Conventions in the United States in 2000 and 2001 and found a total injury rate of 170 per 100,000 jumps and a hospital admission rate of 18 per 100,000 jumps [25]. The Swedish 1999–2003 national skydiving statistics, in which a "personal injury" was defined as an "injury requiring care of a physician" [26], had a reported nonfatal injury event rate of 48 per 100,000 jumps [24], but when the reporting system itself was examined, it was found to have an overall sensitivity of only 37 %, meaning that the true injury rate was closer to that found at those World Freefall Conventions [27].

Skydiving has suffered injuries related to the parachute opening [24]. The opening shock of a typical civilian parachute is believed to expose its user to around 3–5G [11], though the literature on this subject is scarce. The cumulative effect of this exposure to a competing skydiving athlete or a professional skydiver, doing some ten jumps a day and several hundreds of jumps yearly, remains to be investigated. Skydiving photographers and videographers usually use helmet-mounted cameras, adding considerable mass to the head and changing the center of mass of the head complex, aggravating the force exposure to the neck.

In conclusion, a typical nonfatal skydiving injury is a fracture of the lower extremities caused by a miscalculated landing of a perfectly functioning parachute, such as a low turn, landing off headwind, or a miscalculated horizontal leveling for landing. Thus, the burden of injury, both fatal and nonfatal, in the sport of skydiving is primarily related to the wing parachute piloting skills of skydivers.

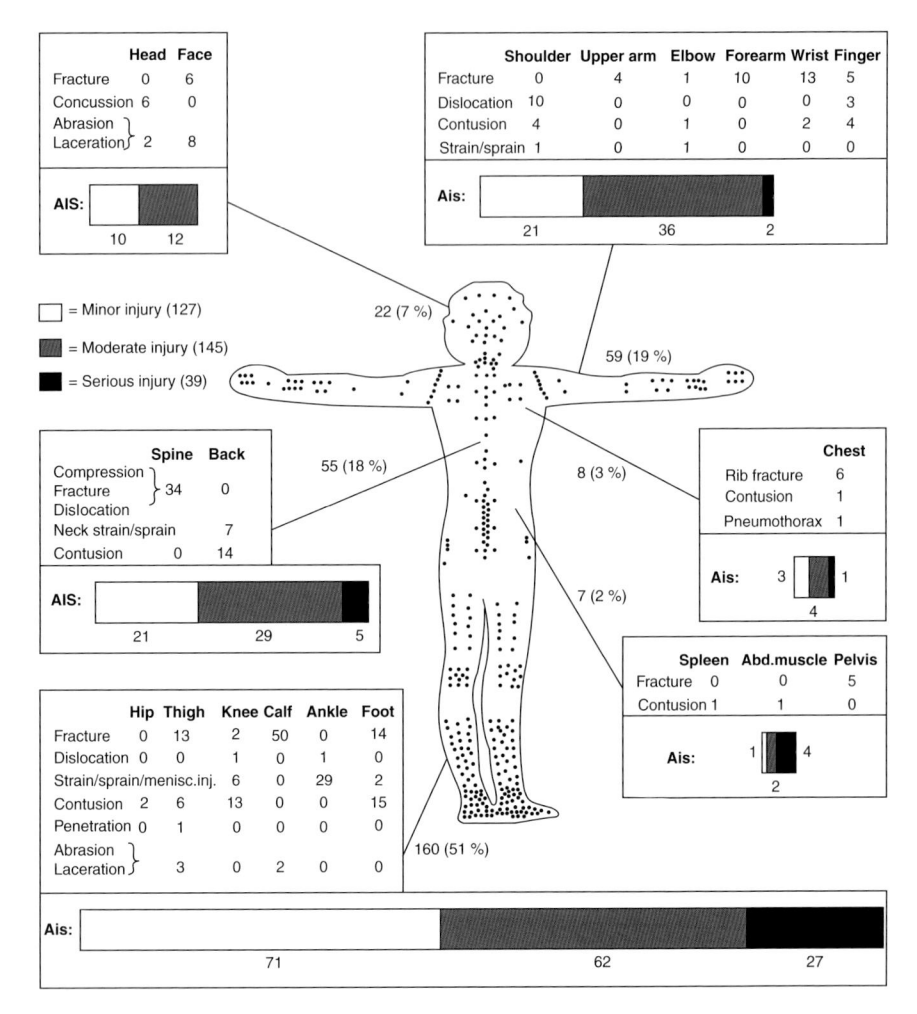

Fig. 4.4 "The injured skydiver." Distribution of injuries ($n=311$) sustained in reported nonfatal skydiving incidents in Sweden in 1999–2003 ($n=257$), every dot representing an injury. Bar diagrams show injury severity categorized with the Abbreviated Injury Scale (AIS) [23]. All numbers are absolute except where stated as percent of total. Anatomical outline from parachute inventor Leonardo da Vinci. Abd, abdominal; menisc inj, meniscus injury (Reprinted with kind permission from the *British Journal of Sports Medicine*; Figure from Westman and Bjornstig [24])

Common Treatments and Relevant Rehabilitation

Local Emergency Services

To the medical layman, a good advice on how to treat a skydiving injury is to call the local emergency services. While some of the sports covered in this book are pursued in a remote wilderness, skydiving drop zones are often located within a

4 Skydiving

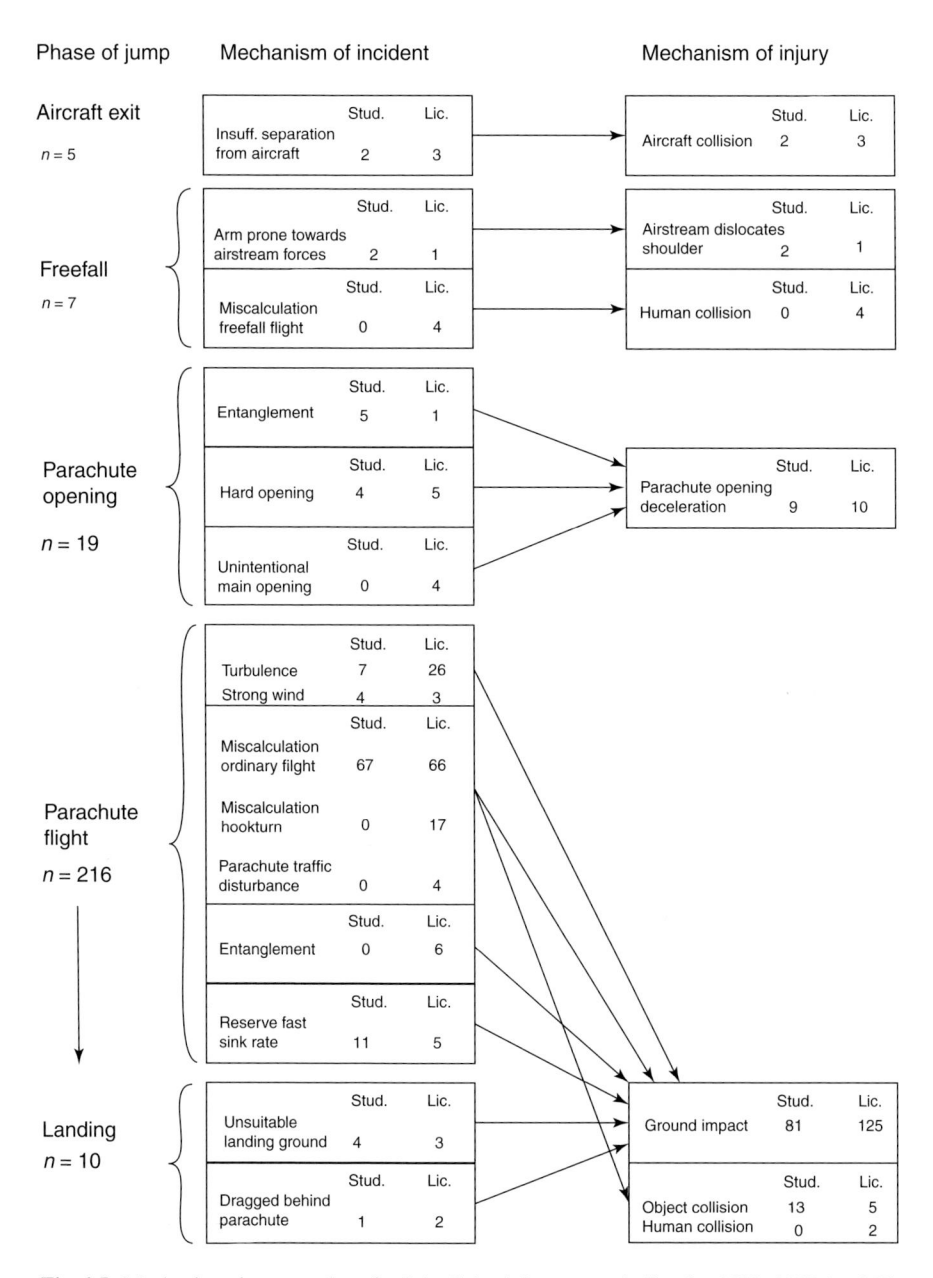

Phase of jump	Mechanism of incident			Mechanism of injury		
Aircraft exit $n=5$	Insuff. separation from aircraft	Stud. 2	Lic. 3	Aircraft collision	Stud. 2	Lic. 3
Freefall $n=7$	Arm prone towards airstream forces	Stud. 2	Lic. 1	Airstream dislocates shoulder	Stud. 2	Lic. 1
	Miscalculation freefall flight	Stud. 0	Lic. 4	Human collision	Stud. 0	Lic. 4
Parachute opening $n=19$	Entanglement	Stud. 5	Lic. 1	Parachute opening deceleration	Stud. 9	Lic. 10
	Hard opening	Stud. 4	Lic. 5			
	Unintentional main opening	Stud. 0	Lic. 4			
Parachute flight $n=216$	Turbulence	Stud. 7	Lic. 26			
	Strong wind	4	3			
	Miscalculation ordinary filght	Stud. 67	Lic. 66			
	Miscalculation hookturn	Stud. 0	Lic. 17			
	Parachute traffic disturbance	Stud. 0	Lic. 4			
	Entanglement	Stud. 0	Lic. 6			
	Reserve fast sink rate	Stud. 11	Lic. 5			
Landing $n=10$	Unsuitable landing ground	Stud. 4	Lic. 3	Ground impact	Stud. 81	Lic. 125
	Dragged behind parachute	Stud. 1	Lic. 2	Object collision Human collision	Stud. 13 0	Lic. 5 2

Fig. 4.5 Mechanisms in reported nonfatal skydiving injury events in Sweden 1999–2003 ($n=257$) in relation to phase of jump and experience level (student (Stud.) vs. licensed (Lic.)). Miscalculations during "ordinary flight" included low turns, landings off headwind, and miscalculated horizontal levelings for landing, but excluded intentional low turns aimed at gaining landing airspeed (i.e., "hook turns" referred to a separate group) (Reprinted with kind permission from the *British Journal of Sports Medicine*; Figure from Westman and Bjornstig [24])

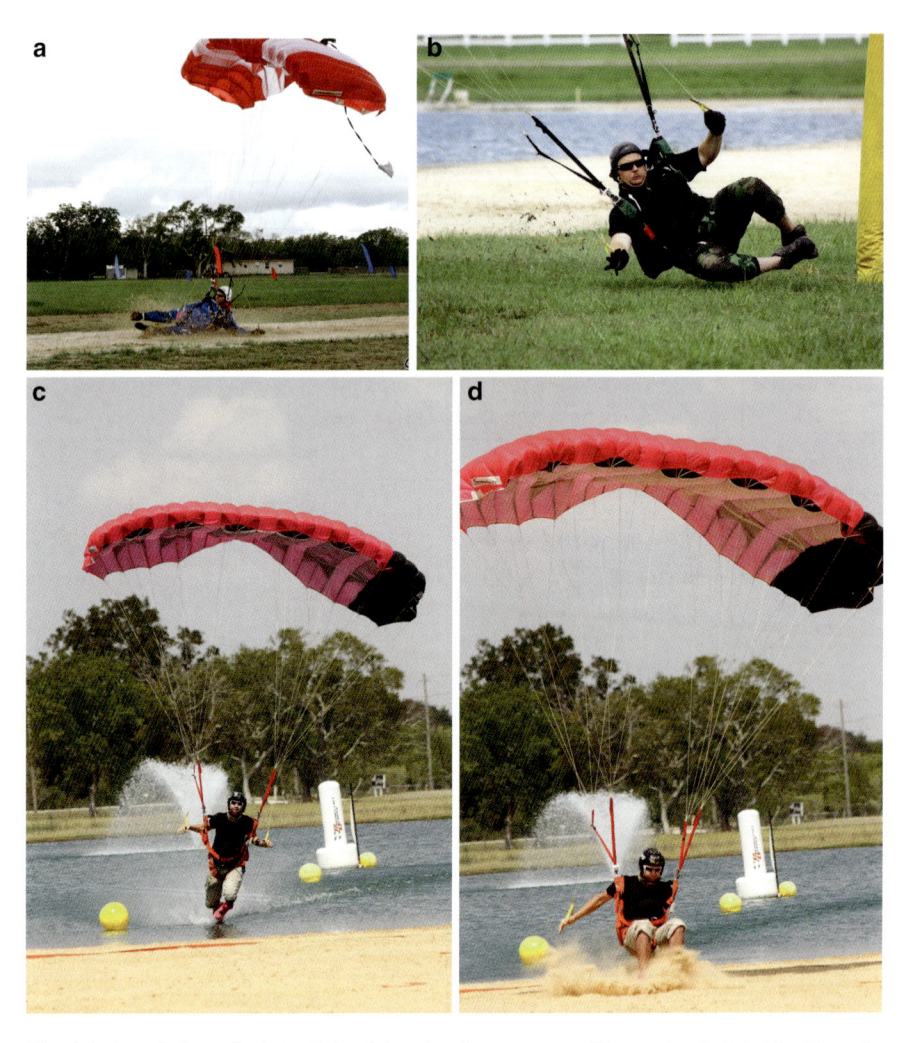

Fig. 4.6 A typical nonfatal skydiving injury is a fracture caused by a miscalculated landing of a perfectly functioning parachute. (**a–d**) show the exposure of extremities (note the extension of elbows and wrists) and spine to impact energy. High-performance main parachutes are regularly flown and landed at forward speeds exceeding 100 km/h (Photos courtesy of Ori Kuper)

reasonable distance from a hospital. Consequently, priorities in drop zone traumas should aim to optimize a smooth and fast transport to a trauma center, by road ambulance or helicopter. The emergency medical dispatcher will ask about basic facts such as location, preferably including Global Positioning System (GPS) coordinates and relevant driving directions, callback number, what has happened, and the condition of the injured person. Both road ambulances and helicopters may need some assistance in their approach, and their personnel will be aided by a clear, structured report containing information about what happened, what care has been provided, and any changes in the condition of the injured. They should also be informed of the magnitude of the energy in the trauma, preferably including speed at impact, if there was a second impact, angles, etc.

"The Golden Hour"

An established keystone of trauma care is the so-called golden hour, emphasizing that the time between injury and treatment should be kept to a minimum. This is an important consideration in off drop zone landings, when there may be an initial lag time until the skydiver has been found and injury established. In one case several years ago, before the implementation of modern trauma care, a skydiver landed off drop zone in a tree and suffered a subsequent fall of 5 m. The skydiver was found conscious complaining about pain in the abdomen, later became unconscious, and died the same night with pelvic fractures and associated internal hemorrhage. It may be suggested that paramedics should be on standby close to the drop zone for all skydiving activities, particularly for activities in which the skydivers themselves consider to have an increased risk of major trauma. Swooping (high-speed landing) competitions or training camps should consider having a road ambulance on site and the nearest trauma center should be notified of the activities beforehand.

Immediate Care

It is outside the scope of this book to teach prehospital trauma life support, but it is recommended to follow the procedures and practices of the Advanced Trauma Life Support course or similar. The ABCDE sequence (Airway maintenance with cervical spine protection, Breathing, Circulation, Disability, Exposure and Environmental control) may also be used for structured communication with the emergency medical dispatcher and the ambulance personnel and for repeated assessment of the patient's condition while waiting for the ambulance. Changes in condition are of paramount importance. Another mnemonic that may facilitate structured communication is MIST– Mechanism of injury, Injuries at scene, Symptoms at scene, Treatment at scene.

　　A special concern is the manual technique for cervical spine protection while removing a full-face helmet, which may be necessary for airway maintenance. It may be advisable for skydiving instructors, expecting to be first responders in future skydiving traumas, to take a course to learn manual techniques such as helmet removal and basic fracture stabilization. The medical layman must realize that A comes first in the ABCDE sequence because it is the most important: Airway maintenance may be a matter of minutes.

Initial Hospital Care

To the admitting emergency department health-care provider, a skydiving trauma may initially be considered as somewhat similar to a motorcycle crash with a largely unprotected rider. Critical care unit admission should be considered. If the patient's needs exceed local capabilities, further transport to definitive care must be arranged. If other skydivers who were present at the scene come in to the hospital, additional information about speed, angles, and the magnitude of the trauma energy may be obtained. Note the accumulation of lower back injuries in Fig. 4.4. Electronic devices found on the injured should be kept safe for later jump data analysis.

Rehabilitation

Basic concepts in rehabilitation of extreme sports injuries are covered in a separate chapter of this book, but a few considerations particular to skydiving may be noted. As mentioned above, the biomechanics of sport parachute openings are not well known, but if the estimates found in literature of circa 3–5G hold true, a skydiver having suffered a spinal injury and wishing to get back into the sport must undergo relevant surgery and rehabilitation, possibly including neck and back muscle exercise regimens, with this cumulative force exposure in mind. Joint stability is an important concern in skydiving. In wing parachute landing, the ankle joint in effect serves as the undercarriage of an aircraft, and a physiotherapist rehabilitating a skydiving athlete having suffered trauma to her fragile landing gear must obtain a clear understanding of the speeds and angles in an uneventful landing, as well as in a miscalculated landing. An excellent level of functional recovery must be obtained before returning to the sport, as a graded return to parachute landing cannot be obtained. It is not uncommon for skydivers flying fast parachutes to run a few steps during landing, especially on no-wind days. As with the opening sequence, the biomechanics of sport parachute landing sequences are not well known.

A joint of special concern in skydiving is the shoulder since reserve parachute emergency procedures require bilateral hand and arm function [28]. Therefore, a shoulder joint dislocated midair can be life-threatening, especially if the incapacitated hand is that used for main parachute activation. In addition, a nonfunctional arm can render an inexperienced skydiver unable to maintain a stable body position in free fall, with subsequent risk of entanglement at parachute deployment. Unfortunately, the very nature of skydiving (swimming around in thick, fluid airstreams) poses a threat to shoulder joint stability. Newcomers to the sport with shoulder problems and skydivers having suffered injuries related to the shoulder joint must undergo relevant training, rehabilitation, and if necessary, surgery. Vertical wind tunnel training is a possible option for testing shoulder joint stability in a skydiving context without exposure to a life threat.

Proposed Prevention Measures

Aviation School Considerations

Parachuting is piloting. Flying the human body, a wingsuit, or a wing parachute requires specialized aviator skills. This is obvious in advanced wing parachute maneuvers such as the steeply diving "hookturn" high-speed landing approach but holds true for all aspects of the sport, not at least learning the basics of free fall and wing parachute flight. Historically, parachuting beginners have learned the sport solo from their first jump. Today, tandem skydiving offers a chance to experience the medium for the first time without operator responsibilities, and student training programs with free fall instructors alongside can offer a helping hand when needed, though the student still must handle malfunctions and learn wing parachute flight (including landing) alone. An aviator who came to experience the safety benefits of free fall instructors was George H.W. Bush, 41st President of the United States. After his presidency, Bush went skydiving, and on his second jump he unintentionally flipped over on his back in free fall [29]. In contrast to the previously mentioned Swedish student skydiver, Bush had free fall instructors alongside who turned him back right again. If available, vertical wind tunnel training of free fall flying techniques, before actual jumping, may be an option. Ground-to-student radio instruction regarding wing parachute flight may be considered to minimize the risk for landings outside the drop zone and give some aid in the landing, the student following ground instructor commands in order to navigate his parachute to a safe drop zone landing. Filmed landings may offer a student a chance to receive detailed feedback from instructors and learn faster. Experienced skydivers training advanced wing parachute maneuvers often film their landings and sometimes use air-to-air radio.

Parachute Flight and Landing

It may be assumed that if licensed skydivers used reserve or BASE type of parachutes for main parachutes, skydiving would probably become substantially safer. However, the trend seems to move in the opposite direction with ever faster wing parachutes. To a skydiver progressing in parachute piloting skills, it is important to realize that upgrading from a slow and large beginner main parachute to a fast and small high-performance parachute entails a shift from potential landing speeds that are injurious to potential speeds that are deadly. Various training programs are available but can only protect a parachute pilot willing to protect himself. High-speed parachute flight creates traffic implications, especially over busy drop zones. Ideally, high-speed landing approaches should be separated from other parachute traffic. Mixing heavily loaded high-performance main parachutes and lightly loaded main parachutes in the same airspace may be compared to having bicycles and racing motorcycles in the same velodrome.

There may be a discrepancy between a rapidly increasing free fall flight skills level in the sport, not at least thanks to the vertical wind tunnels, and parachute flight skills lagging behind. If so, paragliding courses for skydivers may be an option to improve parachute flight skills and also learn more about wind and weather.

Medical Fitness

In addition to exemplifying the value of free fall instructors, the parachuting career of George H.W. Bush may be worth some consideration for another reason: his age. Bush commemorated his 75th, 80th, and 85th birthdays skydiving [30]. A recent survey of the age distribution of the active Swedish skydiving population revealed a large proportion of elderly jumpers, as well as a peak of new students entering the sport at the age of 40 [27]. Allowing skydiving to be a sport not exclusively for the young and completely healthy, but a sport that can offer the sky to a great many people of various ages and medical conditions, raises questions about health and safety. One example may be the forces during parachute opening in relation to elderly skydivers, and another example may be insulin-dependent diabetes mellitus. Some countries, for instance, Sweden, Norway, Italy, and the United Kingdom, generally prohibit people with this condition from entering the sport, while other countries, for instance, the United States, do not. Given a lack of internationally recognized requirements or recommendations regarding skydiving medical fitness, medical doctors doing pre-course examinations are advised to consult their national parachuting associations and civil aviation regulatory authorities.

Hypoxia

Hypobaric hypoxia may be of some significance in respect to skydivers of various ages and medical conditions. Current Swedish regulations for sport parachuting require in-aircraft supplemental oxygen to be used on jumps from above 4,000 m (13,000 ft) and self-contained free fall supplemental oxygen to be used on jumps from above 6,000 m (20,000 ft) [31]. Skydivers jumping from above 4,000 m (or, in fact, staying above 3,000 m for a prolonged time) should be made aware that early signs of low-grade hypoxia are subtle and may include delayed reaction time, impaired judgment, impaired muscle coordination, and visual impairment such as tunnel vision and disturbed color/night vision. When jumping from above 6,000 m (e.g., in future world record Big Way attempts), it should be noted that the estimated time of useful consciousness for an unacclimatized person breathing ambient air at 7,600 m (25,000 ft) is only 3–5 min [32].

Skydiving After Subaquatic Diving

The risk of decompression sickness after subaquatic compressed gas diving increases if, after surfacing, the diver is subject to further decompression. Ambient pressure in the atmosphere decreases in a nonlinear manner with increased altitude, due to the compressibility of air. At the regular skydiving exit altitude of 4,000 m (13,000 ft), ambient pressure is around 0.6 bar, that is, 60 % of the ambient pressure at sea level. A minimum 24-h abstinence from skydiving after repetitive, multiple day or decompression diving has been suggested. Though there is a considerable body of literature on flying after diving, details regarding parachuting after diving remain to be investigated (R. Cali-Corleo, 2011, Skydiving after SCUBA diving – textbook chapter, Personal Communication) [11, 33, 34]. A military parachuting concern that under rare circumstances may also apply to sport parachuting is HALO jumps after diving. Before jumps from above 5,486 m (>18,000 ft) following compressed gas diving, the US Air Force requires a minimum 24-h surface interval and oxygen breathing for a minimum of 30 min prior to ascending above 3,000 m and throughout the high-altitude exposure. Breathing oxygen before the ascent reduces the risk of decompression sickness by increasing the gradient for inert gas to move from tissues into the lung and subsequently out of the body. Civilian sport parachutists planning HALO jumps after diving are advised to contact military experts on the subject. The threshold altitude associated with a risk of developing decompression sickness in aviation without a previous subaquatic exposure is estimated between 4,900 m (16,000 ft) and 6,400 m (21,000 ft) [32].

Water Landings

Personal flotation devices and rescue boats should be available when a deepwater landing is possible. Swimming pool training with parachute equipment, getting out from under parachute and out of harness while treading water, is advisable. Weight vests used to match free fall rates must be configured for a quick release in the case of a deepwater landing (N.W. Pollock, 2011, is mandatory in United States Air Force, Personal Communication).

Impact Energy

While water landings entail risk, water can also provide a partial remedy for the high-speed landing death epidemic. So-called swoop ponds are shallow bodies of water over which high-speed landings are executed, providing a liquid cushion in the case of a miscalculated approach, wetting and perhaps lightly injuring the wing parachute pilot, instead of killing him as a penalty for not achieving level flight. In addition to using swoop ponds as impact energy absorbers, some skydivers flying high-performance parachutes use various pieces of body armor such as backplates. The use of helmets appears to be widely accepted in the sport today. The military paratrooper boot is obsolete in civilian sport parachuting, but military studies showing the effectiveness of outside-the-boot ankle braces in preventing landing injuries have motivated a current explorative trial of protective ankle braces for skydiving students in Sweden [35].

An extreme example of the effectiveness of impact energy absorbers was provided on May 23, 2012, when Gary Connery landed a wingsuit into a runway of some 18,500 cardboard boxes at Mill End Farm in the United Kingdom, without deploying a parachute, unharmed. In addition to a helmet, Mr. Connery also wore a neck brace. The jump was made from a helicopter, and the exit altitude was 730 m (2,400 ft) (G. Connery, 2012, Book chapter, Personal Communication).

The Human Factor

As both the IPC world statistics and in-depth studies of skydiving traumas indicate human factors to be of greater safety importance than equipment or environment factors, an athlete may conclude that the injurious agent to fear is the man in the mirror. In sports such as track and field athletics, pushing the edge, the farther boundary of one's capabilities, may be a desirable mentality, but in sports involving a risk of high-energy trauma, sport psychology and sport sociology need to address not only athlete performance but also survival. Skydiving's old creed "Blue Skies Black Death" has been perceived by some as an expression of recklessness, but skydivers active in the pre-1980s era say that "BSBD" originally expressed the opposite: "Lovely up there… watch out" [35]. In other words, "while in the blue sky, remember the black earth."

Acknowledgments The author would like to thank Liam McNulty, Petter Alfsson-Thoor, Jan Wang, Neal W. Pollock, Linda Persson, Stane Krajnc, Johan Hansson, Sven Mörtberg, John Carter, Björn Äng, Michael Nekludov, Henrik Jörnvall, Pär Forsman, Svante Holmberg, Eva Schmidtke, Ann Lindberg, Ola Jameson, Uno Asker, Anders Lindberg, Peter Lindholm, Johan Jendle, Mohammad Yousef, James Cumberland, Zoltan Hübsch, Kjell Påhlsson, Brian Germain, Eddie Keogh, and Gary Connery.

References

1. Lucas J. The silken canopy: a history of the parachute. Revth ed. Shrewsbury: Airlife; 1997. p. 173, [16] p of plates.
2. Encyclopaedia Britannica Parachute. 2008 [cited 27 Oct 2008]. Available from: http://search.eb.com/eb/article-9058369.
3. Vinci LD. Paracadute. In: Ambrosiana B, editor. Codice Atlantico f 1058. Milano; [c 1485].

4. White L. The invention of the parachute. In: Technology and culture. Chicago: The University of Chicago Press Society for the History of Technology; 1968. p. 462–7.
5. Hearn P. The sky people: a history of parachuting. Shrewsbury: Airlife; 1997. p. 168.
6. Guard J. Airborne: World War II paratroopers in combat. Oxford/New York: Osprey; 2007. p. 304.
7. Poynter D, Turoff M. Parachuting: the skydiver's handbook. 9th ed. Santa Barbara: Para Pub; 2003. p. 408.
8. Jalbert D. Multi-cell wing type aerial device. U.P.a.T. Office, editor. USA; 1966.
9. International Parachuting Commission Technical and Safety Committee. Safety report 2009. In: IPC safety reports. McNulty L, editor. Fédération Aéronautique Internationale; 2010.
10. ISSA. GSSDB hall of fame. 2009 [cited 18 Jan 2009]; Available from: http://gssdb.speedskydiving.eu/hall_of_fame.php?links=off.
11. Davis JR. Fundamentals of aerospace medicine. 4th ed. Philadelphia: Lippincott Williams & Wilkins; 2008. p. xxvii, 724 p.
12. Riksinstruktören, 402:01 Grundläggande bestämmelser, in Swedish regulations for sport parachuting [SFF Bestämmelser Fallskärmsverksamhet; in Swedish]. Svenska Fallskärmsförbundet; 2011.
13. Airtec GmbH. Cypres user's guide. Wünnenberg: AIRTEC; 1991, 53 p.
14. Pecnik R. VAMPIRE 2 wingsuit user manual. Gorica, Croatia: Phoenix Fly; 2006.
15. Royal Thai Air Force. Royal sky celebration. 2006 [06 Oct 2011]; Available from: http://www.theworldteam.com/06RTAF.htm.
16. Record File n 13052. Fédération Aéronautique Internationale World and Continental Record Claims – Class G (Parachuting) 2011 [cited 10 Oct 2011].
17. Westman A, Bjornstig U. Fatalities in Swedish skydiving. Accid Anal Prev. 2005;37(6): 1040–8.
18. WHO. Maternal deaths per 100000 live births. 2011 [06 Oct 2011]; Available from: http://data.euro.who.int/hfadb/tables/tableA.php?w=1024&h=768.
19. Sitter P. A decade of landing deaths. Parachutist. 2004. p. 36–45.
20. Hart CL, Griffith JD. Rise in landing-related skydiving fatalities. Percept Mot Skills. 2003;97(2):390–2.
21. Airtec GmbH. Cypres user's guide. 06/2001 ed. Germany: AIRTEC; 2001.
22. Lasczkowski G, et al. An unusual airplane crash – deadly life saver. Unintentional activation of an automated reserve opening device causing airplane accident. Forensic Sci Int. 2002;125(2–3):250–3.
23. Committee on Injury Scaling. The abbreviated injury scale 1998 revision. Des Plaines: Association for the Advancement of Automotive Medicine; 1998.
24. Westman A, Bjornstig U. Injuries in Swedish skydiving. Br J Sports Med. 2007; 41(6):356–64.
25. Barrows TH, Mills TJ, Kassing SD. The epidemiology of skydiving injuries: world freefall convention, 2000–2001. J Emerg Med. 2005;28(1):63–8.
26. Riksinstruktören, 408:01 Parachute report [408:01 Fallskärmsrapport; in Swedish], in Swedish regulations for sport parachuting [SFF Bestämmelser Fallskärmsverksamhet; in Swedish]. Svenska Fallskärmsförbundet; 2000.
27. Westman A, et al. The SKYNET data: demography and injury reporting in Swedish skydiving. Accid Anal Prev. 2010;42(2):778–83.
28. Westman A. Shoulder injuries have been noted as a recurring problem in skydiving. J Trauma. 2005;59(4):1033.
29. George HW Bush. Salute to the skydiver. United States Parachute Association: United States; 2006.
30. AP, At 85, Ex-president Bush skydives over Maine coast, in *USA TODAY*; 2009.
31. Riksinstruktören, 402:14 Höghöjdshoppning, in Swedish regulations for sport parachuting [SFF Bestämmelser Fallskärmsverksamhet; in Swedish]. Svenska Fallskärmsförbundet; 2011.

32. Pollock NW. Human physical stresses at normal and abnormal cabin pressures. In: Handbook of environmental chemistry. Heidelberg: Springer; 2005. p. 87–109.
33. Divers Alert Network Europe. Skydiving after diving. 2011 [09 Oct 2011]; Available from: http://www.daneurope.org/web/guest/readarticle?p_p_id=web_content_reading&p_p_lifecycle=0&p_p_mode=view&p_r_p_-1523133153_groupId=10103&p_r_p_-1523133153_articleId=16834&p_r_p_-1523133153_articleVersion=1.0&p_r_p_-1523133153_articleType=General+Web+Content&p_r_p_-1523133153_commaCategories=&p_r_p_-1523133153_commaTags=answers%2Cdoctor%2Cenglish&p_r_p_-1523133153_templateId=GENERIC_TEMPLATE_NO_IMG.
34. Pollock NW, et al. Risk of decompression sickness during exposure to high cabin altitude after diving. Aviat Space Environ Med. 2003;74(11):1163–8.
35. Amoroso PJ, et al. Braced for impact: reducing military paratroopers' ankle sprains using outside-the-boot braces. J Trauma. 1998;45(3):575–80.
36. Works P. What does "blue sky, black death" mean to you? In: Skydiving magazine. 2003. p. 34–5.

Chapter 5
BASE Jumping

Omer Mei-Dan

Contents

The Origins of the Sport and Its Development to the Current Stage	92
The Birth of a New Sport	92
The Concept	94
BASE Events and Records	96
The Equipment Used	97
Parachuting Systems	97
Protective Gear and Assisting Equipment	99
Injury and Fatality Rates	100
Injuries in BASE Jumping	100
Fatalities	102
How Dangerous Does It Get?	103
Comparison to Skydiving	104
Wingsuits and Proximity Flying	105
Unique Medical Aspects to Consider	107
Emergency/Prehospital Care	107
Hospital Care	108
Rehabilitation	108
Return to Fly	108
Prevention Measures	109
BASE Courses	109
Specific BASE Environment Issues	109
Weather Conditions	110
Mental Aspects	110
Takeaway Messages	111
References	111

O. Mei-Dan, M.D.
Division of Sports Medicine, Department of Orthopaedic Surgery,
University of Colorado School of Medicine,
Aurora, CO 80045, USA

CU Sports Medicine,
Boulder, Colorado, USA
e-mail: omer@extremegate.com, omer.meidan@ucdenver.org

O. Mei-Dan, M.R. Carmont (eds.), *Adventure and Extreme Sports Injuries*,
DOI 10.1007/978-1-4471-4363-5_5, © Springer-Verlag London 2013

The Origins of the Sport and Its Development to the Current Stage

The Birth of a New Sport

BASE jumping is a sport that evolved out of skydiving while using specially adapted parachutes to jump from fixed objects.

The first documented fixed object parachuted jumps date back to the early days of the previous century and go hand in hand with the development of the modern parachute. On February 4, 1912, Franz Reichelt, a French tailor and parachuting pioneer, conducted the first (fatal) fixed object jump off the Eiffel tower's first platform, testing a wearable parachute he designed. A year later, the first reported successful fixed object parachute jump was performed by Štefan Banič, a Slovakian immigrant to the USA. Banič constructed a prototype of his parachute and tested it in Washington, D.C., in 1913, in the presence of US Patent Office and military representatives, by jumping off a 15-story building. This military-devised parachute was the first to be deployed in actual use, saving the lives of many American Air Force aviators during World War I.

Several parachuted fixed object jumps were made during the following decades stimulated by the rapid development of parachute designs, materials, and the sport of skydiving. However, these sporadic incidents were usually one-off experiments, not the systematic pursuit of a new form of parachuting.

The acronym "B.A.S.E." (now more commonly referred to as "BASE") was coined only as late as 1981 by filmmaker Carl Boenish, his wife Jean Boenish, Phil Smith, and Phil Mayfield. It stands for the four categories of fixed objects that participants can jump from. These are Building, Antenna, Span (a bridge, arch, or dome), and Earth (a cliff or other natural formation) (Fig. 5.1a–d). Carl Boenish was the real catalyst behind modern BASE jumping sport with his 1978 film documenting the first BASE jumps using ram-air parachutes from Yosemite National Park El Capitan cliff. This activity was the effective birth of the sport. Boenish continued to publish films and informational magazines on BASE jumping until his death in 1984, while BASE jumping off the Norwegian Troll Wall.

During its early days, most BASE jumps were made using standard skydiving equipment, being conducted mainly from high cliffs. These "borrowed" skydiving parachuting systems included two parachutes (main and reserve), completely different than the established concept of a "single canopy sport" BASE jumping evolved to be. Specialized equipment and techniques, designed specifically for the unique needs of the sport, were developed later toward the 1990.

In 1997, the newly founded Cliff Jumpers Association of America (CJAA) published *The CJAA Guidelines*, outlining BASE standards and practices, coming from the respected and established manufacturers of the time. In parallel, legal events and competitions began to emerge; the first BASE jump courses were initiated and equipment reached safety levels never before thought possible. With

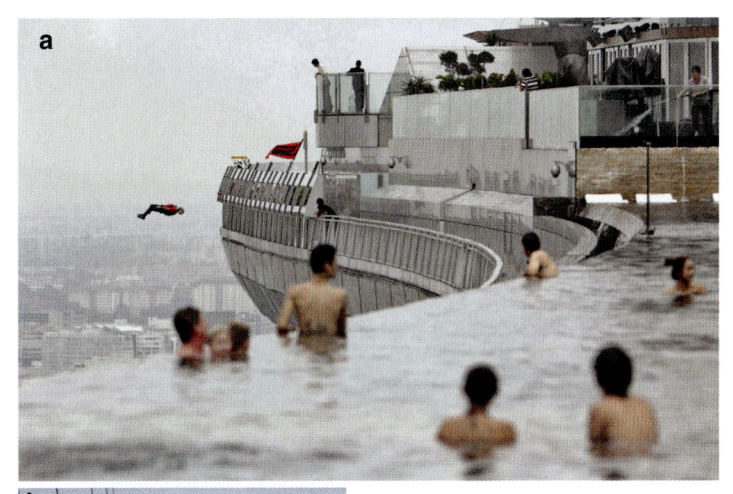

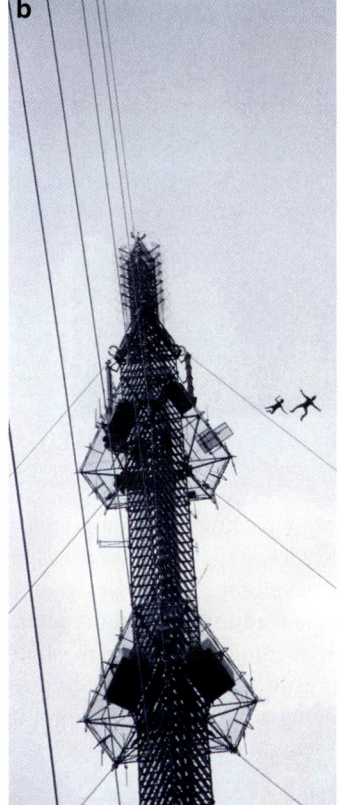

Fig. 5.1 (**a**) A jumper leaps off Marina Bay Sands building in Singapore. (**b**) A two-way jump from a high wire tower. (**c**) The author in a quadruple back gainer off the New River Gorge bridge, during Bridge Day, West Virginia. (**d**) The author jumps into the 512 meters vertical Mexican cave, Sotano the Los Golondrinas

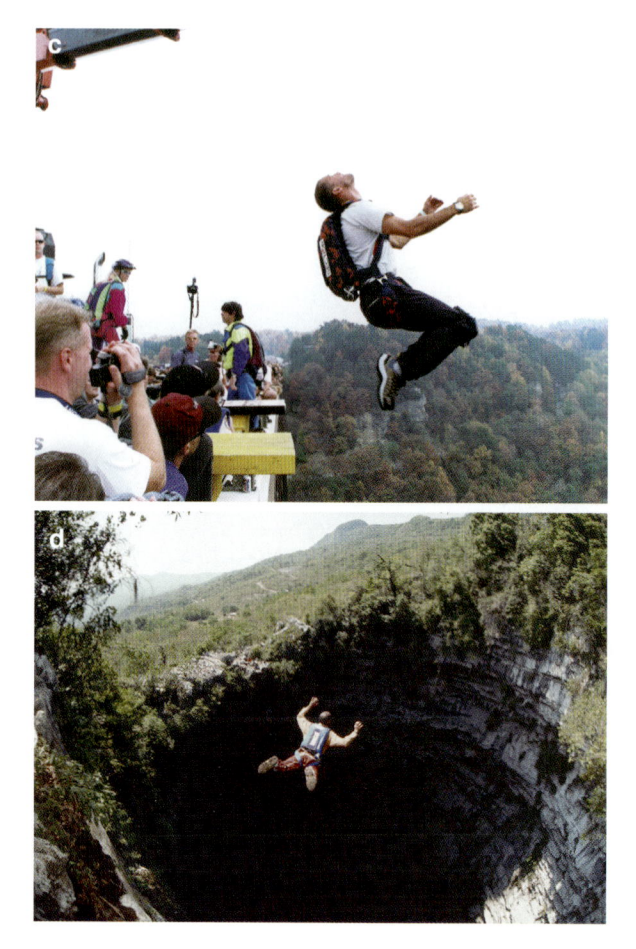

Fig. 5.1 (continued)

this development of specific equipment, canopy packing, and jumping technique, the unacceptable injury and death rate of the early days of the sport has improved remarkably. Nevertheless, as a constantly developing sport, designated BASE parachuting systems keep on evolving, and new adjustments, modifications, and materials improve the reliability of canopy openings and jumpers safety. Many times these "new ideas" are an unfortunate result of an analyzed equipment malfunction, or suboptimal performance, following a jumping mishap or a fatality.

The Concept

In order to understand why BASE jumping is so much more dangerous than skydiving, we must appreciate first the major differences in the physics and aeronautics principles working on the BASE jumper, alongside the various aspects of the equipment used and environmental factors involved.

BASE jumps are made from much lower altitudes than skydives, often less than 500 ft above the ground, while taking place close to the object one leaps from. Skydivers use the air flow surrounding them to stabilize their position, allowing the parachute to deploy cleanly. BASE jumpers generally fall at lower speeds than skydivers (a BASE jumper rarely achieves terminal velocity), have far less aerodynamic control, and may contend with significant flying instability. As so, the attitude of the body at the moment of jumping determines the stability of flight in the first few seconds before sufficient airspeed has built up to enable aerodynamic stability. Moreover, on low BASE jumps, parachute deployment takes place during this exact early phase of the flight. If a poor "launch" leads into a tumble or is markedly asymmetric, the jumper may not be able to correct his body position, before having to deploy his chute, leading to high risk of entanglement or malfunction. Uncontrolled deployment may result in off-heading (facing the object) opening which while being irrelevant in skydiving can lead to a collision with the fixed object in BASE jumping. This "object strike" is the leading cause of serious injury and death in BASE jumping [1, 2].

By contrast, higher falling airspeeds provide jumpers with more aerodynamic control of their bodies, as well as quicker parachute deployment process, which in turn would result in more consistent on-heading opening (a canopy which inflates and flies away from the object one jumps from). This is the case with most high-cliff BASE jumps.

BASE jumps from high cliffs are found in wilderness areas, often hours of hiking away from civilization. In these jumps, a significant trauma following a jump may result in a consequent fatality, due to the time constraints of the rescue and recovery involved. Understanding winds, clouds, and possible turbulence behavior is another crucial skill, which can determine the ability to assess the feasibility of a jump. Weather changes, which can happen in a split second, may turn the whole journey into a real survival mission if proper equipment or knowledge is not available. And that is before adding the actual BASE jump into the equation.

Additionally, most BASE jumping exit points, whether urban or in nature, have very small, hazard-free areas in which to land. Good canopy skills are of real essence in this sport where one commonly needs to navigate between parking cars, electricity street cables, and poles, trees, or boulders, often at night, to a small open space where he can stall his canopy to stand.

BASE jumpers who have jumped from all four object categories may apply for a "BASE number," which are awarded sequentially. BASE #1 was awarded to Phil Smith of Houston, Texas, in 1981. As of January 2012, over 1,600 BASE numbers have been issued [3]. However, some jumpers elect not to apply for a "BASE number" even after completing the four objects jumps, so relying on this data to assess world jumping population would be a mistake. Also, more than a few jumpers who achieved a "BASE number" have ceased jumping due to injury, fatality, or a personal (or forced) decision to retire from the sport.

Calculations within the BASE jumping community, backed up by the very few companies manufacturing BASE jumping equipment and running BASE jumping courses, estimate that less than 1,000 active jumpers are currently operating worldwide.

Legality of BASE jumping has tended to be a well-discussed issue in the media, usually following high-profile object jumps, some more successful than others. Although BASE jumping is banned at many potential jump sites, it is legal in many countries and locations worldwide and many places in the United States [2]. The main reason behind banning BASE jumps lays in liability issues which might follow an unsuccessful jump, whether in a state national park or a city skyscraper. The ability to control and order such a potential jumping site is also a major parameter, which has led to the ban of BASE jumping in many locations. Nevertheless, no specific law presently exists against BASE jumping as a sport, while the two felonies which are usually being used against unauthorized jumpers are trespassing and reckless endangerment.

These relative barriers of the sport did not stop BASE jumping from experiencing a major growth in the past decade with many new evolving subdisciplines. Some of these have pushed the boundaries of the sport so far that a "regular BASE jump" might seem almost too ordinary. These "extreme BASE jump" subdisciplines may involve complex aerobatic maneuvers, similar to the ones conducted by the pool high divers, or wingsuit flying off next to high cliffs (proximity flying). Proximity flying is one of the commonest causes of recent BASE jumping fatalities.

BASE Events and Records

In some extreme sports, the elimination of official events has been adopted. This is to try to prevent increased fatalities as athletes try to push their limits for prizes, audience, or fame. Having said that, there are some BASE jumping events which do occur and are well established and organized. Some are annual events, multi or single, while others would be high-profile one-off professional demonstrations.

The most famous of them all is the Bridge Day.

Once a year, on the third Saturday in October, permission to BASE jump has explicitly been granted at the New River Gorge Bridge (297 m high), in Fayetteville, West Virginia, USA. This annual event, celebrating first and for all the bridge "day" itself, attracts about 450 BASE jumpers and nearly 200,000 spectators. If weather permits, during the 6 h that it is legalized, there may be over 1,000 jumps. This event has a very small competition portion to it while being mainly a great celebration of the sport and an opportunity to gather jumpers from all over the world, exchange experience and information, and have fun. For many skydivers who would like to get a taste of the sport in a relatively safe manner but with proper training, this will be the only fixed object from which they ever jump. Nevertheless, fatalities did occur also from this bridge and during Bridge Day.

Real BASE competitions have been held since the early 1980s. These include landing accuracy and free fall aerobatics as the judging criteria. Recent years have seen a more "formal" competitions held at the 452-m-high Kuala Lumpur's Petronas

Towers, the 321-m-high Colorado's "Royal Gorge Bridge" (the GoFast games), and other venues around the globe.

The evolution of wingsuit BASE flying has also led to the establishment of a formal circuit known as "The BASE Race," where wing-suited BASE jumpers compete head to head flying off high cliffs, mainly in Europe.

In 2010, Northern Norway celebrated with a world record of 53 BASE jumpers jumping from a high fjord cliff. A 15 jumpers simultaneous building jump was recorded off China's Jin Mao, while the tower jump record belongs to 30 jumpers simultaneously jumping off Ostankino Tower in Russia in 2004.

The Equipment Used

Parachuting Systems

A BASE jumper, or a human body for that matter, who jumps from a 150-m object has about 5.6 s of free fall to ground impact and only 10–15 s of a canopy ride if deployment takes place after 2 s following jumping. In comparison, a skydiver, after parachute deployment, may have 2–3 min of canopy ride to the ground.

On a typical BASE jump, the parachute must open at a much lower airspeed than during a skydive and much quicker while covering a shorter vertical distance as possible. Standard skydiving parachute systems are not designed to stand for these prerequisites, so BASE jumpers use specially designed parachuting systems, based on the "single canopy" concept. Although it is hard to believe and understand, a single canopy system may actually be much more reliable and safer than a parachuting system containing two separate canopies packed in the same container. Having two canopies on ones back will dictate some compromises in packing and fitting characteristics while raising the susceptibility for malfunction of the two canopies becoming entangled. Most air force fighter pilots evacuation systems comprise a single canopy only. In addition, many BASE jumps would have little time to utilize a reserve parachute, being conducted from very low altitudes or intending to deploy their chute very close to the ground (Fig. 5.2).

In very low jumps (below 60 m/200 ft), the parachute must open almost instantly, leaving the jumper with less than a few short seconds to release his canopy's brakes or/and stall his canopy to land. One way to achieve this goal is to use a static line or direct bag deployments. These devices form an attachment between the bridle attached to the packed canopy and the jump platform, bypassing the normally used pilot chute. The technique would stretch out the parachute and suspension lines as the jumper falls before separating and allowing the parachute to inflate. This method is similar to the army paratrooper's deployment system (Fig. 5.3).

Due to the major variability in objects a jumper would jump from, the parachuting system is built to be highly versatile. That is to say that in lower jump the pilot chute used would be a larger one and the canopy would be packed differently.

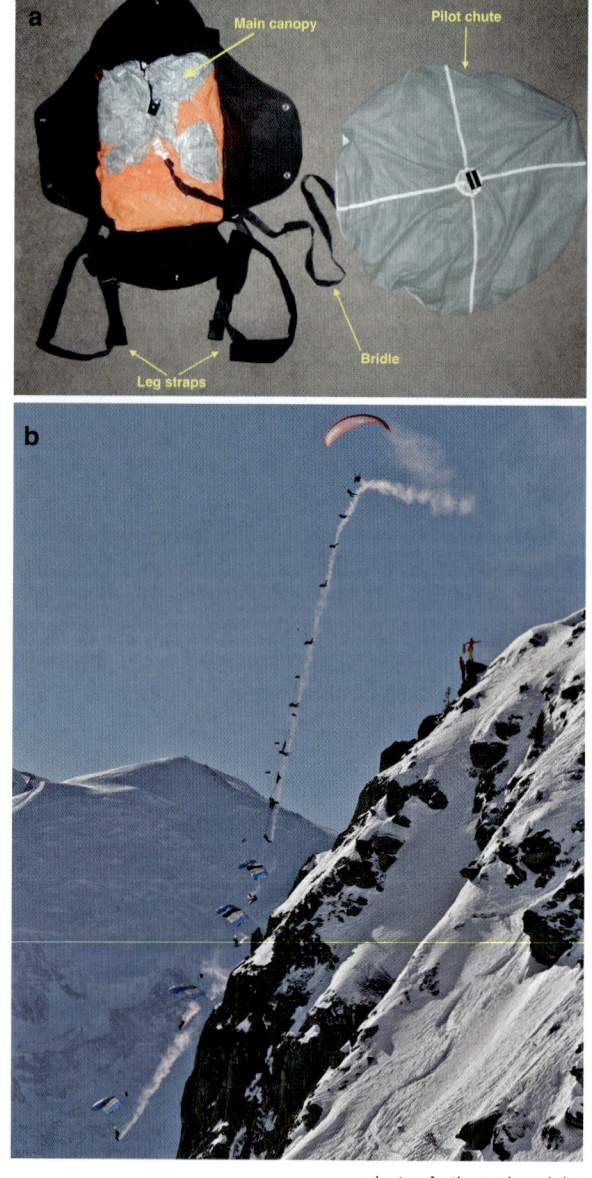

photo: Anthony Lamiche

Fig. 5.2 Main components of a common BASE jump parachuting system are presented in (**a**). (**b**, **c**) In order to initiate a deployment process in a BASE jumping, the jumper must throw his pilot chute, which then pull out the main canopy out of the container

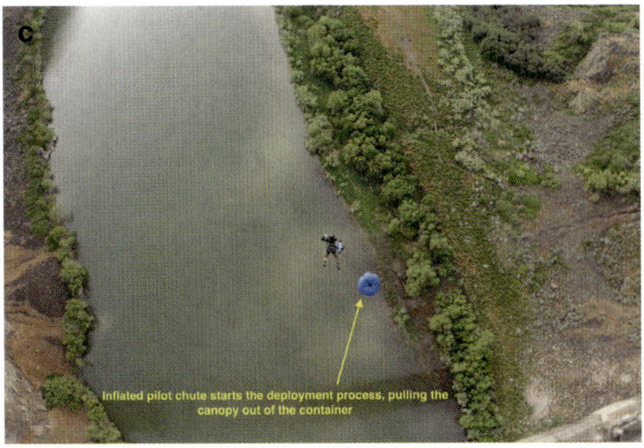

5 BASE Jumping

Fig. 5.2 (continued)

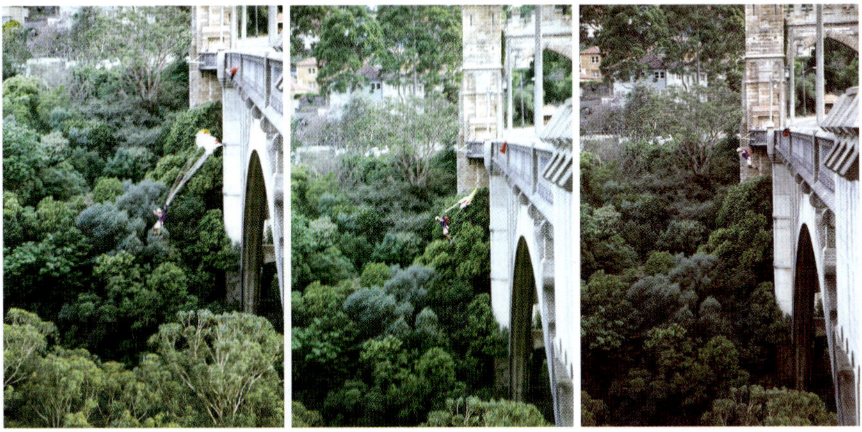

Fig. 5.3 The author jumps off "Northbridge" in Sydney, Australia. This jump is only 47 m above the ground, so automatic deployment (static line) is used

A lower speed upon deployment would need a larger surface area of a pilot chute to generate the same pull force required to deploy the canopy of its container. Finally, most BASE jumping systems would have a "cutaway" function which will enable the jumper to release himself from the canopy, if accidentally landed on a tall tree.

Protective Gear and Assisting Equipment

In a recently published study, all BASE jumpers reported as using various protection devices with the majority wearing helmets for all jumps [4]. The other commonly worn protection devices reported to be used were ankle soft braces, knee hard pads, and spine or elbow protection in jumps with very bad landing areas. Shoulder and spine protection, shin guards, and gloves are also used commonly in BASE jumping.

In order to maintain constant communication between jumpers and their ground crew, which may be crucial to the decision-making stage prior to a jump, almost all jumpers carry two-way small radio devices with them. These are used to report or receive data regarding weather conditions in the landing area or get technical tips and recommendations from jumpers who have just completed the index jump.

Injury and Fatality Rates

Participation in BASE jumping has increased dramatically over the past decade, mainly due to the web-based video content forums, as YouTube or Vimeo. The development of small portable high-definition cameras enabled the wide release of breathtaking footage of unique jumps made by professional athletes. Nevertheless, the number of participants still remains relatively small. The sport is known to have a high dropout rate from fatality, injury, and the increased awareness of risk over time. In 2002, the total number of BASE jumpers worldwide was estimated at 700 participants [5] and the current estimate is around 1,200–1,500 participants (personal communication with BASE equipment manufacturers). Very few formal studies have been conducted on the BASE jumping population. The numbers of jumpers are relatively small, and by its very nature the sport rarely participated in groups making it hard to access these athletes and get them to respond or follow proper methodology research. The author has been a BASE jumper for many years and has facilitated access to a heterogenic group of jumpers and enabled the determination of new data on jumpers' demographics, injuries, fatalities, and mental and physiological aspects. These research projects were initiated 5 years ago and involve also the studies of jumpers' mental characteristics and physiology (stress hormones around a jump, etc.). We have also ran a prospective longitudinal study to assess injuries and fatalities within the sport.

Injuries in BASE Jumping

A comprehensive assessment of accidents and their sequelae in BASE jumping was published recently by the author and colleagues (Table 5.1) [4]. This study had captured 68 active jumpers, which represents around 5 % of the total world BASE jumping population with a balanced coverage of age, gender, experience, and countries of origin. The subjects conducted 19,497 jumps with an average 0.2 % severe injury rate (2 severe injuries per 1,000 jumps). Accordingly, jumpers spend a total of 15,000 jumping days leading to an injury per 384 jumping days or 2.6 significant injuries per 1,000 jumping days.

5 BASE Jumping

Table 5.1 Type of injury and injury score from a study on BASE jumping injury characteristics [4]

Type of injury	No. of incidents	AIS
ICU related, multi trauma (pneumothorax, ACLS required, head injury, cervical spine)	3	5
Head injury\concussion	2	4/3
Fx Thoraco-Lumber-Scaral spine	6	4/3
Fx Ribs	5	4/3
Fx\Dx upper limb (arm, forearm, Scapula)	4	4/3
Fx upper limbs (hand\wrist)	4	3/2
Fx femur	2	3
Fx Dx\open Fx, of ankle\tibia fibula	3	3
Fx ankle (simple)	9	3/2
Fx talus	2	3
Fx calcaneus	2	3
Fx foot (mid\forefoot)	7	3/2
Tear achilles	1	2
Head major laceration	1	2

This is only half the rate of a previous study concluding an injury rate of 0.4 % (4 per 1,000 jumps, 75 % moderate to severe) which was found in a considerably smaller survey of 35 jumpers completing 9,914 jumps [6]. Soreide et al. studied jumps made off a single jump site in the Norwegian fjords and reported an identical rate (0.4 %), but injuries were generally minor [1]. The difference is likely to be due to the fact that the Scandinavian study drew their study population from a 1,000-m-high cliff that allows greater speed of fall and distance from the wall before parachute deployment, longer reaction time for possible malfunctions, with a clear landing area and a safer water landing option.

Analyzing the injury mechanism in the sport is not an easy task. The two main reasons for BASE jumping injuries and fatalities are object strike and bad landing, but the two are very hard to distinguish. That is mainly due to the fact that a cliff strike, if survived by the jumper, would increase the chance of a bad, unplanned landing, so many times both would occur simultaneously. In the 68 jumper series described above, 25 % of injuries were a result of an object strike, while 75 % occurred on landing. Westman et al. [2] also found object strike to be a major fatality factor. Although this was considered by them to be an equipment related problem, it is often a combination of human error and environmental factors, which often cannot be distinguished. These can be an unstable or asymmetric body position upon canopy deployment, a canopy which was packed improperly with relation to specific object characteristics or the misjudgment of a strong side wind, all which might result in uneven canopy inflation and object strike.

Exact injury demographics and characteristics are still lacking for BASE jumping, being a relatively new sport and not yet well studied. The author's group's study [4] has indicated that 61 % of BASE jumping accidents involved the lower limbs, 20 % involved the back/spine, 18 % were chest wall injuries, and 13 % were a head injury. As a result of these injuries, jumpers were sidelined from the sport for an average of 4.5 missing months (range 2 weeks to 60 months). The mean Abbreviated Injury Score (AIS) was 3.2, and more than half of the injured jumpers (52 %) required an acute surgical intervention.

The above study documented and analyzed only injuries involving fractures, critical organs trauma, or severe soft tissue injuries [4]. The reason is that ankle sprains, knee sprains, bruises, or lacerations are very common in BASE jumping and would not be considered a real injury by most jumpers. These "minor" to "moderate" incidents usually form the majority of reported injuries in most studies [7]. This lack of standardized injury severity and rate scales makes it difficult to compare studies directly. Moreover, most studies report relative injury rate as a number per 1,000 h, or activity days, according to the sports examined. This method has less relevance to BASE jumping, when the risk period is generally a few seconds to several minutes per jump.

When considering the role of experience in respect to injury occurrence, it was shown that 30 % of reported injuries occurred when jumpers had performed less than 50 jumps, 25 % of injuries occurred around the 100 jumps mark, and 31 % between 200 and 500 jumps [4]. This suggests that the injury rate per jump is usually higher in the early days of the jumper's career, when less experience and judgment are present. The high incidence rate peaks around the 100 jump mark (between 90 and 130) and is most probably related to the stage where jumpers have acquired enough experience to feel confident, maybe too confident, to step up to a higher level of performance. Typically, this involves aerobatic jumps, less forgiving jumping objects, or wingsuit BASE flights. Having said that, it is important to note that most jumpers studied reported turning back on a jump if their "gut feeling" (i.e., experience, judgment) told them it was too dangerous (even in jumps that they have jumped many times before), usually due to strong or inconsistent winds, lack of proper visibility, or general discomfort with the jump environment [4].

Fatalities

As expected, and documented, fatalities are an integral part of BASE jumping, maybe more than with any other extreme sports field. The fact that most of the experienced jumpers in the sport have witnessed at least one such incident [4] supports the claim that BASE jumping withholds a significant risk of mortality.

The relatively small number of BASE jumpers worldwide and their streamline communication enabled the precise documentation of fatality data. Since 1985, BASE jump fatalities were documented by the jumper Nick Di Giovanni and this register, known as "BASE fatality list," is updated regularly and serves as an open source containing reports on the attributable factors leading to the incident described for the benefit of future participants [8]. "BASE fatality list" was recently analyzed by Westman et al. [2]. Their calculation of the approximate overall BASE jumping annual fatality risk during the year 2002 was of one fatality per 60 participants per year (1.7 %) and is based on Mæland's appraisal of 700 active BASE jumpers worldwide that year [5] and 12 reported fatalities. Westman's study was unable to record actual number of BASE jumps made during 2002, and therefore the fatality rate in relation to number of jumps (exposure) was not made. The fatality rate of BASE jumps made from a single cliff, known as the Kjerag massif in Norway, has been found to be 0.4 per 1,000 jumps [1], but, as mentioned earlier in the injury section, this object is not a representative of the sports as whole, being a relatively forgiving jumping site.

Since 1981 to date (April 2012), there were 183 BASE jumping documented fatalities [8] attributed to a population of presumably less than 1,500–1,800 jumpers indicating an estimated 10 % overall fatality rate since its evolution. Fatality rates for BASE jumping seem to be consistent as 2009, 2010, and 2011 resulted in 15, 16, and 20 fatalities, respectively, but these come together with the growing numbers of jumpers [8].

We must appreciate that the mortality associated with participating in BASE jumping changes significantly if we consider only active jumpers or include also subjects which have conducted few BASE jumps in the past but are no longer active in the sport. If we consider as a BASE jumper every person who has experienced only a single jump but who has never really perused the sport, this rate would obviously reduce. On the other hand, looking only into jumpers, which would consider themselves as active BASE jumpers, performing minimum of several jumps per year, would increase this rate dramatically.

How Dangerous Does It Get?

Our recent study [4] reported that 72 % of the jumpers had witnessed death or serious injury of other participants in the sport, 43 % jumpers had suffered a significant BASE jump injury, and 76 % had at least one "near miss" incident (an incident which would most probably result in serious injury or fatality but was avoided). Only 6 % of the jumpers in this series have never sustained an injury, never had a near miss, and never witnessed a fatality or critical injury in BASE jumping. The average time in the sport for these "untouched" jumpers group was 2 years, compared with 5.8 years for the rest of the jumpers in the study. The number of jumps made by these "untouched" jumpers averaged only 23, compared with 286 jumps with all others. These numbers suggest that if you have not injured or almost killed yourself while jumping or have not seen a jumper die yet, you are probably new to the sport of BASE jumping. This finding was then further supported by a positive correlation ($p<0.001$) between number of jumps made and the amount of time participating in the sport and witnessing an accident or fatality or suffering a significant BASE jump injury. Another interesting and statistically significant finding was that older jumpers have spent less days BASE jumping and made less jumps per year while still maintaining activity in the sport.

Assumption was made that this is due to family- and work-related commitments or a natural maturation in the sport, understanding its inherent risks. These parameters would then lead to less time in the sport overall but with greater preparation for unique jumps.

Comparison to Skydiving

The literature has tended to compare BASE jumping to skydiving as they both share the same general equipment. This is, however, a poor comparison on account of the risks of injury from object strikes, ground strike (due to low parachute deployment), and the confined landing areas rather than effectively a mistimed landing with skydiving. Nevertheless, in order to put BASE jumping injuries and fatalities in perspective, skydiving probably provides the best reference. Skydiving is a commercial sport involving many worldwide participants. It can be performed safely, if one follows all accepted rules and working practices in the common drop zones and uses jumping equipment suited to the jumpers' ability. As outlined in more detail in the skydiving chapter, the major and universally accepted reason for the drastic increase in fatal skydiving incidents is the introduction of fast wing and small-sized canopies (20 % in the USA and 31 % internationally in 2006) which tend to produce more malfunctions, high-impact landings, and air collisions [9–11]. That is in contrast to the relatively slow flying canopy used in BASE jumping. Skydiving provides a similar measure of exposure, which relates to incidents per jump rather than activity hours or days.

Barrows et al. [7] documented skydiving incidents during two consecutive world free fall skydiving conventions in 2000–2001. During the study period 8,976 skydivers made 117,000 skydives resulting in a total injury rate of 1.7 per 1,000 jumps. However, 66 % of those injuries were considered minor, requiring minimal simple first aid, while fewer than 30 % (0.6/1,000 jumps) had to visit the ER. Of these, 21 skydivers (0.18/1,000 jumps) had to be hospitalized and 20 fractures were diagnosed (12 lower and 3 upper limbs, 5 spinal) indicating a rate of 0.17 fractures per 1,000 jumps. This data suggests BASE jumping, with the injury rates outlined above, has 12 times the fracture rate and 16 times the hospitalization rate of skydiving.

Westman evaluated the skydiving injury rate during five consecutive years and more than half a million jumps in Sweden [12]. He found the incidence of nonfatal events to be 0.48 per 1,000 jumps when 88 % of these occurred around the landing. Eliminating 41 % of these injuries which were categorized as minor, the resulting moderate to severe injury rate would be 0.28 per 1,000 jumps, seven times less than in BASE jumping. Moreover, if we consider only AIS 3 injuries from the Westman paper, being the basic score of the injuries documented in this recent comprehensive BASE jump study [4], then BASE jumping injury rate is 30 times higher. Interestingly, women were over-presented among injured skydivers (RR 1.4–2.7), and they also had a higher proportion of landing injuries than men. This was not observed or reported in BASE jumping, where the number of female jumpers is relatively low, comprising only 13 % [4].

BASE jumping fatalities are well documented at the "BASE fatality list" already mentioned. Westman estimated a fatality risk during the year 2002 of one death per 60 participants per year (1.7 %) [2]. The fatality rate associated with skydiving from 1994 to 2009 has gradually increased during periodic analysis from 0.008 to 0.01 per 1,000 jumps or per 3,600–4,000 solo jumpers per year [9–11, 13]. These skydiving fatality rates suggest that the overall annual fatality risk in BASE jumping is approximately 40–65 times higher than in skydiving.

Wingsuits and Proximity Flying

The latest "big thing" in the skydiving and BASE jumping worlds is wingsuit flying.

This refers to the sport of flying using a special jumpsuit, which modifies the body area exposed to wind, to increase the desired amount of lift. The glide ratio of most wingsuits is 2.5. This means that for every meter dropped, two and a half meters are gained moving forward. Modern wingsuits, first developed in the late 1990s, create the surface area with fabric between the legs and under the arms (Fig. 5.4a). The jumper deploys the parachute at a planned altitude and unzips the arm wings, if necessary, so he can reach up to the control toggles and fly to his designated landing spot. During a flight, the jumper can manipulate his flying characteristics by changing the shape of his torso, arching or bending at the shoulders, hips, and knees, by changing the angle of attack in which the wingsuit flies relative to the wind, and by the amount of tension applied to the fabric wings of the suit. But, flying a wingsuit also adds considerable complexity to the jump. Poor flying technique can result in a spin that requires active effort on the part of the jumper to stop. A spin or uncontrolled flight next to an object, as in BASE jumping, is usually detrimental.

The "extreme" version of wingsuit flying, within BASE jumping, is known as "proximity flying." Here, jumpers fly as close as possible to the cliffs, trees, or other natural formations, sometimes only couple of feet away from a potential impact (Fig. 5.4b–c). The unparalleled visuals of this wingsuit version have resulted in an increase of interest within the community, an interest which has surpassed the usual acquisition of adequate experience.

Wingsuit was introduced into BASE jumping on late 1999 and was initially used by only a few experienced jumpers. With the advancement of wingsuit's designs and materials, its popularity and commercialism increased, mainly in the skydiving world. As a result wing-BASE had also started to become more common with an immediate increase in mortality. The first wing-BASE fatality took place in 2002 [8]. That year, 3 of 12 BASE fatalities were attributed to wingsuit use. The following years have seen relatively low percentage of wing-BASE fatalities in relation to "normal" fatalities in the sport, with an average of 15 % (except 2004, 50 %). Major

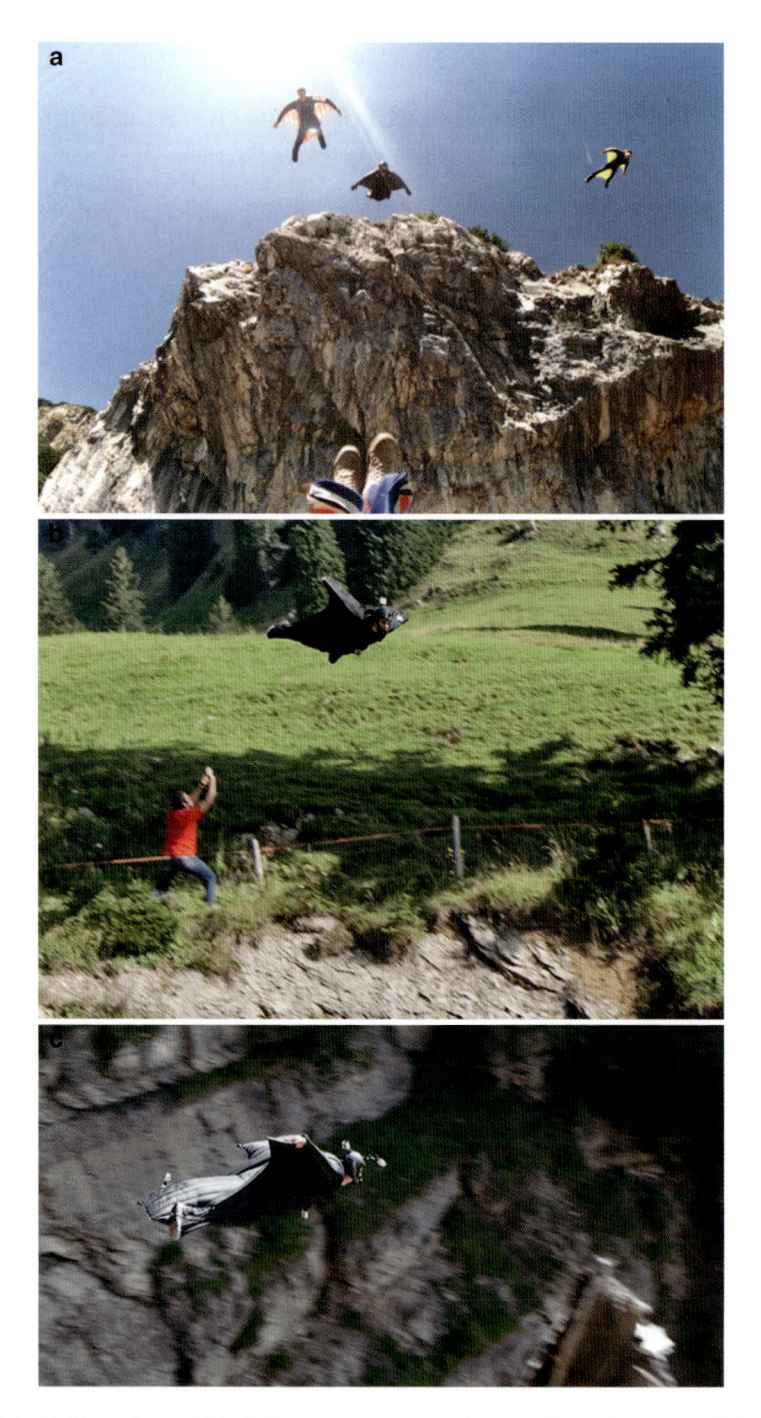

Fig. 5.4 (**a**) The author and friends jumping one of the early wingsuits versions, off a cliff in Italy, year 2000. (**b–c**) Jeb Corliss, Proxy flying "the crack" in Switzerland

increase in wing-BASE and proximity flying popularity had occurred in the past 4 years. From 2008 (six wing-BASE fatalities, 75 %) to date, wing-BASE fatalities are on the raise, with a consistent 50 % rate of general annual fatalities or more (ten wing-BASE fatalities in 2011) [8]. Most of these incidents are due to misjudgment of the proximity to the ground during wingsuit flight or inability to maintain the planned gliding ratio in order to outfly rock formations. Only one jumper, Jeb Corliss, survived such a misjudgment and managed to recover from a cliff impact during a wingsuit flight, just on time to deploy his parachute and crash to the ground with both lower limbs broken.

Unique Medical Aspects to Consider

Emergency/Prehospital Care

Section 4.4 in the Skydiving chapter outlines the various aspects of first aid and evacuation of the injured skydiver, most of which apply also to BASE jumping. Nevertheless, as opposed to skydivers, BASE jumpers usually tend to relay on air rescues rather than land ones. By its very nature, BASE jumping involves high mountains, sheer vertical cliffs, high antennas, and long tall bridges over fast flowing rivers. These are found in remote locations far away from habitation and settlements. The extraction of an injured BASE jumper, relying on local and government assistance, may take a considerable period of time, and an element of recovery may be required before surgical fixation can be achieved. When injury occurs, this typically results in multiple injuries with high Injury Severity Scores and urgent rescue, and transfer to high level trauma center is required. Some geographical locations where BASE jumping have evolved and is considered common and legal have become very popular, and local services have developed into designated rescue teams, usually air ones, to answer this needs. Examples for these are the Norwegian fjords, just out of the port city of Stavanger, and the Swiss cliffs around Lauterbrunnen village overlooking the Eiger, both of which attract many BASE jumpers year round.

In these locations it is well accepted that jumpers would call the air service to let them know of the intended jump prior to its performance. That is to make sure the team is available if needed and also to reassure no helicopters are flying or training within the same air zone. In an organized BASE drop zone, as in Norway, this act would be controlled by the local drop zone team. In some other areas, as the Perrine Bridge in Twin Falls, Idaho, the jumpers are requested to report of the intended jump to local police. That is mainly due to the fact that the bridge also serves as a major traffic route, and passing vehicles might report on "suicide acts" off the bridge or might be distracted with it.

When jumping in the remote locations, it is crucial for jumpers to carry proper communication devices (e.g., satellite phone) as cellular reception is usually absent. Global Positioning System (GPS) coordinates and personal knowledge and understanding local environment and weather characteristics may assist helicopters' search, approach, and rescue when these are required. Nevertheless, as these forms of rescue might take a while to contact and arrive, jumpers should have a fair bit of confidence with trauma principles and equipment, including spinal protection and limb splintage. Many jumpers, being involved in the outdoors for many years, are also climbers and have a good rope handling understanding and skills, which may be required, when a fellow jumper is stuck on a cliff ledge after surviving a cliff strike.

Hospital Care

Many BASE jumping cliff strikes or mislandings will end up as a fatality on impact or within the next hour or days. The energy sustained by the jumper once hitting the cliff or landing away from designated spot would not leave him much chance, and if survived, significant injury is to be expected.

Upon arrival to the ER, usually with a search and rescue air team, a multitrauma scenario and working hypothesis should be considered. Proper data should be retrieved from the helicopter doctor, especially if this was documented in person, from the jumper, prior to intubating him or altering his consciousness with pain medications. Proper ER triage work should be followed from head to toes. If the patient's needs exceed local capabilities, further transport to definitive care must be considered. Due to the significant trauma sustained by the jumper, many of the surgical procedures performed in the initial stage would involve temporary fixation and/or soft tissue work. That would enable a proper systemic stabilization of the subject, and at times, the follow-up permanent fixation would take place upon return to country of residence. Fixation, whether temporary or permanent, should take into account expected level of function and activity-related goals.

Rehabilitation

Return to Fly

Like with other extreme sports fields, BASE jumpers do return to active jumping once rehabilitation from injury is completed, even after life-threatening and disabling injuries [4]. Adventure sports athletes see injuries as integral part of the sport and are very keen on getting back on their feet and cope with the mental aspects involved in the incidence which have put them off.

The ability to be able to respond immediately to an equipment malfunction or a "mishap" stands as a basic prerequisite for survival in BASE jumping and should be achieved prior to sport resumption. Simulation exercises must be performed in a reduced risk environment prior to full return, especially if this is pushed into a short time period, as clearing a BASE jumper to pursue his activity, before body and mind are fully ready, may result in life-threatening injuries. For example, a lax shoulder prone to dislocation in the BASE jumper can result in inability to deploy the single parachute on time, which would most probably result in a fatality. Following a shoulder stabilization surgery and rehabilitation program, the jumper would be better off testing his shoulder stability and function primarily in a wind tunnel environment prior to resuming his BASE activity.

Most BASE jumps require good level of overall musculoskeletal function. Symmetrical flight is a crucial aspect in the sport, both for stability and proper canopy opening, and would not be achieved if subject has not completed proper rehabilitation. Also, a typical BASE jump landing would involve small restricted areas with many boulders and uneven terrain which require good lower limb coordination and proprioception.

For more specific rehabilitation principles, we would recommend to refer to the chapter on Rehabilitation.

Prevention Measures

BASE Courses

BASE jumping was initially taught in a "one-on-one" format. That was usually an experienced jumper who was willing to take the responsibility on a new comer, usually a friend, which he knew well enough and trusted his skills. No one wants to introduce into the sport someone with very low chances to survive it. With time, established course was introduced, mainly by the few BASE gear manufacturers, which wanted to make sure they were selling equipment to subjects who have the (minimal) skills to use it as safely as possible. Nowadays, it is almost a universal standard that no subject would take up BASE jumping without going through a proper guided course, and companies would usually do not sell equipment to inexperienced jumpers who have not been qualified by a BASE instructor. The dropout rate of subjects who have completed this course is very high and according to the largest BASE manufacturing and guiding company (Apex BASE, Boulder, Colorado, USA) is ranging around $x\%$.

Through these courses, experienced skydivers who prove to be skillful canopy flyers and have the ability to confront the involved stress/fear and the reaction time needed can become BASE jumpers. This training progresses in a well-planned, gradual manner, starting from "easy and safe" bridge jump and advancing to the more complicated and dangerous ones.

Specific BASE Environment Issues

A famous BASE jumping expression states, "it dries faster than it heals…." This is to suggest that if you jump from a cliff over water and plan on getting into a small restricted rocky landing area, be ready to modify your plans while under canopy and prepare for a water landing, if there is a doubt you will make it there safely. Although being a major hassle needing to clean and dry the equipment afterward, this is clearly better than an unplanned landing on a rocky area leading to injury. Equipment has to be cleaned if a salt water landing occurs.

Another BASE expression emphasizes the above, "every jump you walked out of is a good jump!"

Weather Conditions

Many BASE jumps take place in the high mountains where weather conditions are very unpredictable. Similar to the dilemmas mountain climbers are facing, BASE jumpers also might have to take tough decisions to back out from a jump, after putting much efforts and time to get to the exit point. A common wrong decision in that instance, which have resulted in several known fatalities of very experienced jumpers in the past [8], is to jump into still or moving clouds with no direct visual contact with the designated landing area. It is very "easy" to lose orientation (vertigo) when one flies under canopy inside a cloud, which can result in a cliff strike. It is easy to fly into the cliff wall when disorientated in cloud. Some jumpers would trust their experience and skills, using a person on the ground (ground crew) to tell them where the cloud base ends, so they can be reassured that if maintaining a perfect flight line, away from the cliff, they will be deploying their chute after passing through the cloud base. Needless to say, this method has also resulted in several mishaps. It is crucial for BASE jumpers to consider weather condition and their dynamic nature.

A few fatalities have been attributed to jumping in cold weather. Cold, stiff, numb, and insensate fingers make deployment hard and the use of gloves makes it fiddly to grab the pilot chute.

Lastly, several known BASE injuries and fatalities are thought to be attributed to lack of sleep and/or to use of access/forbidden substances [8]. Both which can alter the crucial reaction time needed to complete a safe BASE jump.

Mental Aspects

The author and colleagues have studied BASE jumpers mental characteristics, and this data is presented with more detail in the chapter dedicated to this topic. In summary, temperament trait scores of BASE jumpers found to differ significantly when compared to normative population [14]. When BASE jumpers were assessed based on a temperament score of harm avoidance, they actually found to have much lower scores than a non-jumping population. A subject which has scored low in this temperament trait would be defined as carefree, relaxed, daring, courageous, outgoing, bold, optimistic even in situations which worry most people, and confident in the face of danger and uncertainty. As temperament traits are thought to be neurochemically regulated and moderately heritable, it is likely that to some extent engagement in these sports is genetically determined and "hardwired." However, no tightly defined personality profile among BASE jumpers was found [14].

Takeaway Messages

1. BASE jumpers report an average of one severe injury for every 500 jumps, resulting in a 0.2 % severe injury rate, 2 severe injuries per 1,000 jumps, or 2.6 severe injuries per 1,000 jumping days.
2. BASE jumping carries 10 % overall fatality rate since its evolution.
3. Wing-BASE is responsible for major portion of BASE fatalities in the past 5 years.
4. Almost all active BASE jumpers have witnessed death or severe injury of a participant and yet continue in their sport.
5. BASE jumping has a much higher risk than skydiving, with around ten times higher injury rate and 40–66 times higher fatality rate.
6. It dries faster than it heals!

References

1. Soreide K, Ellingsen CL, Knutson V. How dangerous is BASE jumping? An analysis of adverse events in 20,850 jumps from the Kjerag Massif, Norway. J Trauma. 2007;62(5):1113–7.
2. Westman A, Rosén M, Berggren P, Björnstig U. Parachuting from fixed objects: descriptive study of 106 fatal events in BASE jumping 1981–2006. Br J Sports Med. 2008;42(6):431–6.
3. http://www.basenumbers.org/ui.asp
4. Mei-Dan O, Carmont MR, Monasterio E. The epidemiology of severe and catastrophic injuries in BASE jumping. Clin J Sport Med. 2012;22(3):262–7.
5. Mæland S. Basehopping – nasjonale selvbilder – sublime opplevelser. Norsk Antropologisk tidsskrift. 2004;1:80–101.
6. Monasterio E, Mei-Dan O. Risk and severity of injury in a population of BASE jumpers. N Z Med J. 2008;121(1277):70–5.
7. Barrows TH, Mills TJ, Kassing SD. The epidemiology of skydiving injuries: world freefall convention, 2000–2001. J Emerg Med. 2005;28(1):63–8.
8. Di Giovanni N. World BASE fatality list. http://www.blincmagazine.com/forum/wiki/BASE_Fatality_List. Accessed on April 2012.
9. International Parachuting Commission, FAI. Technical and safety committee. Safety report. 2006. http://www.paracaidismo.org.ar/SYT/Textos/FAI%20Reports/Safety%20Report%202006.pdf
10. International Parachuting Commission, FAI. Technical and safety committee. Safety report. 2009. http://issuu.com/delta3x/docs/safety-report-2009

11. Paul S. The 2008 fatality summery – "back to the bad old days", USPA parachutist magazine. April 2009, Volume 50, Number 04(594):30–5
12. Westman A, Björnstig U. Injuries in Swedish skydiving. Br J Sports Med. 2007;41(6):356–64.
13. Westman A, Björnstig U. Fatalities in Swedish skydiving. Accid Anal Prev. 2005;37(6):1040–8.
14. Monasterio E, Mulder R, Frampton C, Mei-Dan O. Personality variables in a population of BASE jumpers. J Appl Sport Psychol. 2012;24:391–400. doi: 10.1080/10413200.2012.666710.

Chapter 6
Whitewater Canoeing and Rafting

Jonathan P. Folland and Kate Strachan

Contents

Origins and Development of Whitewater Paddle Sports	114
Craft, Equipment, and Safety Recommendations	117
Overview of Whitewater Accidents and Injuries	121
Acute Injuries	124
Fractures, Lacerations, and Abrasions	124
Acute Muscle Strains and Joint Sprains	124
Shoulder Dislocation	125
Major Traumatic Injuries	125
Chronic Injuries	126
Hand, Wrist, and Forearm Injuries	126
Elbow Injuries	128
Chronic Shoulder Injuries	128
Back Injuries	129
Rib Fractures	129
Pelvic and Lower Limb Injuries	130
Environmental Injuries and Illnesses	130
Skin	130
Illnesses	131
Cold/Heat Illness	131
Prevention of Accidents, Injuries, and Illness	131
Whitewater Accidents	132
Injury Reduction	132
Illness Reduction	133

J.P. Folland, Ph.D., FACSM (✉)
School of Sport, Exercise and Health Sciences,
Loughborough University, Sir John Beckwith Centre for Sport,
Loughborough, Leics, LE11 3TU, UK
e-mail: j.p.folland@lboro.ac.uk

K. Strachan, MBChB, MRCGP, M.Sc., DRCOG FFSEM(UK)
English Institute of Sport – East Midlands, EIS/Loughborough Performance Centre,
1st Floor, Loughborough University, Loughborough, Leics, LE11 3TU, UK

O. Mei-Dan, M.R. Carmont (eds.), *Adventure and Extreme Sports Injuries*,
DOI 10.1007/978-1-4471-4363-5_6, © Springer-Verlag London 2013

Treatment and Rehabilitation 133
    Abrasions, Lacerations, and Contusions 133
    Skin and Blisters 133
    Fractures 134
    Shoulder Dislocation 134
    Muscular Strains 136
    Chronic Shoulder Injury 137
    Elbow, Wrist, and Forearm Tendinopathies 137
    Gastrointestinal Illness 138
Summary 138
References 139

Origins and Development of Whitewater Paddle Sports

The development of whitewater canoeing both as a sport and recreation began with the navigation of upland European rivers in a variety of craft, including canoes, kayaks, and rafts, during the late nineteenth and early twentieth centuries. The first documented whitewater competition was a downriver (wildwater) race in foldboats held on the river Isar in Germany on July 16–17, 1921. The first whitewater canoe slalom took place on the river Aar in Switzerland in 1933, rapidly leading to international competition and the first World Championships in Geneva in 1949. Canoe slalom was first incorporated into the Olympic Games in 1972, but not regularly featured until 1992. After more than a century of river exploration, the majority of the whitewater rivers in the developed world have been paddled extensively, although river exploration of more remote, less developed regions is continuing. An International Scale of River Difficulty is used to classify rivers and individual rapids, from grade I to VI (Table 6.1).

Modern canoeing is a diverse sport, and the International Canoe Federation (ICF) oversees competitive canoeing across 11 disciplines that encompass a wide range of different craft, paddles, and water conditions. The principal ICF competitive whitewater disciplines are canoe slalom, wildwater canoeing, and canoe freestyle (Table 6.2; in this context canoeing is the overarching term for all canoe and kayak activities, although most of the disciplines have specific canoe and kayak classes). In addition, the water conditions in some canoe marathon and ocean racing (surfski) events include whitewater paddling depending on the course and prevailing weather conditions. The disciplines of rafting and surf/waveski also take place on whitewater.

The essence of these competitive disciplines is practiced extensively at recreational level and often described as playboating, whitewater touring, or river running. The most challenging and extreme whitewater paddling involves descending grade V and VI rapids, including shooting waterfalls (Fig. 6.6a, b), as well as exploring new or seldom-navigated rivers typically in remote wilderness locations. In addition, recreational rafting is an extensive commercial adventure tourist activity in many mountainous parts of the world. In the year 2000, it was estimated that that

6 Whitewater Canoeing and Rafting

Table 6.1 International scale of river difficulty

Grade	Water conditions
I	Moving water with riffles and small waves. Few obstructions, all obvious, and easily missed with little training. Risk to swimmers is slight; self-rescue is easy
II	Straightforward rapids with wide, clear channels. Occasional maneuvering required, but rocks and medium-sized waves are easily avoided
III	Moderate rapids that include irregular waves, strong eddies, and a powerful current. Good boat control and regular maneuvering required to avoid obstacles (boulders & small drops). More pronounced obstacles (large waves or strainers) may be present but are easily avoided
IV	Intense, powerful, turbulent, but predictable rapids often featuring large, unavoidable waves and holes. Requires precise boat handling and fast maneuvers under pressure. Scouting may be necessary the first time down. Risk of injury to swimmers is moderate to high, and a strong eskimo roll is highly recommended
V	Extremely long, obstructed, or very violent rapids that expose a paddler to added risk. Frequent large, unavoidable waves, and holes or steep, congested chutes with complex, demanding routes. Few eddies that are small, turbulent, and difficult to reach. Scouting is recommended but often difficult. Swims are dangerous, and rescue is difficult even for experts. A very reliable eskimo roll, proper equipment, extensive experience, and rescue skills are essential
VI	These runs have almost never been attempted and often exemplify the extremes of difficulty, unpredictability, and danger. The consequences of errors are very severe, and rescue may be impossible. For teams of experts only, at favorable water levels, after close personal inspection and taking all precautions

Adapted from American Whitewater

Table 6.2 Competitive whitewater disciplines

Discipline	Description of competition
Canoe slalom	Timed completion of up to 25 gates while negotiating a ~300 m course of whitewater rapids (Fig. 6.1a, b)
Wildwater canoeing	Descent of a section of whitewater rapids in the fastest time. Classic race >3 km, sprint race <1 km (Fig. 6.2)
Canoe freestyle	Acrobatic tricks/maneuvers performed on a specific whitewater river feature, e.g., wave or hole (Fig. 6.3)
Rafting	Racing with four to eight people in raft. The World Championships have sprint, head-to-head, slalom and downriver events (Fig. 6.4)
Surf/waveski	Stunts/maneuvers performed while surfing a wave into shore (Fig. 6.5a, b)

there were ~10 million rafting participants and ~2 million whitewater canoe/kayak paddlers in the USA annually [35].

This chapter will primarily consider whitewater accidents, injuries, and relevant illnesses. The prevention and treatment of the most prevalent will be reviewed with some reference to flatwater paddling injuries, due to their relevance. While canoeing is the overarching term for all canoe and kayak activities, for precision in the remainder of this chapter, the terms canoeing (propelled with a single-bladed paddle typically from a kneeling position) and kayaking (propelled with a double-bladed paddle from a seated position) will be used in their more specific sense.

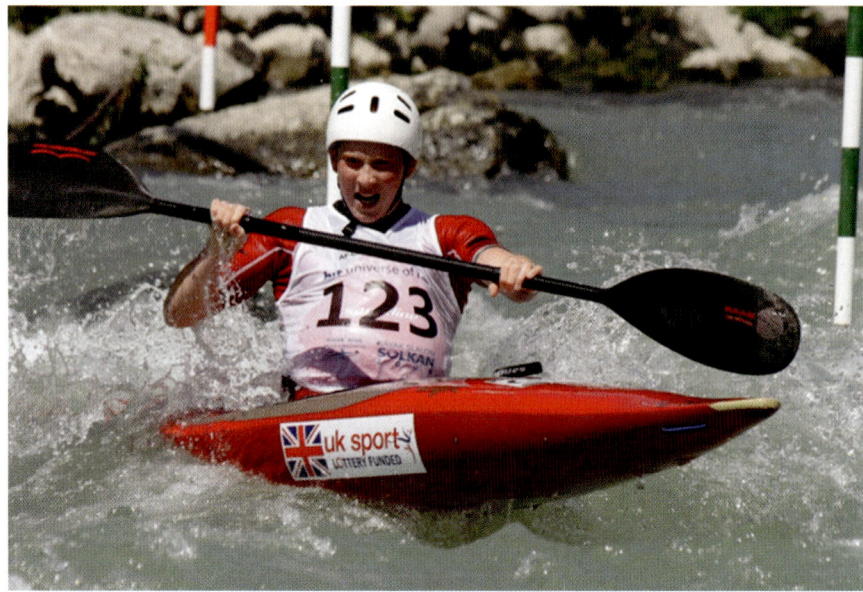

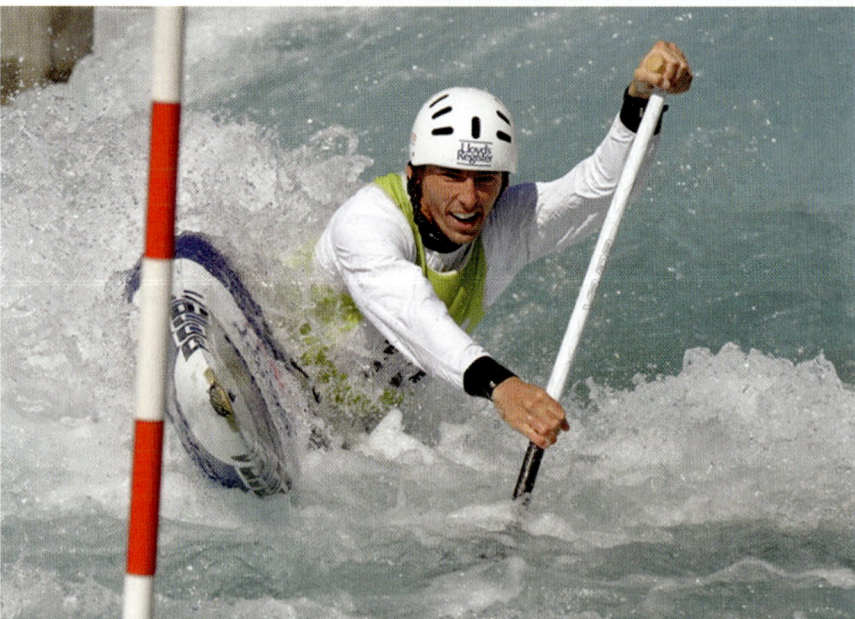

Fig. 6.1 Canoe slalom competitors in the Men's K1 (*top*) and C1 classes (*bottom*). The crossbow stroke shown by the C1 paddler requires considerable flexibility and balance. These craft are designed for maneuverability and stability being relatively short with a flat-bottomed hull (Pictures courtesy of Andy Maddock (*top*) and Jon Royle (*bottom*))

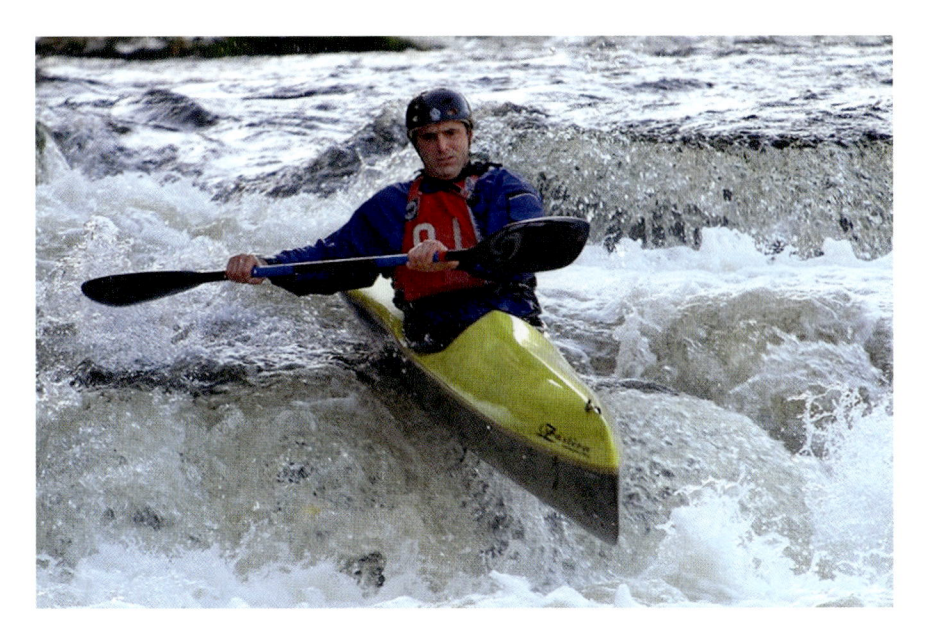

Fig. 6.2 A paddler in the Men's K1 class of a wild-water canoeing competition (one of the ICF competitive disciplines) descends a grade III fall. Note the long sleek craft that is designed for speed when descending whitewater as fast as possible (Picture courtesy of Jon Royle)

Craft, Equipment, and Safety Recommendations

Whitewater canoes and kayaks come in different shapes and sizes, depending on the purpose of the craft and expected water conditions. Craft designed with an emphasis on linear speed are long and sleek to reduce drag, e.g., wildwater, touring, or marathon kayaks (3.5–5.2m). Slalom, freestyle, and surf craft are typically shorter for increased maneuverability (3 m and <2 m, respectively) and flat bottomed for greater stability. For higher grade whitewater (III+), decked craft are the norm. Those designed for "heavy" (highly aerated) whitewater are higher volume compared to those intended for smaller whitewater, with an extreme being squirt boats – a form of freestyle kayak that can perform subsurface maneuvers even on flatwater. Competition canoes and kayaks are constructed from composite materials to minimize weight and maximize performance. Modern recreational canoes and kayaks are constructed from polyethylene plastic in order to maximize durability, although this comes at the cost of increased weight. These stronger plastic boats have led to the exploration of smaller steeper creeks, the running of waterfalls, and the evolution of the modern playboat that is shorter than more traditional canoes and kayaks. Playboats have also evolved to have highly rounded ends in order to reduce the risk of pinning the craft in a dangerous manner. Inflatable and sit-on-top canoes and

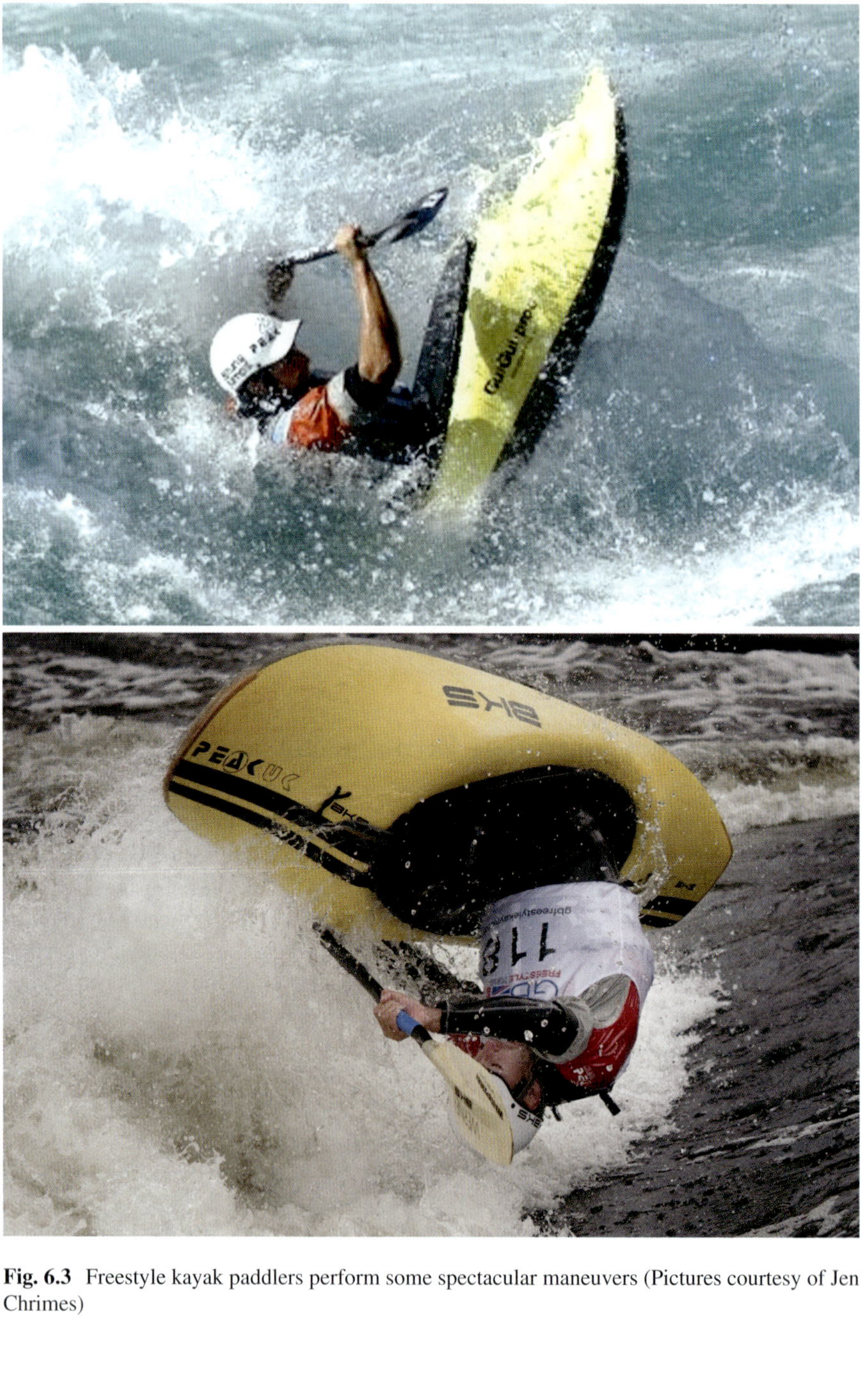

Fig. 6.3 Freestyle kayak paddlers perform some spectacular maneuvers (Pictures courtesy of Jen Chrimes)

6 Whitewater Canoeing and Rafting

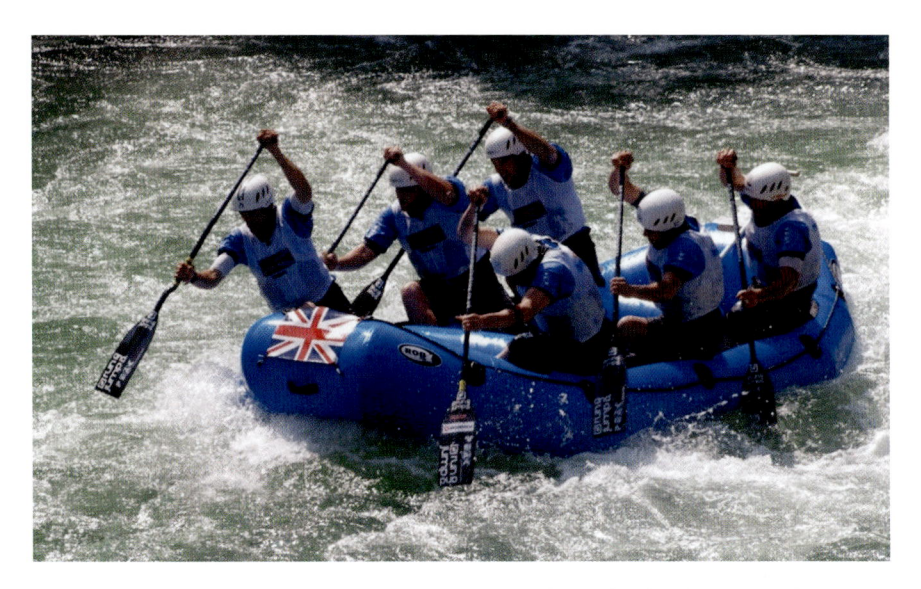

Fig. 6.4 A six-person raft in competition. Commercial rafting often involves larger eight to ten-person rafts with the raft guide seated at the back from where they can see all of the paddlers and the river ahead, as well as steer the raft (Picture courtesy of Lawrence Harris)

kayaks have also become increasingly popular, particularly with novice paddlers and for grade I–II water. Modern rafts are constructed from inflatable rubber with multiple chambers aiding buoyancy (even if one chamber is punctured). Raft paddlers sit perched on the outer tube with both legs in the raft and use a longer paddle to reach the water (Fig. 6.4).

In the event of capsize, sufficient boat buoyancy is an important safety feature as upturned canoes or kayaks filled with water are extremely heavy and difficult to extract from a fast flowing river. In contrast a buoyant capsized boat can provide an excellent flotation aid to a swimmer struggling to stay on the surface of turbulent water. For this reason, removable air bags placed inside the craft are a standard requirement for Whitewater competitions and strongly recommended for recreational paddling.

Paddle design is largely dependent on the craft and canoeing discipline plus the physique and ability of the paddler (Fig. 6.7). Craft with greater linear speed tend to be propelled with longer paddles that have a larger blade area. For these faster craft, kayak paddles with a greater feather angle (45–85°) and winged blades ("spoon" shaped with a distinct upper lip) are commonly used. Cranked shaft paddles are popular among slalom kayakers and have been suggested to improve performance and reduce injury risk.

Personal flotation devices (PFD) or buoyancy aids are essential personal equipment for all Whitewater paddle sports. This is reinforced by statistics from two

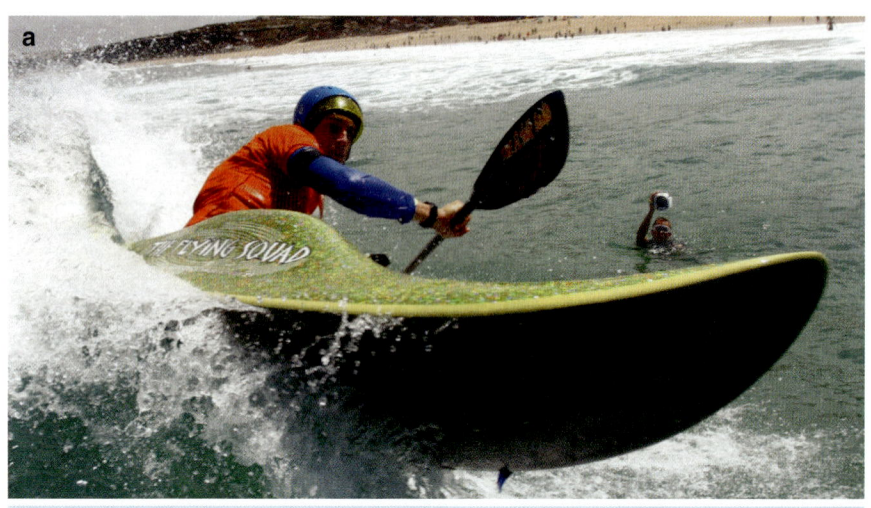

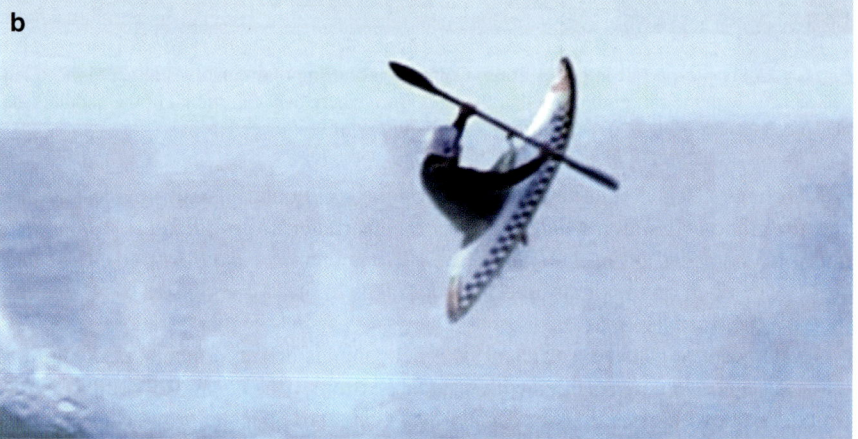

Fig. 6.5 Surf paddlers perform a top turn high on a wave (**a**) and an aerial maneuver (**b**) (Pictures courtesy of Stephen Bowens)

surveys where a high proportion of fatalities (68 and 92 %) were not wearing a PFD [9, 11]. The minimum competition standard is 60 N of buoyancy (EN/ISO 12402-5), but for more severe conditions/river grades, higher levels of buoyancy are recommended and may be crucial in helping to keep a swimmer on the surface. A helmet is also essential personal equipment. Approved helmets (e.g., CE EN 1985) are recommended for all Whitewater activities. For more extreme Whitewater helmets incorporating jaw and/or face protection may also be appropriate. Face guards are more relevant for rafters due to the higher incidence of reported facial injuries.

The water temperature of alpine or mountain rivers is often just a few degrees above freezing; therefore, even in warm/hot air temperatures, wet or dry suits can be an important safety precaution, mitigating the risk of hypothermia during a prolonged capsize and swim. Wet suits also provide other advantages, increasing

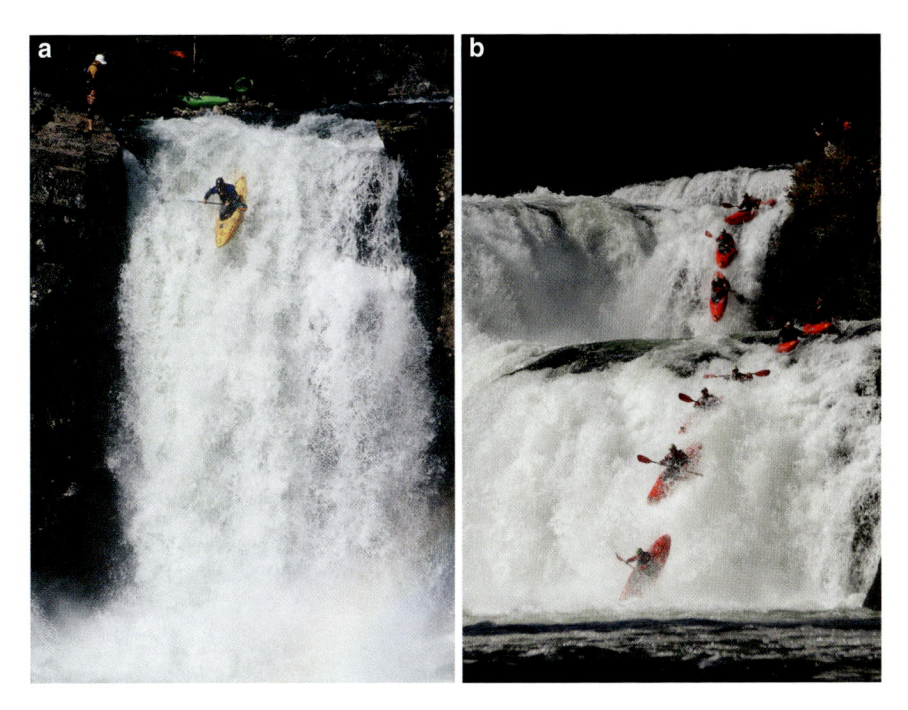

Fig. 6.6 (**a**) A kayak paddler, in a typical playboat, descends a substantial waterfall (Picture courtesy of Omer Mei-Dan) (**b**) A kayak paddler picks up the best "line" down a "2-stage" waterfall (Picture: David Carlier)

personal buoyancy and reducing abrasion/impact injuries if a paddler should be separated from their craft. Watertight clothing and equipment, including a spraydeck, help to maintain body temperature and prevent craft becoming water logged, which causes a rapid loss of paddler control.

Throw bags are an important piece of equipment when there is a significant chance of capsize. A throw bag thrown from a stable position into swift water or rapids enables a swimmer to grab the rope and be pulled to safety.

Many paddle sport organizations (clubs, federations, etc.) offer courses, tuition, and extensive information on safe Whitewater paddling. Table 6.3 contains a summary of important safety advice for all Whitewater paddlers issued by American Whitewater.

Overview of Whitewater Accidents and Injuries

Accidents and injuries in Whitewater paddle sport are relatively rare, but due to the unpredictable nature of the Whitewater environment, the consequences can be severe. Most river fatalities are thought to occur in inexperienced paddlers attempting rivers

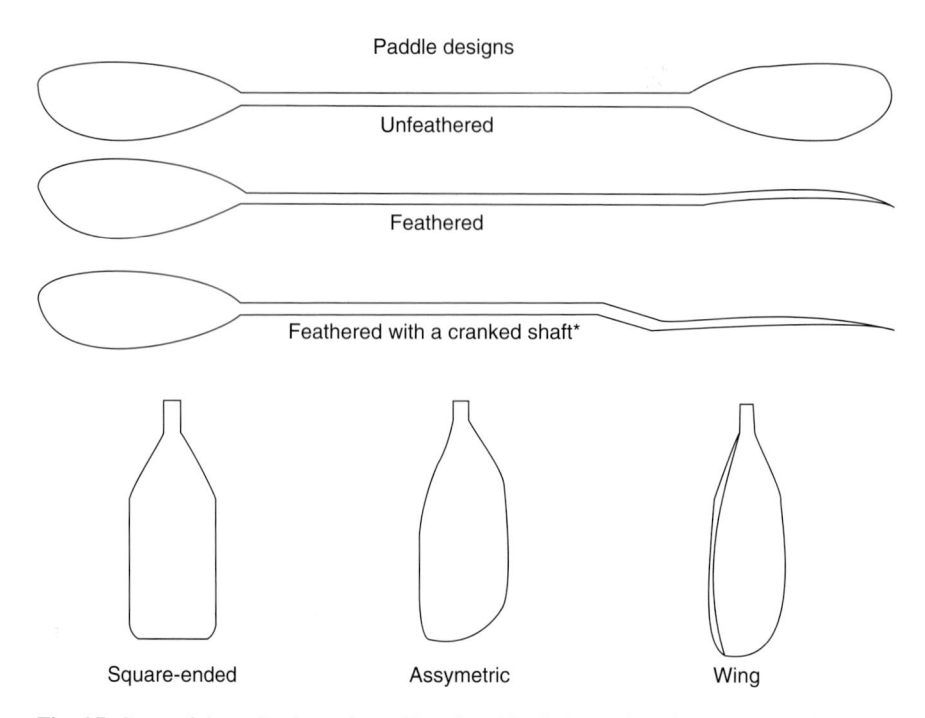

Fig. 6.7 Some of the main alternatives of kayak paddle design. *Note that cranked shaft paddles have a crank where both hands grip the shaft

Table 6.3 A summary of the Whitewater Safety Code of American Whitewater

Whitewater safety advice
Know your limitations
Be able to swim at least 50 m
Know the water/course and weather conditions
Always wear a buoyancy aid/life jacket/personal flotation device
Always have a float plan (i.e., others know where you are going and when you'll be back)
Have the appropriate clothing/equipment for the conditions, e.g., helmet
Paddle in a group
Avoid drugs and alcohol prior to paddling
Know what to do in the event of a capsize

The full safety code can be accessed at: http://www.americanwhitewater.org/content/Wiki/safety:start

beyond their skill, in adverse weather or high water conditions, and without appropriate safety gear [8]. Submersion accidents are the primary life-threatening hazard, possibly accounting for ~1/3 of all Whitewater injuries [27] that include drowning, near drowning, and impact-related trauma while submerged. Fortunately fatalities are relatively rare, occurring at a rate of 8.7 per 1,000,000 user days for rafters, canoeists, and kayakers [50], which is similar to trekking [42]. The primary causes of drowning in whitewater are entrapment, blunt head trauma, or hypothermia leading to disorientation or loss of consciousness. Sudden immersion in cold water can

Table 6.4 Common acute traumatic, chronic overuse, and environmental injuries/illnesses in whitewater canoeing, kayaking, and rafting

Acute traumatic	Chronic overuse	Environmental
Lacerations/abrasions	Tendinopathies of the wrist, forearm, elbow, and shoulder	Drownings/near drownings
Contusion/hematomas	Muscle strain of the lower back and vertebral disk degeneration	Blisters/calluses on hands
Shoulder dislocations	Rotator cuff impingement	Fungal and bacterial skin infections
Fractures	Rib stress fractures	Gastroenteritis
Head and face injuries		Otitis media and otitis externa
Muscle strains and joint sprains		Cold/heat injury
		Leptospirosis

cause hyperventilation, bronchospasm, and even cardiac arrest [4]. Therefore, all participants should be prepared for a capsize (as it is an integral part of the sport) and advised to wear appropriate watertight clothing with sufficient insulation (e.g., spray deck, waterproof jacket/cagoule, wet/dry suit). Submersion accidents and injuries primarily occur during a capsize or when a paddler is swimming downriver separated from their craft. Capsized paddlers and swimmers are also susceptible to hematomas, contusions, abrasions, and lacerations from contact with rocks and other objects, as they are carried downstream.

The incidence of Whitewater injuries has been estimated as 4.5 and 5.2 injuries per 1,000 paddler days among recreational [41] and competitive slalom [28] canoeists and kayakers. This is a similar injury incidence to alpine skiing, but higher than cross-country skiing or windsurfing [22, 34]. The injury incidence in commercial rafters appears to be lower at 0.26–0.44 injuries per 1,000 paddler days [49]. As with most sports, the incidence of Whitewater injuries rises with increased exposure [41] and is substantially greater during competition than training (ten times higher in competitive slalom paddlers [28]). The etiology of injuries/illnesses sustained by paddlers can be divided into acute trauma, chronic overuse, and environmental (Table 6.4). There are relatively few detailed reports in the scientific and medical literature regarding specific Whitewater injuries. Previous studies have typically been retrospective surveys relying on self-reporting, rather than any professional diagnoses.

Unsurprisingly for a predominantly upper body sport, the majority of injuries in canoeists and kayakers involve the wrist, forearm, elbow, and shoulder. Rafters have a different pattern of injury with more face (33 %) and knee injuries (15 %) and fewer shoulder injuries (6 %) [7].

The only evidence on severity of Whitewater injuries is from the surveys observing that 42–51 % of all injuries reported required medical attention [16, 41]; one survey showed that the severe injuries were similar in nature to milder injuries, i.e., 47 % acute versus 36 % chronic [41]. The shoulder was the most common site for severe injury in canoe/kayak paddlers, with 15 % of respondents in one survey reporting at least one dislocation [28] and more than half a cohort of elite slalom paddlers reporting a history of shoulder injury [15].

More than 50 % of all rafting injuries occur on the raft and include collisions with other rafters, impacts from paddles or other equipment, and entanglement of extremities within the raft. 40 % of rafting injuries occur when paddlers are ejected from the raft [49]. In Whitewater kayakers, 87 % of injuries occurred while in the boat, 8 % when in the water having abandoned their craft, and 5 % while walking or portaging [16].

Acute Injuries

The majority of Whitewater injuries are of an acute traumatic nature, accounting for 57–61 % of all injuries [28, 41]. The most common acute injuries in canoe/kayak paddlers were sprains (35 % of acute injuries) and tendonitis (20 %) in one survey [28] and sprain/strain (26 %), lacerations (17 %), and contusions (17 %) in another [41]. In rafters the most common acute injuries are similar: lacerations (33 %), strains and sprains (23 %), fractures (23 %), and contusions/bruises (10 %) [49].

Fractures, Lacerations, and Abrasions

The predominant cause of fractures, lacerations, contusions, and abrasions is direct impact with rocks, the river bed, or other paddlers/equipment [41]. Fractures can vary from the minor undisplaced finger fractures to life- or limb-threatening injuries, the more severe injuries being more frequent on higher grade whitewater. Surveys of paddlers, both amateur and elite, have reported similar fracture occurrence rates 5–9 % of acute injuries [28, 41]. There is no detail on the exact diagnoses, but 19 % of acute ankle/foot injuries and back/chest/hip injuries were fractures. 14 % of acute wrist and forearm injuries were also reported as being fractures [41].

Acute Muscle Strains and Joint Sprains

While the etiology of these acute injuries has not been documented, they are likely to result from sudden overload of a muscle group or joint. The mechanical limits of the muscle or joint tissues may be exceeded when making a very forceful movement to negotiate an object/gate or performing a "last-ditch" support stroke or roll. With the shoulder and lower back thought to be at greatest risk of acute strain or sprain.

In the canoe class of paddlers, although not reported in the literature, hip flexor muscle strains and quadriceps/hamstring strains can occur due to the kneeling position and consequent loading of these structures.

Shoulder Dislocation

In one survey of canoe and kayak paddlers, 15 % of respondents reported at least one shoulder dislocation [28]. This is a severe injury that typically results in several weeks of shoulder immobilization and a prolonged absence from paddling. Dislocation and subluxations are mostly due to anterior displacement of the humeral head that commonly occurs when a paddler is forced to brace strenuously to avoid capsize. Extreme bracing or support strokes inevitably involve a high degree of shoulder abduction, which if pronounced and combined with simultaneous external rotation and extension can lever the humeral head out of the glenoid fossa. In this position the musculature that typically spans the anterior of the joint (subscapularis, biceps brachii, anterior deltoid, and pectoralis major) is lifted above the joint, and there is limited anterior stabilization. An extended elbow can also help to transmit force along the arm wrenching the humeral head from the glenoid fossa. Good technique with high brace support strokes conducted with limited shoulder abduction, extension, and external rotation is thought to reduce the risk of this injury (Fig. 6.8). In practice this involves keeping the elbow in front of and below the shoulder, the hand in front of the elbow, and with the elbow flexed. It has been suggested that the potential for this injury is greater in female paddlers who have less upper body muscle mass to help stabilize the shoulder [8], but as yet there is no definitive evidence that this is the case.

Major Traumatic Injuries

While there are no systematic scientific reports of the injuries incurred during more extreme grade V and VI descents and waterfall jumping, there are numerous press reports and online databases (e.g., American Whitewater) that provide some information about the more extreme injuries that can occur during higher grade descents where drops/falls are often involved. These injuries can include vertebral compression fractures, long bone and pelvic fractures, abdominal/chest trauma, and head injuries. Paddling high waterfall appears to involve an inherent risk of spinal compression and/or a broken spine due to the potential for high impact forces on landing particularly if the boat lands flat [3]. These injuries frequently cause temporary or permanent paralysis.

Where individuals attempt jumping falls, reports in the media suggest that they do so with medical back up to manage any of these potential injuries, with personnel trained in rescue from the water, as well as managing multiple traumatic injuries in a prehospital setting.

In general, the number of accidents reported in the press and online is very low, with a higher proportion of drownings. However, the reports do not often have the formal cause of death, so whether death has been due to drowning primarily or secondary to another injury is not clear.

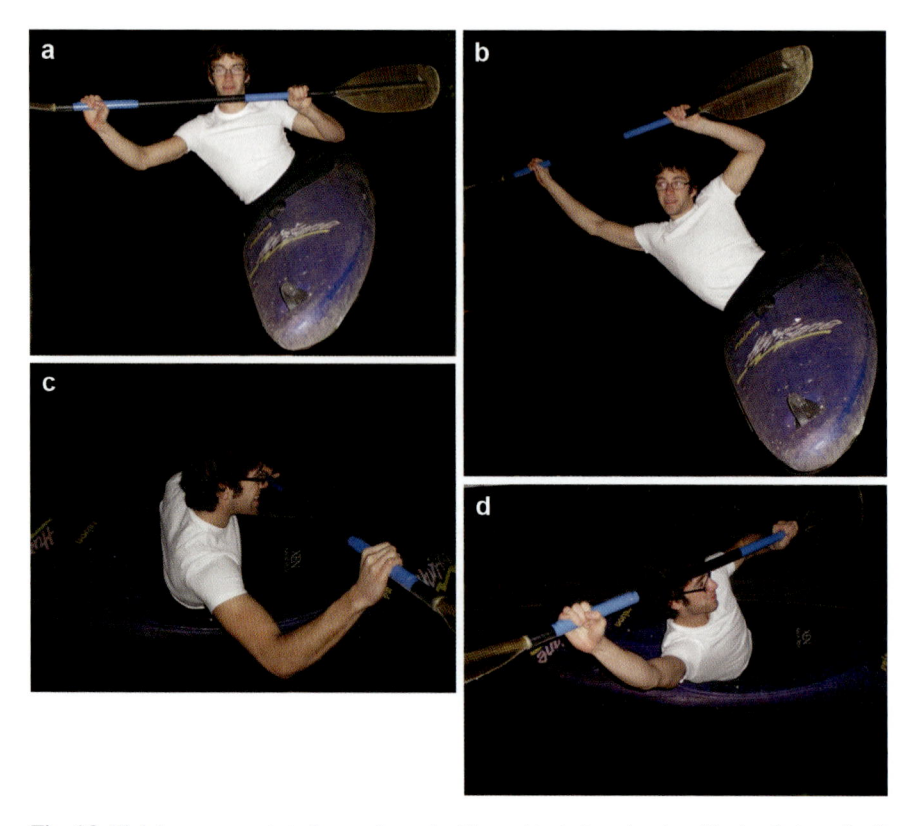

Fig. 6.8 High brace support strokes performed with good technique (**a, c**) and bad technique (**b, d**) with respect to the risk of shoulder dislocation injury. Note the highly abducted and externally rotated shoulder position (with the elbow above and behind the shoulder) indicative of bad technique. In this position the elbow is almost straight, and any force along the arm will tend to wrench to humeral head from the glenoid fossa. In addition, with the wrist behind the elbow and both behind the shoulder, there is no musculature spanning and stabilizing the front of the joint, thus leaving it prone to anterior dislocation. In contrast with good technique, the shoulder is less abducted and externally rotated (with the elbow kept below and in front of the shoulder) and the elbow is flexed

Chronic Injuries

Chronic injuries are fairly common in canoeists and kayakers, accounting for 25–40 % of all injuries [16, 41], but are less frequent in rafters (13 %) likely due to the single or occasional participation of commercial rafters. The most common types of chronic injuries among recreational canoe and kayak paddlers are "tendinitis" (44 %) and sprain/strain (27 %) [41].

Hand, Wrist, and Forearm Injuries

As the hand, wrist, and forearm channel the power developed by the paddler to the blade and water, it is unsurprising that this area is at risk of injury. All forms of

Whitewater paddling necessitate stabilization of the paddle in order to execute fine paddle control in turbulent water. Kayak paddlers are especially prone to overuse forearm and wrist injuries due to the combination of repetitive wrist flexion and extension with intense gripping.

Perhaps the best known forearm injury is tenosynovitis of the wrist extensor tendons, characterized by inflammation of the sheath lining surrounding the tendons within the dorsal aspect of the wrist/forearm (Fig. 6.9). It is an overuse injury that typically occurs in the control hand of kayakers [14], has been reported to be the most common injury in Olympic kayakers and canoeists [47], and is also common among marathon kayakers, 23 % reporting symptoms in one study [14]. Surprisingly the incidence of tenosynovitis in these events has not been related to the feather angle of the paddle, but to the surface water and wind conditions [14]. Flexor "tendinitis" is thought to be more common in single canoe paddlers who may have to "J" stroke extensively to maintain their course [5] (Fig. 6.10). Other conditions such as carpal tunnel syndrome, median nerve entrapment (due to flexor tendon hypertrophy), and tenosynovitis/tendinitis of the wrist flexor tendons (from overgripping the paddle shaft) also occur. De Quervain syndrome, a tenosynovitis of the sheath or tunnel surrounding the abductor pollicis longus and extensor pollicis, has also been reported in the literature.

Forearm exertional compartment syndrome, typically of the wrist flexors and adductors, can occur with intense paddling. It results in painful, tight, hard muscle compartments during and immediately postexercise that usually resolves within a

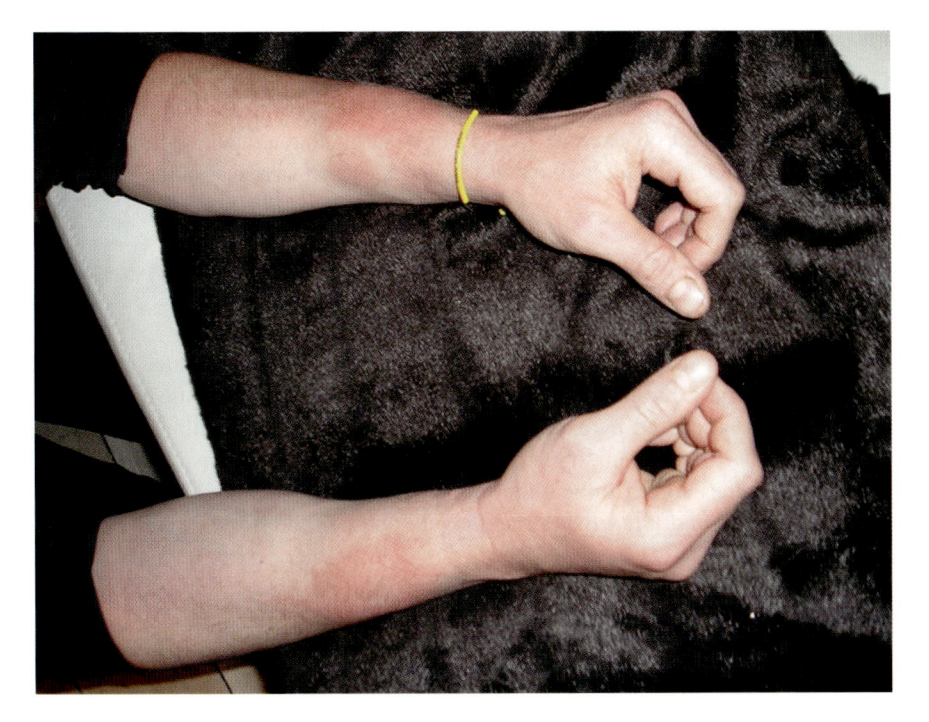

Fig. 6.9 A severe case of wrist extensor tenosynovitis following the Devizes to Westminster canoe race. Not the redness and swelling of the wrist extensor tendon, particularly of the left control hand (Picture courtesy of Mike Carmont)

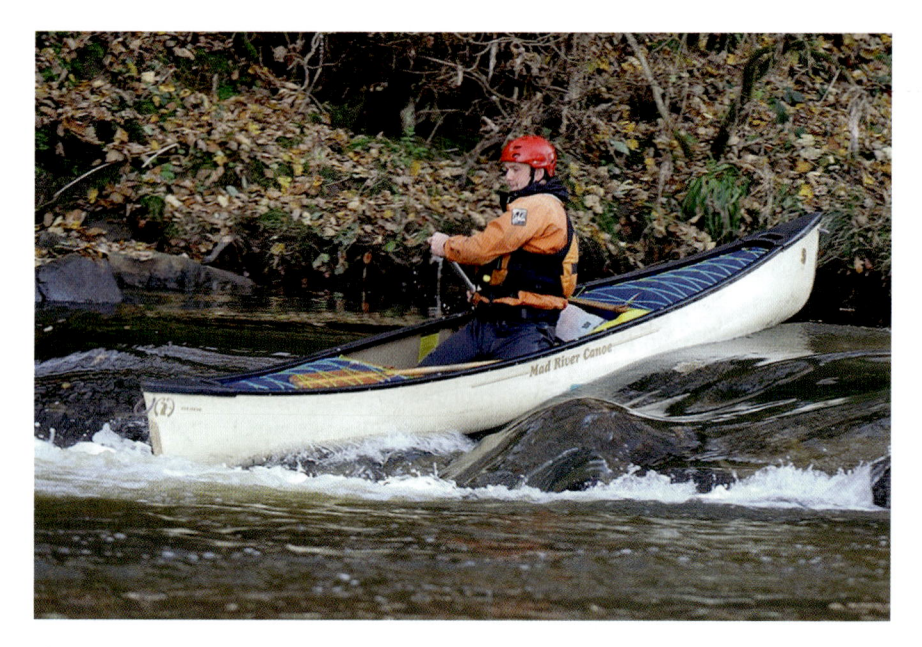

Fig. 6.10 A recreational open canoeist descending a grade II rapid (Picture courtesy of Jon Royle)

few minutes of rest. However, for some competitive paddlers this condition can recur incessantly during hard paddling limiting performance. This form of chronic exertional compartment syndrome tends to be unresponsive to conservative treatment, but can be alleviated by surgical fasciotomy that prevents the buildup of intramuscular pressure during exercise [51]. Prior to surgical treatment it is important to assess the kinetic chain and look for secondary causes of overload in the forearm.

Elbow Injuries

Tendinopathy and epicondylitis are the most common injuries to the elbow. Triceps tendinopathy can occur particularly at the distal insertion of canoeists. Medial epicondylitis can be caused by excessive wrist flexion during the pulling action and therefore tends to occur in single canoe paddlers due to repetitive "J" stroking, although this does appear to be quite rare [47]. Lateral epicondylitis is caused by repetitive extension of the wrist during the pull phase of the stroke.

Chronic Shoulder Injuries

Rotator cuff tendinopathy is caused by a multifactorial combination of environmental, intrinsic, and extrinsic factors [6, 30]. In canoe paddling impingement of the supraspinatus is a common overuse injury in the top arm due to the continually abducted and internally rotated position [5] impinging the supraspinatus tendon and subacromial bursa against the acromion and coracoacromial ligament. Similar injuries occur less frequently in kayakers as the paddle shaft is not normally placed in such a vertical position so requires less abduction at the shoulder. The exception appears to be highly experienced marathon kayakers with 42 % of a cohort of 52 complaining of shoulder pain, and 87 % of these injuries considered chronic overuse [18]. These authors associated rotator cuff injury with secondary impingement, such as the growth of acromioclavicular bony spurs impinging the supraspinatus, rather than primary impingement due to restricted subacromial space. The biceps brachii and pectoral muscles are also thought to be at particular risk of strain, but there has been little or no detailed investigation of these injuries.

Back Injuries

Due to prolonged sitting and repetitive, heavy rotational and shear loads, kayakers are prone to paraspinal fatigue and lumbosacral strain. In competitive canoeists and kayakers, predominantly flatwater paddlers, 23 % experienced low back pain, limited back movement, or numbness [25]. Among elite competitors the incidence of lower back problems has been reported similarly at 20 % [15] plus a significantly higher 52 % [25]. The detailed report of Kameyama et al. [25], which found this high incidence, also included diagnoses of spondylolysis (17 %), myofascial pain syndrome (16 %), and spondylosis deformans (13 %). Upon X-ray examination 42 of these elite flatwater paddlers (86 %) had concave vertebrae and assumed ballooning of the intervertebral disks (vs. <30 % in male athletes generally [44]), due to vertebral degeneration/stress fracture, although this typically occurred without any displacement of the disks.

A high proportion (78 %) of commercial raft guides reported back pain at some point during their guiding career, with 21 % experiencing current back pain lasting >1 week [23], which is similar incidence to the normal population (5–30 %). Only 7.4 % of these guides reported missing work because of back pain compared to 9–29 % in other industries. Excessive sagittal plane spinal curvature [21] and limited hamstrings extensibility [24] are said to predispose to back injuries in a range of sports, including canoeing and kayaking [29].

Rib Fractures

Rib fractures have been reported more in the surveys of outrigger canoe paddlers [19]. It seems likely that this is due to chronic bone stress, and evidence from rowing suggests that they tend to occur following a sudden increase in training load or a change of equipment [26, 48]. Due to their lower volumes of paddling, recreational and competitive Whitewater paddlers are less likely to develop this problem. Diagnosis is clinical but ultrasound can help identify periosteal reaction and cortical breaches. XR can be unhelpful particularly in the early stages but MRI scan can give a definitive diagnosis and show any associated muscle injury.

Pelvic and Lower Limb Injuries

Ischial tuberosity bursitis and hamstrings tendinitis have been reported in kayakers, and prolonged sitting and rotating on a hard seat provide a logical inciting mechanism. Sciatica has also been recognized as a common complaint in Olympic [47] and marathon kayakers [10]. Preliminary evidence indicates no influence of seat height on the incidence of sciatica in one study [10], but changing the shape and pressure distribution across the seat has been found to help alleviate this problem [47].

Environmental Injuries and Illnesses

Thirty-three percent of all injuries in competitive canoe/kayak paddlers were related to exposure or environmental stresses [28]. These injuries include medical complaints associated with exposure to the water (skin complaints and gastrointestinal illnesses) and extremes of temperature.

Skin

In Whitewater sports, mild skin infections are common due to prolonged contact with water or moist clothing. Folliculitis secondary to bacterial infection can occur where tight dry suits cause mild skin irritation from rubbing. Similarly, fungal infections arise in similar areas where skin is frequently moist and abraded (including groin and axillae). Most cases are self-limiting and require only regular cleaning and careful drying. However, frequent minor integumentary trauma, repeated immersion in water, and close contact with others who may also have wounds predispose regular paddlers to an increased rate of wound infections. It is not surprising that outbreaks of skin infections (e.g., *Staphylococcus aureus* [13]) have been reported in Whitewater paddlers. Otitis media and otitis externa are relatively common complaints in paddlers, with one survey reporting a 5 % frequency [39]. The problems arise due to contaminated water being driven into the ear canal where it can cause infection or canal irritation.

Hand blisters, caused by abrasion from gripping the paddle shaft, are the most common injury among Whitewater paddlers afflicting 65 % [12] and 94 % [41] of respondents in two surveys. The most common site is base of thumb. Blisters can occur in novice paddlers who have not developed calluses or in more experienced paddlers who change their paddle.

Illnesses

Gastrointestinal illness is a fairly common complaint, and water cleanliness is the main contributing factor, combined with exercise-induced lowered immunity. Surveys of competition paddlers have found 13 % of slalom paddlers [28] and 14 % of Duzi marathon competitors [2] were suffering with diarrhea. Giardiasis infection, a cause of persistent diarrhea and increased flatulence, has been reported in 14 % of paddlers [27, 49]. This protozoal infection is often self-limiting, but if persistent should be treated with antibiotics, following a stool sample to confirm diagnosis and sensitivity. High concentrations of *E. coli* and other bacteria are also likely causes of gastrointestinal distress and diarrhea [2].

Leptospirosis (Weil's disease) is a rare but important cause of illness in paddlers. It is a bacterial infection resulting from exposure to the Leptospira interrogans resulting in flu-like symptoms and a fever. While mild symptoms are quite common, only occasionally does the infection progress to become Weil's disease (~50 cases in UK annually), presenting as jaundice and hemorrhagic illness that can quickly lead to multiorgan failure, fatal in ~3 cases in the UK annually. Infection is caused by direct or indirect contact with animal urine, specifically from rodents that carry and excrete leptospires. A blood test is the only reliable diagnostic tool. Prompt treatment with antibiotics (e.g., oral doxycycline) is important to prevent deterioration.

Upper respiratory tract infections are commonly reported in all elite level sports, Whitewater kayaking being no exception. 34 % reported upper respiratory infection and 13 % sinusitis when elite paddlers were surveyed [28].

Cold/Heat Illness

If the warning signs of hypothermia (shivering, numbness of extremities followed by apathy, confusion, lethargy, and slurred speech) are recognized, then it is important to get the paddler off the water, dried, and their core warmed. Being prepared with warm drinks, blankets, and other sources of heat is vital in remote places. Heat stroke again requires the paddler being taken off the water, stripped appropriately, rehydrated, and if possible externally cooled (cold drinks, ice packs, etc.). For both conditions, recognizing the need for hospital treatment is vital.

Prevention of Accidents, Injuries, and Illness

Whitewater paddling typically takes place in a remote location with limited first aid or emergency assistance available, making the immediate management of Whitewater accidents and injuries problematic and increasing the consequences of any incident. This reinforces the need for individuals to know their limitations and have sufficient skills and physical abilities for the conditions. For all paddlers, a managed progression of relevant skills and experience is clearly important for risk mitigation.

Equipment precautions in particularly remote regions include a first aid kit and having at least one registered first-aider in the group, spare clothing, and paddle.

Whitewater Accidents

Practical prevention measures include education of paddlers on the more specific dangers such as low-head weirs/dams. A number of fatalities and near drownings have been reported when paddlers have shot apparently innocuous weirs/dam only to get caught in a hydraulic that pulls them under [1]. Where there have been a number of accidents on a particular part of a river, lowering the risk by increasing the visibility of warning notices may be practical.

Injury Reduction

Injury prevention aims to raise the resilience of the paddler and/or reduce the external stress. Well-maintained equipment, appropriate for the individual and the conditions, will reduce the stress on the paddler and therefore the risk of injury. Due to the high proportion of rafting injuries occurring while on board on the raft, reducing the number of paddlers on each raft improving the design and ergonomics of the ropes and straps may reduce injuries. In addition, considering the high proportion of facial injury in rafting (33 %), face protection may be warranted; however, increasing helmet weight also increases the risk of submersion accidents including drowning [49].

Appropriate physical capability for the paddling trip, event, or competition is important. For example, extensive training (>100 km per week) in the weeks prior to long-distance kayaking events appears to reduce the risk of tenosynovitis [14]. Furthermore, strengthening synergist and joint stabilizing tissues through strength and conditioning is recommended for paddlers at all levels and should specifically include exercises for the scapular, glenohumeral, and core stabilizers. The resilience of body regions at high risk of injury can be increased through specific strength training [38].

Competitive paddlers should undergo regular health screening including both clinical (health) and kinesiological (musculoskeletal) investigations. Potential muscle or biomechanical imbalances should be identified and addressed, as well as any preexisting medical conditions. Following assessment, where necessary a period of individualized prehabilitation can then be undertaken. Prehabilitation involves specific conditioning exercises with the aim of reducing injury risk by correcting functional weaknesses, imbalances, poor posture, or malalignment and may entail reduced paddling until weaknesses are addressed. This is particularly pertinent around the shoulder and anecdotally is reported to reduce dislocation rates in paddlers. Published studies are lacking in the literature, but prehabilitation is a widely accepted method of risk mitigation [38]. Clearly this level of support is often only available to elite level competitors. Careful monitoring of training load throughout the season with a systematic progression of intensity and volume is important for prevention of overuse injuries.

Overgripping the paddle and poor technique (excessive or unnecessary wrist flexion or extension as opposed to a neutral wrist position) are risk factors for forearm injury. These injuries may be prevented by development of the forearm musculature through specific gym training. A more flexible paddle shaft, cranked paddles, and reduced angle of feather of kayak paddles could all help with these injuries. One survey found that 13 % of respondents ($n=41$) reported decreasing the feather angle of their kayak paddles due to wrist problems, and 73 % of these felt this change had been beneficial to their wrist complaint [41].

Illness Reduction

Basics of good hand hygiene should be adopted to reduce levels of GI Tract upset. In a competitive environment, isolation of infectious cases from others helps to reduce the spread of illness. Probiotic use has been studied in the general population. Reviews have found they reduce duration of diarrheal illness and may prevent occurrence [32].

Treatment and Rehabilitation

Abrasions, Lacerations, and Contusions

For clean superficial lacerations/abrasions, cleansing, dressing, and a check of tetanus vaccination status are all that is needed. Dirtier wounds or deeper lacerations may require fluid irrigation (with >250 ml of regular saline) and scrubbing to remove debris. The dressing should be appropriate to the individual (i.e., having checked for allergies), nonadherent and should be reexamined 48-h post injury. Deeper lacerations may require wound opposition and medical treatment (e.g., stitching) and rarely surgical repair of underlying structures or further investigation of penetrating injuries. Prophylactic broad spectrum antibiotics are required for some wounds (e.g., co-amoxiclav or if penicillin allergic, a combination of doxycycline and metronidazole), particularly those over 6-h old on presentation and where there is an underlying fracture. With facial lacerations requiring treatment, chloramphenicol ointment is often applied four times daily while the wound heals.

Skin and Blisters

For skin infections topical antibiotic creams are used, and for widespread areas or severe cases, oral antibiotics. Topical antifungal creams should be applied to fungal infections, sometimes in combination with hydrocortisone to reduce itching/inflammation.

The priority with blisters is keeping them clean and free from infection, preferably by keeping the blister intact to protect the underlying skin. However, lancing and draining may be necessary if the blister is causing too much pain or if infection is suspected. Antibiotics should be used only if there are signs of infection, e.g., pus or redness. Strapping and taping of the hand may be required to alleviate the pain of continued paddling. Nonadherent and hydrocolloid dressings are most appropriate for protection and promotion of healing, but with exposure to water additional taping is required.

Fractures

Standard principles of fracture treatment should be applied. Assessment of neurovascular status distal to the suspected fracture site determines the urgency of treatment and whether manipulation is required prior to onward transfer to hospital. Altered sensation, loss of pulse, and skin tenting all require more urgent treatment, prehospital if possible. Immobilization to reduce pain and prevent displacement is a priority, as is analgesia. Further management is then determined by appearance on X-ray. Surgical reduction ± fixation may be required. Following immobilization, if possible, the site should be elevated to reduce swelling.

Depending on the fracture, fitness and function may be maintained with dryland training. Once movement is allowed, gentle range of motion work is started immediately followed by a progressive low-level strengthening program. To return to the water, an individual must have full pain-free range of motion and minimal strength deficit. They would then follow the flow chart in Fig. 6.11.

Rib fractures are initially treated with relative rest and avoidance of pain-provoking activity. Analgesia is used if the pain is severe, avoiding NSAIDs due to their potential to interfere with bone healing. Physiotherapy to aid normal breathing patterns and strapping to provide some support can be helpful for pain relief. Addressing the cause of overload is important – both during paddling and other activities, e.g., strength and conditioning. In competitive paddlers training within pain limits is allowed as this does not seem to impair the healing process [46].

Shoulder Dislocation

The priority when a dislocation occurs is getting the individual off the water, to prevent further injury while they are incapacitated. Support for the shoulder and analgesia in the form of Entonox help alleviate some of the distress. Initial treatment involves reduction of the dislocation as soon as possible to minimize stretching of the capsule and other soft tissues. However, presence of other injuries and neurovascular

6 Whitewater Canoeing and Rafting

```
Initial phase:
NO PADDLING
Consider cross training to maintain aerobic/anaerobic
and cardiovascular fitness as required.
Consider continuing strength training for unaffected
body areas.
```

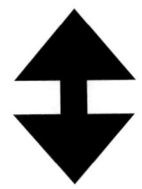

⇕

```
Return to flatwater:
Water with little or no flow.
Initial light pressure through paddle, straight lines,
minimal turns.
Increase in power through strocke, straight lines,
Re-introduce turning skills
Next step is the above on moving flatwater.
```

⇕

```
Return to whitewater
Initial work in straight lines.
Build back in direction changes/turns in slower
moving sections building back to faster water.
Re-introduce upstream paddling and work on
manoevres needing specific attention due to nature of
injury.
```

Fig. 6.11 Progression of rehabilitation toward whitewater paddling following injury

compromise should be ascertained first as these could be exacerbated by attempts at reduction. Any evidence of impaired distal circulation or neurological function would prompt the need for urgent treatment. Whether reduction is done prehospital versus hospital should be decided on a case-by-case basis and may well be easier in a recurrently dislocated joint than a first-time dislocation of a paddler with well-developed musculature, although Hill–Sachs lesions on the humeral head of recurrent dislocators may complicate reduction. If reduction is done in the prehospital setting, an X-ray is needed to ensure correct relocation. In hospital, it is a common practice to use a combination of benzodiazepines and/or intravenous opiates to aid muscle relaxation prior to reduction. There are a number of different reduction techniques, but their success depends on relaxation of the patient and experience of the medical personnel. In the acute situation if relocation fails, then surgical treatment, specifically reduction under general anesthetic, will be required. Primary surgical repair of the soft tissues after reduction has undergone a Cochrane Review [20] that supported primary surgical repair for young, active males, although the best method of repair has not been identified. After surgical repair the recurrence rate is still higher than the general population, although significantly lower than when treated conservatively [20]. Depending on the mechanics of the injury, shoulder dislocation is often accompanied by soft tissue damage such as Bankart lesions (both anterior capsule and labrum are separated from glenoid rim), Hill–Sachs lesions (humeral head compression fracture), and subscapularis dysfunction. Surgical treatment for these injuries aims to repair the disrupted anatomy and may also strengthen/tighten other structures to improve stability.

Immobilization in a brace or a sling with a strap to prevent external rotation or abduction is applied for 3–4 weeks. An example of a standard rehabilitation protocol is gentle elbow range of motion exercises while in the sling, plus (pain allowing) gentle passive pendulum exercises. When out of the sling, active assisted range of motion and low-level strengthening exercises are done but with abduction limited to <90° and external rotation to <30°. At 6 weeks post injury, movement restriction is lifted, and rehabilitation focuses on strengthening. (Please refer also to Chap. 17.)

Muscular Strains

Treatment for muscle strains is conservative for the majority of injuries. Conservative management follows the usual soft tissue injury principles with use of ice over the affected muscle and rest from pain-provoking activity. Compression and elevation are not as relevant in the trunk, but pain can be reduced with supportive taping. Analgesia is appropriate only if the pain causes dysfunctional movement patterns and may help to reduce any associated spasm in surrounding muscles. Analgesics should be stopped prior to the return to activity so pain is not masked. Nonsteroidal anti-inflammatory drugs (NSAIDs) would not be the first choice as there is no evidence that they improve outcome and may have detrimental affects; paracetamol could be considered as it has the analgesic effect without the theoretical increase in leukotriene production leading to tissue damage [37]. Where possible, early phase physiotherapy should focus on maintenance of movement to prevent capsular adhesions and stiffness in the joint. This involves gentle flexibility and strengthening movements before progressing to a greater range of motion and increasingly forceful exercises. Common sites of acute muscle strain in paddlers include the lower back and shoulder. For lower back strains, rehabilitation should focus on improving activation and strength of the core-stabilizing muscles to reduce future recurrence. Shoulder injuries may be related to shortened tight pectoral muscles that result in a protracted shoulder girdle and thoracic spine kyphosis and thus poor posture. It is important to address these issues with postural reeducation and scapular setting exercises.

Chronic Shoulder Injury

On early presentation, treatment for rotator cuff tendinopathy involves rest from provocative activities, NSAIDs, and gentle range of motion exercises with flexibility work to maintain shoulder movement and to begin lengthening tight muscle groups. If pain is persistent, then injection under ultrasound guidance is sometimes needed to reduce pain and facilitate physiotherapy. Substances injected range from corticosteroids to hyaluronic acid derivatives and platelet-rich plasma (PRP). Corticosteroid injections have been shown to improve pain in the short-term but not longer term. In younger age groups, hyaluronic acid derivatives have been used for their anti-inflammatory properties and better side effect profile [40]. Surgical treatment is only considered for those who fail conservative treatment. Subacromial decompression involving bursectomy, acromioplasty, and coracoacromial ligament release is one of the more common procedures undertaken in the general population. In athletes it is not the treatment of choice as it may compromise function, and in these cases aggressive conservative treatment or a stabilization procedure is more appropriate. Rehabilitation involves correcting the common postural problems that are considered an important intrinsic risk factor, scapular setting, and rotator cuff strengthening.

Elbow, Wrist, and Forearm Tendinopathies

Treatment as with the other tendinopathies involves rest from provoking activities, RICE principles with an emphasis on cryotherapy, as well as NSAIDs in the acute phase. Rehabilitation involves flexibility work, range of motion exercises followed by strengthening (with emphasis on eccentric contractions), with a focus on functional positions. Assessing the kinetic chain with correction of imbalances around the shoulder girdle is recommended. Treatment should also encompass a holistic assessment of technique, training loads, and equipment (e.g., paddle length, type of shaft, and feather angle).

A range of other medical treatments have also been used with some success. Injection of a mixture of local anesthetic and corticosteroid has been found to promote significant short-term improvements, but no long-term benefits over physiotherapy [43]. Injections of autologous blood and platelet-rich plasma (PRP) have a growing evidence base [12, 33], with some studies showing improvements in pain and function scores with PRP being advocated as superior [17, 45]. Glyceryl trinitrate (GTN) patches have also been used (off-license) in extensor tendinosis to provide nitric oxide that has been postulated to modulate tendon healing and found to produce better outcome for pain and function scores than a placebo [36]. In contrast, topical nonsteroidal anti-inflammatory gels do not seem to alleviate the symptoms or pain of wrist extensor tenosynovitis during multiple-day long-distance kayaking events [31]. Surgery is now only rarely undertaken for recalcitrant cases of tendinopathy. For extensor tendinopathy, degenerative tissue within the extensor carpi radialis brevis tendon is excised along with the release of the tendon from the lateral epicondyle. Percutaneous as opposed to an open procedure has reported faster return to activity.

Gastrointestinal Illness

Treatment is symptomatic, ensuring adequate oral hydration. Switching to food that requires less digestion, such as the BRAT diet (Bananas, Rice, Applesauce, and Toast – plain with no spreads or sauces), can speed recovery once vomiting settles. Antidiarrheals can often cause more abdominal symptoms, and their anticholinergic actions can cause a dry mouth and reduce sweating, increasing the risk of heat illness in warmer climates. Further investigations are only necessary when symptoms are prolonged or if diarrhea is bloody. When oral rehydration is failing, intravenous fluids should be administered in a hospital setting. In elite paddlers subject to doping legislation, this requires therapeutic use exemption within competition.

Summary

The majority of injuries in canoeists and kayakers involve the upper limb, while rafters also suffer from facial and lower limb injuries. The majority of Whitewater injuries are of an acute traumatic nature, and the most common acute injuries are sprains, strains, tendonitis, lacerations, and contusions. Shoulder dislocation is a common severe injury in canoe and kayak paddlers, and preemptive shoulder strengthening exercises and a greater awareness of good technique are strongly recommended. Initial treatment involves reduction of the dislocation as soon as possible, and following a full dislocations, primary surgical repair appears to reduce recurrence compared to conservative treatment. "Tendinitis" and sprain/strain are the most common types of chronic injuries, with the wrist and forearm, and the lower back being the most common sites of these injuries. Overgripping the paddle, poor technique, and suboptimal equipment may all contribute to wrist and forearm complaints. Environmental injuries and illnesses are common in paddlers and encompass skin complaints, gastrointestinal disturbance, and extremes of body temperature.

References

1. American Whitewater Accident Database. Available at: http://www.americanwhitewater.org/content/Accident/view/ Accessed Sep 2012.
2. Appleton CC, Bailey IW. Canoeists and waterborne diseases in South Africa. S Afr Med J. 1989;78:323–6.
3. Baker S. The 'ultimate' waterfall. Canoeist. 1990 Jan:51.
4. Baker S, Atha J. Canoeists' disorientation following cold immersion. Br J Sports Med. 1981;15:111–5.
5. Berglund B, McKenzie D. Injuries in canoeing and kayaking. In: Renstrom PAFH, editor. Clinical sports medicine. Oxford: Blackwell Scientific Publications; 1994. p. 633–40.
6. Bigliani L, Levine W. Current concepts review: subacromial impingement syndrome. J Bone Joint Surg. 1997;79-A:1854–67.
7. Bureau of Land Management and Colorado State Parks. Arkansas headwaters recreation area end of the season report 1997. Boulder: Bureau of Land Management and Colorado State Parks; 1998.
8. Burrell CL, Burrell R. Injuries in whitewater paddling. Phys Sportsmed. 1982;10:119–24.
9. California Department of Navigation and Ocean Development. Whitewater fatalities (rivers only). Sacramento: California Department of Navigation and Ocean Development; 1973. p. 1973–4.
10. Carmont MR, Baruch MR, Burnett C, Cairns P, Harrison JWK. Injuries sustained during marathon kayak competition: the Devizes to Westminster race. Br J Sports Med. 2004;38:650.
11. Centre for Disease Control. Paddle sport fatalities. Maine 2000–2007. MMWR Morb Mortal Wkly Rep. 2008;16:524–7.
12. Connell DA, Ali KE, Ahmad M, Lambert S, Corbett S, Curtis M. Ultrasound-guided autologous blood injection for tennis elbow. Skeletal Radiol. 2006;35:371–7.
13. Decker MD, Lybarger JA, Vaughn WK, Hutcheson Jr RH, Schaffner W. An outbreak of staphylococcal skin infections among river rafting guides. Am J Epidemiol. 1986;124:969–76.
14. Du Toit P, Sole G, Bowerbank P, Noakes TD. Incidence and causes of tenosynovitis of the wrist extensors in long distance paddle canoeists. Br J Sports Med. 1999;33(2):105–9.
15. Edwards A. Injuries in kayaking. Sports Health. 1993;11:8–11.
16. Fiore DC, Houston JD. Injuries in whitewater kayaking. Br J Sports Med. 2001;35(4):235–41.
17. Gosens T, Peerbooms JC, van Laar W, den Oudsten BL. Ongoing positive effect of platelet-rich plasma versus corticosteroid injection in lateral epicondylitis: a double-blind randomized controlled trial with 2-year follow-up. Am J Sports Med. 2011;39:1200–8.
18. Hagemann G, Rijke AM, Mars M. Shoulder pathoanatomy in marathon kayakers. Br J Sports Med. 2004;38:413–7.
19. Haley A, Nichols A. A survey of injuries and medical conditions affecting competitive outrigger canoe paddlers on O'ahu. Hawaii Med J. 2009;68:162–5.
20. Handoll HH, Almaiyah MA, Rangan A. Surgical versus non-surgical treatment for acute anterior shoulder dislocation. Cochrane Database Syst Rev. 2004;CD004325.
21. Harrison DE, Colloca CJ, Harrison DD, Janik TJ, Haas JW, Keller TS. Anterior thoracic posture increases thoracolumbar disc loading. Eur Spine J. 2005;14:234–42.
22. Hartung HG, Goebert DA. Watersports injuries. In: Caine D, Caine C, Koenraad L, editors. Epidemiology of sports injuries. Champaign: Human Kinetics Publishers; 1996. p. 29–39.

23. Jackson DM, Verscheure SK. Back pain in whitewater rafting guides. Wilderness Environ Med. 2006;17(3):162–70.
24. Jones MA, Stratton G, Reilly T, Unnithan VB. Biological risk indicators for recurrent non-specific low back pain in adolescents. Br J Sports Med. 2005;39:137–40.
25. Kameyama O, Shibano K, Kawakita H, Ogawa R, Kumamoto M. Medical check of competitive canoeists. J Orthop Sci. 1999;4:243–9.
26. Karlson K. Rib stress fractures in elite rowers. A case series and proposed mechanism. Am J Sports Med. 1998;26:516–9.
27. Kizer KW. Medical problems in whitewater sports. Clin Sports Med. 1987;6(3):663–8.
28. Krupnick JE, Cox RD, Summers RL. Injuries sustained during competitive Whitewater paddling: a survey of athletes in the 1996 Olympic trials. Wilderness Environ Med. 1998;9(1):14–8.
29. Lopez-Minarro PA, Alacid F, Rodriguez-Garcia PL. Comparison of sagittal spinal curvatures and hamstrings muscle extensibility among elite young paddlers and non-athletes. Int Sports Med J. 2010;11:301–2.
30. Lyons P, Orwin J. Rotator cuff tendinopathy and subacromial impingement syndrome. Med Sci Sports Exerc. 1998;30:S12–7.
31. May JJ, Lovell G, Hopkins WG. Effectiveness of 1 % diclofenac gel in the treatment of wrist extensor tenosynovitis in long distance kayakers. J Sci Med Sport. 2007;10:59–65.
32. Marteau P, Seksik P, Jian R. Probiotics and intestinal health effects: a clinical perspective. Br J Nutr. 2002;88:S51–7.
33. Mishra A, Pavelkro T. Treatment of chronic elbow tendinosis with buffered platelet rich plasma. Am J Sports Med. 2006;34:1774–8.
34. Nathanson AT, Reinert SE. Windsurfing injuries: results of a paper- and internet-based survey. Wilderness Environ Med. 1999;10:218–25.
35. Outdoor Industry Association. Outdoor recreation participation study for the United States. 3rd ed. Boulder: Outdoor Industry Association; 2000.
36. Paoloni JA, Appleyard RC, Nelson J, Murrell GA. Topical nitric oxide application in the treatment of chronic extensor tendinosis at the elbow; a randomised, double-blinded, placebo-controlled clinical trial. Am J Sports Med. 2003;31:915–20.
37. Paoloni J, Orchard J. The use of therapeutic medications for soft-tissue injuries in sports medicine. MJA Pract Essent. 2005;183:384–8.
38. Pearce PZ. Prehabilitation: preparing young athletes for sports. Curr Sports Med Rep. 2006;5:155–60.
39. Powell C. Injuries and medical conditions among kayakers paddling in the sea environment. Wilderness Environ Med. 2009;20:327–34.
40. Saito S, Furuya T, Kotake S. Therapeutic effects of hyaluronate injections in patients with chronic painful shoulder: a meta-analysis of randomized controlled trials. Arthritis Care Res. 2010;62:1009–18.
41. Schoen RG, Stano MJ. Year 2000 whitewater injury survey. Wilderness Environ Med. 2002;13(2):119–24.
42. Shlim D, Houston R. Helicopter rescues and deaths among trekkers in Nepal. JAMA. 1989;261:1017–9.
43. Smidt N, van der Windt DA, Assendelft WJ, Devillé WL, Korthals-de Bos IB, Bouter LM. Corticosteroid injections, physiotherapy, or a wait-and-see policy for lateral epicondylitis: a randomised controlled trial. Lancet. 2002;359:657–62.
44. Suyama T, Tobimatsu Y, Nihei R. Radiological study of athlete's lumbar spine. J Clin Sports Med. 1987;4:125–8.
45. Thanasas C, Papadimitriou G, Charalambidis C, Paraskevopoulos I, Papanikolaou A. Platelet-rich plasma versus autologous whole blood for the treatment of chronic lateral elbow epicondylitis: a randomized controlled clinical trial. Am J Sports Med. 2011;39:2130–4.
46. Wajswelner H. Management of rowers with rib stress fractures. Aust J Physiother. 1996;42:157–61.

47. Walsh M. Preventing injury in competitive canoeists. Phys Sportsmed. 1985;13:120–8.
48. Warden S, Gutschlag FR, Wajswelner H, Crossley KM. Aetiology of rib stress fractures in rowers. Sports Med. 2002;32:819–36.
49. Whisman SA, Hollenhurst SJ. Injuries in commercial whitewater rafting. Clin J Sports Med. 1999;9:18–23.
50. Wittman L. Kayaking is safer than you think (really!). Am Whitewater. 2000;2000:100–1.
51. Wittstein J, Moorman 3rd CT, Levin LS. Endoscopic compartment release for chronic exertional compartment syndrome. J Surg Orthop Adv. 2008;17:119–21.

Chapter 7
Surfing Injuries

Andrew T. Nathanson

Contents

Surfing: The Sport of Kings – History	143
Demographics	145
Surfing Equipment	147
Surfing, SUP, and Tow-In	147
Bodyboarding and Bodysurfing	147
Wetsuits	148
Injury Rates and Risk Factors	148
Surfing Fatalities	149
Acute Surfing Injuries	149
Acute Injuries and Their Anatomic Distribution	149
Mechanisms of Injury	151
Overuse Injuries	161
Neck and Back Pain	162
Upper Extremity Pain	164
Environmental Injuries	165
Skin, Eyes, and Ears	165
Hazardous Marine Life	166
Wound Care	168
Injury Prevention	169
Basic Safety Recommendations	169
Equipment	169
Personal Protective Gear	170
References	170

Surfing: The Sport of Kings – History

Surfing is perhaps the oldest "extreme sport" in existence, and though its precise origins are unknown, most authorities agree that the sport originated in Polynesia

---

A.T. Nathanson, M.D., FACEP
Department of Emergency Medicine, Alpert School of Medicine at Brown University,
Injury Prevention Center, Rhode Island Hospital,
593 Eddy St., Claverick 2, Providence, RI 02903, USA
e-mail: anathanson@lifespan.org

over 800 years ago. The first written accounts of surfing appear in the journals of English explorer Captain James Cook, who witnessed Tahitians bodysurfing and riding waves in outrigger canoes in 1777 and a year later saw surfers riding waves while standing atop long wooden surfboards in Hawaii. Before the arrival of Westerners to Polynesia, surfing was an important cultural and recreational activity, particularly in the Hawaiian Islands where the chiefs maintained exclusive rights to the best surf breaks while commoners surfed elsewhere. By the early nineteenth century, the sport fell into a rapid decline under the influence of Western missionaries who discouraged surfing as a frivolous pastime [1].

Surfing's revival is widely credited to the charismatic Hawaiian waterman and Olympic swimming champion "Duke" Kahanamoku who introduced the sport to California and Australia in the 1910s. Commercialization of the surfing lifestyle through movies and music in the early 1960s led to rapid growth of the sport along both coasts of the United States and Australia and a gradual spread into Western Europe, Japan, Brazil, and Peru. During this era, the introduction of lighter foam-core fiberglass surfboards and neoprene wetsuits catapulted expansion of the sport beyond a small cadre of rugged individualists and into the mainstream [1].

The 1970s witnessed a revolution in surfboard design, with boards getting ever shorter, lighter, and more maneuverable. Shorter boards led to a new style of surfing which featured aggressive, carving, short-radius turns up and down the face of the wave, in contrast to the straight-line trimming and nose-riding of the past. These boards encouraged surfers to ride steeper, more tubular-shaped waves and allowed the surfer to generate speed along the length of fast-peeling waves. By the mid-1980s, surfers began experimenting with airborne maneuvers above the lip of the wave. A few years later, eleven-time world champion Kelly Slater began routinely landing aerials, giving him a competitive edge in surf contests.

Interest in big-wave surfing, which first developed along Hawaii's North Shore in the 1950s, was rekindled in the late 1980s as surfers ventured out to previously unridden surf breaks such as Maverick's (California), Dungeons (South Africa), and Killers (Todos Santos Island, Mexico) where waves over 10 m in height could be ridden given the right conditions. Catching these swiftly moving mountains of water required fast-paddling, long, tapered surfboards which tended to lack maneuverability and could become dangerously airborne during takeoff due to their large surface area. Though surfers were eager to push the size envelope, there were a few breaks such as Jaws (Maui) that on rare occasion produced even larger, faster-moving, gargantuan-sized surf. These waves appeared to be moving too fast to be caught by conventional means; no matter how daring, it seemed as if a paddling surfer could not generate the speed required to catch these behemoths.

Just when it seemed as if the upper limits of wave size had been reached, Laird Hamilton and others perfected the technique of using personal watercraft (PWC) to tow one another into yet larger waves in the 15+ meter range. Getting slung into waves from a PWC's towrope had a number of distinct advantages. It allowed surfers to ride less buoyant, faster, more maneuverable boards and to drop into the wave early and in optimum position. A system was devised whereby the driver scoots into the white water at the end of the fallen surfer's ride to pull him out of harm's way using a rescue sled affixed to the stern of the PWC to aid in the retrieval process [1].

Though the conventional wisdom of "too big to paddle into" has been recently challenged, and some consider tow-in surfing a bastardization of the sport of kings, this variation of surfing caught on among many big-wave aficionados. Waves nearly 30 m in height have been successfully ridden by tow-in surfers at Cortez Bank, an underwater seamount 160 km off the shore of the California coast.

Stand-up paddle surfing (SUP), which involves standing on a wider, thicker surfboard using a long, single-bladed paddle for propulsion, began to catch on around 2005. SUP's appeal is that it is an excellent full-body workout that can be practiced on any body of water (river, lake, bay, ocean) and is relatively easy to learn. The paddling advantage afforded by a long paddle and the length and stability of the board make catching waves in the surf relatively easy, and the upright stance affords the rider an improved vantage point for spotting incoming swells. SUP has broadened surfing's playing fields and is currently the fastest-growing segment of the sport.

While surfing has always been primarily a recreational pursuit, early Hawaiian chants recount tales of surf contests held between chiefs where the victor would win floral wreaths, land, and other valuables. The 1960s surf boom led to a revival of surf contests with national contests being held in the USA and Australia in the early parts of that decade followed by international contests in the latter part of the decade. Professional contests sprouting up in the early 1970s and a world tour (currently the Association of Surfing Professionals [ASP]) followed shortly thereafter.

Most surfing contests are organized into 20- to 40-min heats of two to four surfers, scored by a panel of judges. The current ASP judging criteria look for the following elements when scoring a surfer's ride: "commitment and degree of difficulty; innovative and progressive maneuvers; combination of major maneuvers; variety of maneuvers; speed, power and flow." The sum of each surfer's top three rides is tallied, and the surfer(s) with the highest score advances into the next round until reaching the final. Currently, there are 65 ASP contests for men and 23 for women held in 6 continents. The top-tier ASP World Tour has 11 events taking place in Australia, South Africa, Brazil, Europe, mainland USA, Hawaii, and Tahiti with a total combined purse of US$9.3 million [2] (Fig. 7.1a, b).

Demographics

Estimates as to the number of surfers worldwide vary greatly. In 2002, Surfing Australia estimated that there were 17 million people who had surfed at least once in the last year, and in 2006 the International Surfing Association put that number at 23 million [3]. A survey by the Outdoor Foundation in 2009 estimated that 2.4 million people in the USA surfed at least once in the last year, with an average of 22

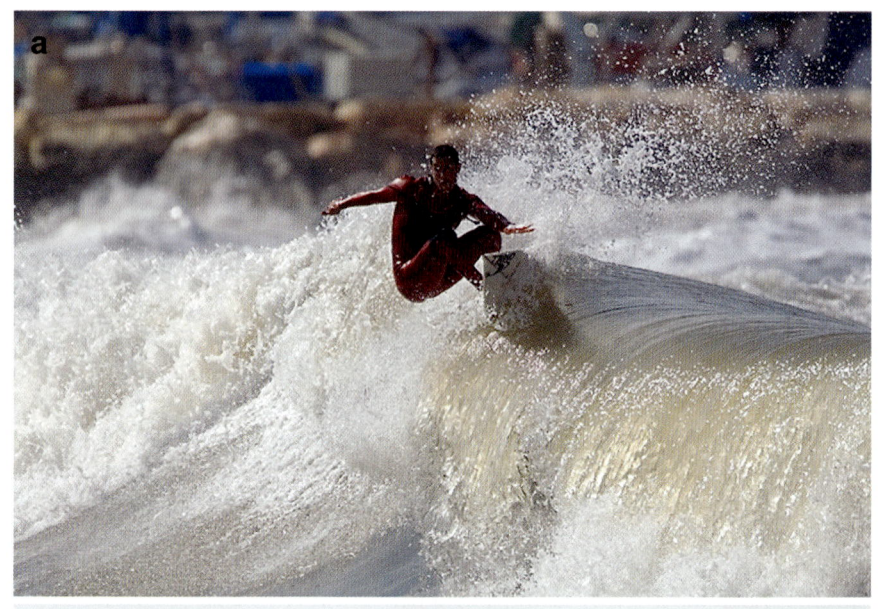

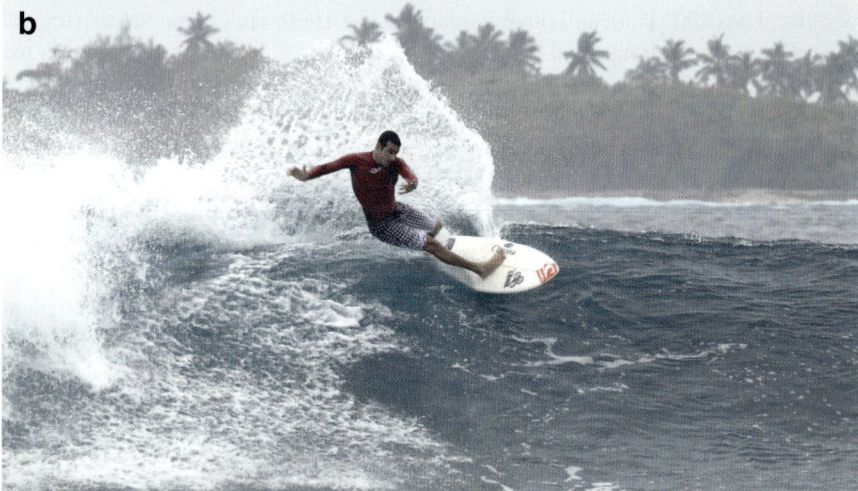

Fig. 7.1 (**a**) A floater is a maneuver where the surfer rides the breaking wave on top of it. Tel-Aviv beach. Surfer: Adi Gluska, (Photo: Roger Sharp). (**b**) A surfer uses a "cut-back" maneuver to get back to the lip of the wave, where most of its energy is concentrated. The Maldives Islands. Surfer: Adi Gluska, (Photo: Navi)

outings per year per surfer. They also found that 23 % were first-time participants, suggesting a continuing high growth rate [4].

Approximately 10 % of surfers are women, and it appears that the average age of surfers in the USA has been increasing over the last decade from the late 20s in 2000 to the mid-30s in 2009 [5, 6].

Surfing Equipment

Surfing, SUP, and Tow-In

Part of surfing's beauty lies in its simplicity. The only necessities are a board and a bathing suit, and the waves are free of charge. Though surfboards vary greatly in size and shape depending on the surfer's weight, ability, and riding style, the basic design and construction of most boards is similar; a foam "blank" is cut to shape and then sheathed in a fiberglass skin to create a lightweight but rigid structure. Polyurethane blanks are strengthened by a longitudinal, glued-in wooden stringer and covered with fiberglass which is saturated with polyester resin, while a more modern technique utilizes a polystyrene foam core and fiberglass saturated with a more durable epoxy resin. Anywhere from one to five fins (skegs) are placed at the tail end of the bottom of the board to give directional stability. The board's deck is coated with nonskid wax or foam pad to provide traction.

Most surfers utilize a leash (tether, leg rope) to prevent their board from being swept shoreward by the waves after a wipeout, thus averting a potentially long swim back to shore. Leashes are made of a thin flexible urethane cord affixed to the tail end of the surfboard's deck at one end and to the rider's ankle via a Velcro strap on the other.

The vast array of surfboard designs can be broken down into four broad categories: longboards, shortboards, SUP boards, and tow-in boards. The overall size (>2.5 M) of longboards makes them relatively stable and efficient to paddle. These characteristics make it easier to catch and ride waves, so these boards are well suited to beginners and favor a graceful, fluid riding style. Shortboards (<2.2 M) are much more maneuverable than longboards and are better suited for steeper, faster breaking waves. SUP boards are thicker, wider, and usually longer than longboards and provide a stable platform on which to stand. SUP boards designed for flat water paddling and racing are up to 5 m in length and relatively narrow, whereas those designed for riding waves tend to be shorter and wider. The single-bladed paddles used to propel an SUP board have a shaft that is approximately shoulder height and are made from rigid, lightweight materials such as carbon fiber. Lastly, tow-in boards, like water skis, are narrow, roughly 2 m in length, and equipped with foot straps so the rider can maintain control when going over chop at high speeds. These boards are heavily built to withstand the forces of the huge waves in which they are ridden and often weighted to prevent them from becoming airborne.

Bodyboarding and Bodysurfing

Bodyboards are used to ride waves in a prone position, with the rider wearing swim fins to aid in propulsion. These short (1.2 m), light, relatively inexpensive boards are made of closed-cell foam and lack fins, so collisions with one's board are relatively harmless. Riding waves is easier than on a surfboard because the rider need not hop up into a standing position, so they are favored by beginners and young children. That being said, there is a cadre of hard-charging expert bodyboarders who ride some of the most technically challenging waves in the world.

Bodysurfing is perhaps the purest and likely the oldest form of surfing. When a meter or so in front of a breaking wave, the bodysurfer swims rapidly shoreward (aided by a short pair of swim fins) and utilizes their elongated body as a planing surface to ride the wave. Experienced bodysurfers extend an arm overhead to create a longer planing surface and increase speed and control.

Wetsuits

Modern neoprene wetsuits are remarkably lightweight, warm, and flexible. They vary in thickness and body coverage according to the water temperature in which they are intended to be used. Advances in wetsuit technology have allowed surfing to be a year-round sport and have expanded the sport's range to include Canada, Northern Europe, as well as the extreme southern latitudes.

In tropical climates, surfers often forgo a wetsuit in favor of a thin nylon "rash guard" which protects against chafe between board and rider and also functions as a sunblock. At the other end of the temperature spectrum, a full-body, hooded, 5–6-mm thick wetsuit, combined with neoprene booties and gloves, can keep a surfer warm for well over an hour in seawater approaching the freezing point. Wetsuits heated by means of a battery pack are now commercially available.

Injury Rates and Risk Factors

Despite its reputation as a dangerous activity, surfing has been found to be relatively safe as compared to more traditional sports. Lowdon's 1983 mail administered survey-based study of self-reported injuries among members of an Australian surfing club found 3.5 "moderate to severe" injuries (those that resulted in lost days of surfing or required medical care) per 1,000 surfing days [7]. More recently, Taylor's 2004 interviewer-administered survey found an injury rate of 2.2 significant injuries per 1,000 surfing days among a convenience sample of surfers at beaches in Victoria, Australia [8].

Lowdon's 1982 interviewer-administered survey of 79 professional surfers found the rate of moderate to severe injuries during practice or competition in that group to be 4 per 1,000 surfing days. He concluded that surfing was safer than professional rugby (55 injuries per 1,000 days), downhill skiing (6 injuries per 1,000 days), and American high school football (5.9 injuries per day) but riskier than men's gymnastics (1.8 injuries per 1,000 days) [9]. Over the period 1999–2005, Nathanson et al. prospectively studied acute injuries sustained at 32 professional and amateur surfing contests worldwide. His group found that the rate of "significant injury" (those that resulted in lost days of competition or required acute medical care) was 6.6 per 1,000 hours of competition. This injury rate compares favorably to those found from studies of American collegiate football (33 per 1,000 hours), soccer (18 per 1,000 hours), and basketball (9 per 1,000 hours) in which similar methods of data collection and definition of injury were used [10].

A logistic regression analysis of Nathanson's data revealed that the relative risk of injury among contest surfers was greater when surfing in wave heights that were overhead or bigger relative to smaller waves (odds ratio 2.4), and that risk of injury was increased when surfing over a rock or reef bottom as compared to a sand bottom (odds ratio 2.6). In a study whose population were predominantly recreational surfers responding to a web-based survey, Nathanson found that the odds-ratios for significant injuries increased with age as well as with self-rated ability, and that there was no difference in injury rates between male and female surfers [10, 11].

Surfing Fatalities

The fatality rate for surfing is unknown. The Hawaii Department of Injury Prevention and Control reviewed the autopsy reports of 306 drowning deaths in the state of Hawaii from 1993 to 1997 and found that bodyboarders and surfers accounted for 17 of 238 ocean-related drownings [12]. During this 5-year period, there were also two fatal shark attacks on surfers. Though surfing is hugely popular in Hawaii year round, there are no reliable estimates of the number of surfers in the state.

An unpublished review of newspaper reports (by this author) searching the Nexus/Lexus database from 1984 to 1998 using the key words "surfer," "surfing," "death," "drowning," and "fatality" found accounts of 95 surfing-related fatalities in which cause of death was reported (though not confirmed). Drowning was stated to be the cause of death in 63 cases. Factors reported to be contributing to these drownings were concussions (11), seizures (4), and leash entanglement (4). Shark attacks were responsible for 12 deaths, lightning strikes for 8, and lacerations from surfboard fins for 2 others.

Acute Surfing Injuries

Acute Injuries and Their Anatomic Distribution

Outpatient studies of surfing-related injuries have found lacerations to be the most common, accounting for 35–46 % of all injuries, followed by sprains and strains, contusions, fractures, and joint dislocations (Table 7.1). Those same studies found the head and lower extremities to be the most commonly injured regions of the

Table 7.1 Acute and chronic surfing-related injuries from outpatient studies

Study	Nathanson [10]	Taylor [8]	Nathanson [11]	Lowdon [9]	Lowdon [7]
Population	Prospective study of surfers in competition	Convenience sample interviewed at beaches in Victoria, Australia	Web-based survey of English-speaking surfers	Survey of International Competitors	Members of Australian Surfing Assoc., Victoria, AU
Average age (SD)	24 (7)	28 (7.9)	29 (10.6)	22 (3.7)	22 (5.7)
Male gender	87 %	90 %	90 %	89 %	95 %
Average #'s of years surfing	Unknown	12	11	11 (5 days per week)	8 (2.7 days per week)
# of acute injuries	116	168	1,237	167	311
Type of acute injury					
Laceration/abrasion	35 %	46 %	42 %	45 %	44 %
Sprains/strains	39 %	29 %	12 %	37 %	29 %
Contusions	9 %	0	13 %	5 %	4 %
Fractures	5 %	9 %	8 %	10 %	16 %
Dislocations	4 %	11 %	2 %	2 %	1 %
Other[a]	9 %	5 %	23 %	1 %	6 %
# Chronic/overuse injuries	Unknown	71	477	20	26

[a]Includes tympanic membrane rupture, tooth fracture/avulsion, concussion, hypothermia, and near drowning

7 Surfing Injuries

Fig. 7.2 Distribution of 572 self-reported surfing-related fractures and lacerations (Photo: Adapted from Nathanson et al. [11])

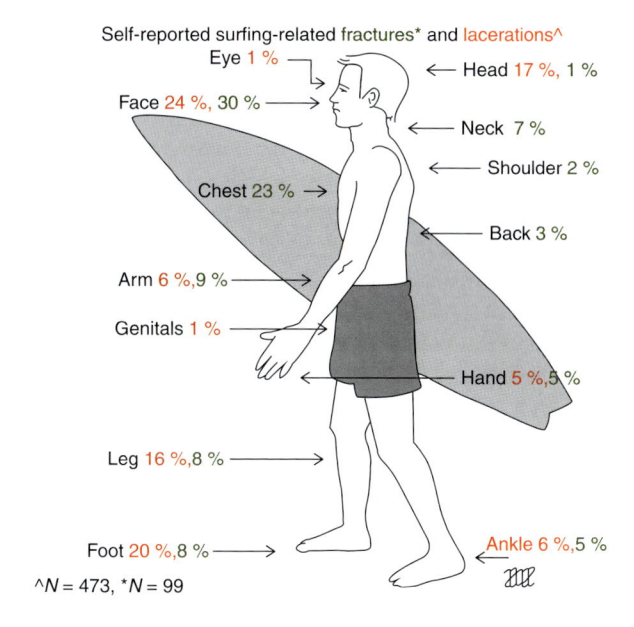

Self-reported surfing-related fractures* and lacerations^

- Eye 1 %
- Face 24 %, 30 %
- Head 17 %, 1 %
- Neck 7 %
- Shoulder 2 %
- Chest 23 %
- Back 3 %
- Arm 6 %, 9 %
- Genitals 1 %
- Hand 5 %, 5 %
- Leg 16 %, 8 %
- Foot 20 %, 8 %
- Ankle 6 %, 5 %

^N = 473, *N = 99

body. Figure 7.2 shows the anatomic distribution of lacerations and fractures from a study of 1,237 self-reported surfing injuries. Hospital-based studies of injured surfers, which in all likelihood consist of higher-acuity patients, show a higher percentage of head injuries and factures, than do outpatient studies (see Table 7.2).

Mechanisms of Injury

Understanding the common mechanisms resulting in surfing-related injuries is useful when caring for an injured surfer and is essential to the development of injury prevention strategies.

Surfboard

Nearly all studies exploring mechanism of injury have found that the majority of acute injuries are caused by collisions between surfer and surfboard (see Table 7.3). Most commonly, surfers are struck by their own boards, but they can also be struck by the boards of others, particularly in crowded surf breaks. Since the near-universal adoption of surfboard leashes, injuries from other surfers' loose boards have become less common, while injuries from the surfer's own board have become more common [7].

Riders collide with their own boards in a number of common scenarios:

- Rider is tumbled into own board by a wave's turbulence.
- During a steep takeoff, the board falls out from under its rider, and the rider inadvertently lands on his/her own board.

Table 7.2 Hospital-based studies of surfing-related injuries

Study	Allen [13]	Chang [14]	Taniguchi [15]	Taylor [8]	Hay [16]	Hay [16]
Population	Hospitalized patients, Kaiser Hospital, Waikiki (includes 12 bodysurfers)	Hospitalized patients, Queens Medical Center (includes 21 bodysurfers)	Emergency Department, Kahului Community Hospital	Emergency Department, Victorian public hospitals	Discharged home, Royal Cornwall Hospital (includes bodyboarders)	Hospitalized, Royal Cornwall Hospital (includes bodyboarders)
Location	Waikiki, Oahu	Oahu	North Shore, Oahu	Victoria, Australia	Cornwall, England	Cornwall, England
Number of subjects	36	47	90	267	190	22
Average age	20	Approximately 27	Unknown	75 % <30 years old	27	27
Male gender	92 %	Unknown	Unknown	83 %	80 %	80 %
Injury type						
Laceration	11 %	13 %[b]	83 %	47 %	38 %	0
Sprain/ligament rupture	5 %	13 %	0	12 %	21 %	0
Fracture[a]	30 %	45 %	7 %	14 %	14 %	64 %
Dislocation	5 %	2 %	3 %	2 %	13 %	10 %
Contusion	3 %	2 %	0	0	14 %	0
Drowning/near drowning	8 %	2 %	0	0	0	4 %
Solid organ injury intra-abdominal bleeding	17 %	2 %	0	0	0	4 %
Concussion/intracranial	3 %	17 %	0	3 %	0	18 %
Tympanic membrane perf.	8 %	0 %	4 %	0	2 %	0
Other	8 %	4 %	0	21 %[b]	0	14 %[d]
Body region						
Head/face	39 %	34 %	49 %	42 %	42 %	18 %

Neck	17 %	21 %	0	3 %	7 %	18 %
Back	5 %	0 %	0	1 %	2 %	4 %
Thorax	0	4 %	12 %	6 %	4 %	0
Upper extremity	8 %	6 %		16 %	12 %	4 %
Lower extremity	6 %	19 %	31 %[c]	23 %	18 %	32 %
Intra-abdominal/Retroperitoneal	14 %	2 %	0	0	0	14 %
Other/unknown	11 %	17 %	0	9 %	3 %	10 %

[a]Includes two tooth fractures
[b]Includes total of four eye injuries
[c]Includes upper and lower extremity injuries
[d]Includes laryngeal fracture and uretheral rupture

Table 7.3 Mechanism of surfing injuries

Study	Nathanson [10]	Taylor [8]	Nathanson [11]	Lowdon [9]	Lowdon [7]
Population	Prospective study of surfers in competition	Convenience sample interviewed at beaches in Victoria, Australia	Web-based survey of English-speaking surfers	Survey of International Competitors	Members of the Australian Surfing Assoc., Victoria, AU
Average age (SD)	24 (7)	28 (7.9)	29 (10.6)	22 (3.7)	22 (5.7)
Male gender	87 %	90 %	90 %	89 %	95 %
Average #'s of years surfing	Unknown	12	11	11 (5 days per week)	8 (2.7 days per week)
# of acute injuries	116	168	1,237	167	311
Cause of acute surfing injury					
Surfboard	29 %	42 %	66 %	47 %	53 %
Seafloor	24 %	18 %	17 %	9 %	13 %
Wave force/"wiping out"	12 %	36 %	7 %	≥4 %	≥6 %
Body motion	16 %	0	5 %	16 %	17 %
Marine animal	2 %	1 %	3 %	0	1 %

Fig. 7.3 Board-related surfing injuries (Photo: Nathanson, Haynes, Galanis [11])

Part of surboard resulting in injury

N = 828 injuries

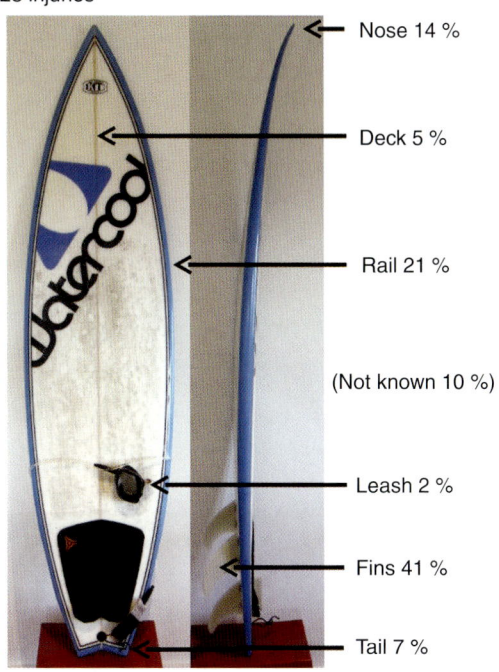

- Nose 14 %
- Deck 5 %
- Rail 21 %
- (Not known 10 %)
- Leash 2 %
- Fins 41 %
- Tail 7 %

- After a wipeout (particularly in offshore winds), the surfboard becomes airborne and comes down on the riders head as he/she surfaces.
- After a wipeout, the board is pulled shoreward by a wave until its leash is pulled taught. The board then recoils back on its leash along the surface, striking rider (often in the face).
- While attempting to "duck dive" under an oncoming wave, the board is forcefully thrust back by the wave's force into the surfer.

Many serious board-related injuries occur when a surfer falls onto or is forcefully struck by sharp parts of the board such as the fin(s) (skeg), nose, or tail (Fig. 7.3). Lacerations obtained from the surfer's own surfboard fins account for as many as 30 % of all significant surfing injuries in some studies and usually involve the lower extremities or head [7, 11] (Fig. 7.4a). Surfboard fins are rigid, have sharp trailing edges and tips, and are capable of inflicting deep lacerations which may involve tendons, arteries, and nerves. Though the majority of fin-induced lacerations are superficial, their potential to cause penetrating trauma should not be underestimated; fatal and near-fatal fin-induced lacerations of the aorta and femoral arteries have been described, as have eviscerations and rectal injuries [17].

Kim et al. reported a series of 11 severe surfboard-related ocular injuries, 5 of which resulted in globe ruptures and permanent monocular loss of vision. Zoumalan described a series of 3 similar injuries. Recoil of the board on its leash causing the

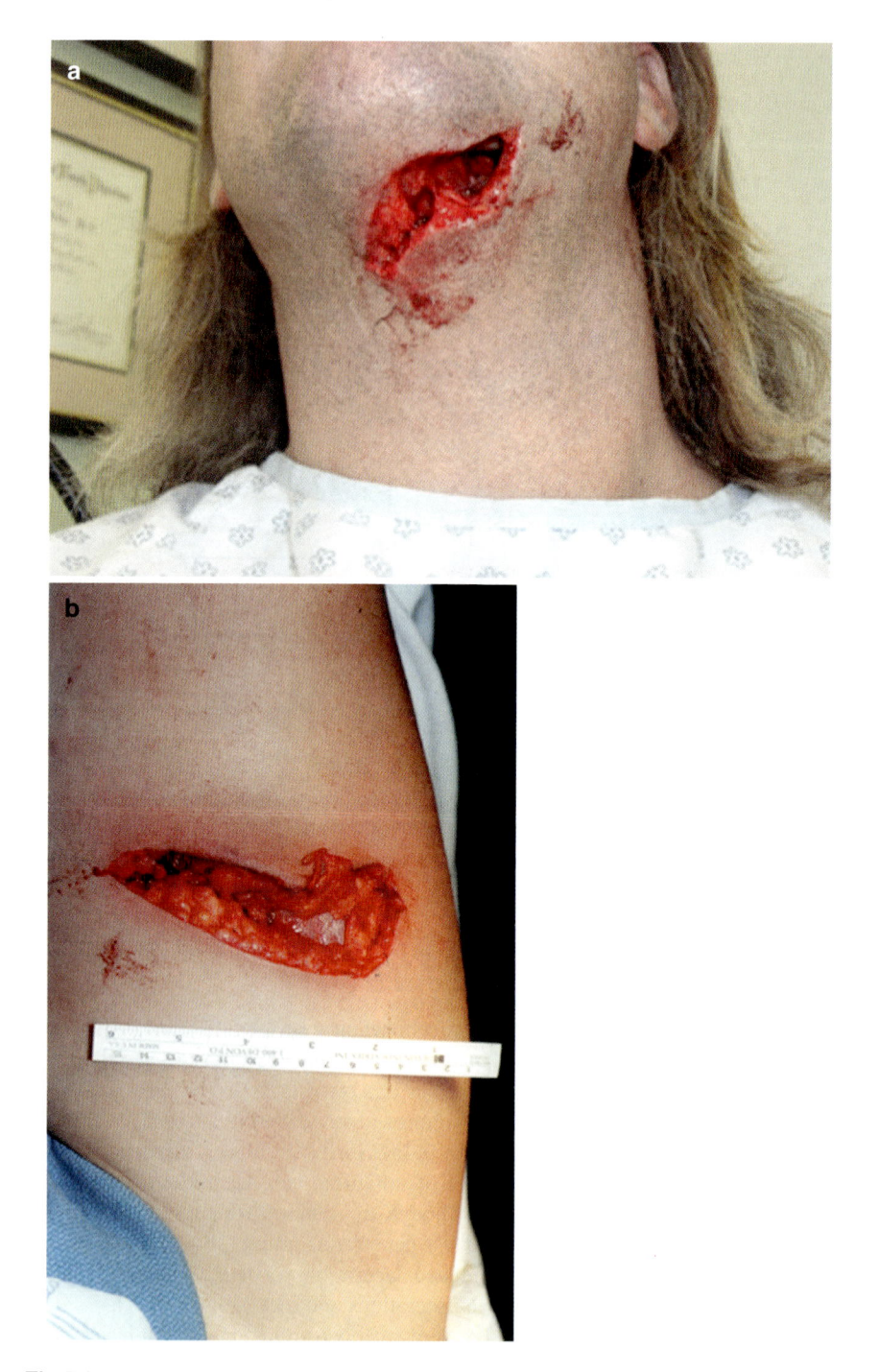

Fig. 7.4 (**a**) Fin induced chin laceration (Photo: SurfCo Hawaii) (**b**). Fin induced thigh laceration (Photo: SurfCo Hawaii)

pointed nose of the board to strike the surfer's eye was cited in both studies as being a common mechanism of ocular injury. Fractures of the orbital wall have also been reported [18, 19].

Blunt trauma from collisions with rounded parts of the surfboard such as the rails and deck is also frequent and usually results in contusions. However, forceful blows to poorly padded parts of the body such as the scalp, face, and shins can cause lacerations and fractures. Nasal bone fractures, tooth avulsions, and other maxillofacial fractures from impact with a surfboard are relatively common. Loss of consciousness secondary to blunt head trauma from a surfboard has led to drowning deaths among beginner as well as elite surfers.

Blunt trauma to the abdomen and chest has been reported to cause splenic rupture and pneumothorax, respectively [8, 13]. Even foam bodyboards have been reported to cause liver and splenic lacerations during wipeouts in which the nose of the board sticks into the sand and the tail is thrust under the rider's ribs [20].

Seafloor

While water is a forgiving surface on which to fall, the same cannot be said of the seafloor. Indeed, some of the most severe surfing-related injuries occur when those riding waves in shallow water fall and hit bottom headfirst.

Because small waves break in shallow water (waves begin to break at a depth of approximately 1.3× the wave's height), striking the seafloor is most common in small surf [21]. However, the large, powerful, tubular waves sought out by expert surfers for "tube riding" also put the rider at significant risk for striking the seafloor. These tube-shaped waves only form in places with a steeply inclined seafloor (e.g., a reef or a ledge), and while these waves begin to wall up in deep water, their lip may come crashing down in the shallows (Fig. 7.5). A surfer falling in the wrong part of such a wave runs the risk of getting carried "over the falls" by the wave's lip and driven onto shallow reef. At Oahu's famed Pipeline, the inner portion of the reef is a mere 1–1.5 m deep, and the fearsome tubular wave at Teahupoo, Tahiti, breaks over an even shallower reef. Experienced surfers have sustained fatal head injuries at both venues.

Abrasions and superficial lacerations obtained from getting dragged by wave action over coral reef are so common among surfers as to have been dubbed "reef rash." These wounds are often embedded with fine particles of coral and are highly prone to infection. Foot lacerations and plantar puncture wounds acquired by stepping on sharp objects are also commonplace, particularly in tropical waters where the seabed is often littered with spiny marine animals, shell fragments, and coral reef. These too are also highly prone to infection and usually occur when entering or exiting the water or while retrieving one's surfboard.

Catastrophic spinal cord injuries due to surfing, bodyboarding, and bodysurfing are well documented and are similar to those seen in shallow water diving accidents. The usual scenario is one in which the surfer wipes out striking bottom headfirst and causing excessive axial loading, hyperextension, hyperflexion, or rotational injury

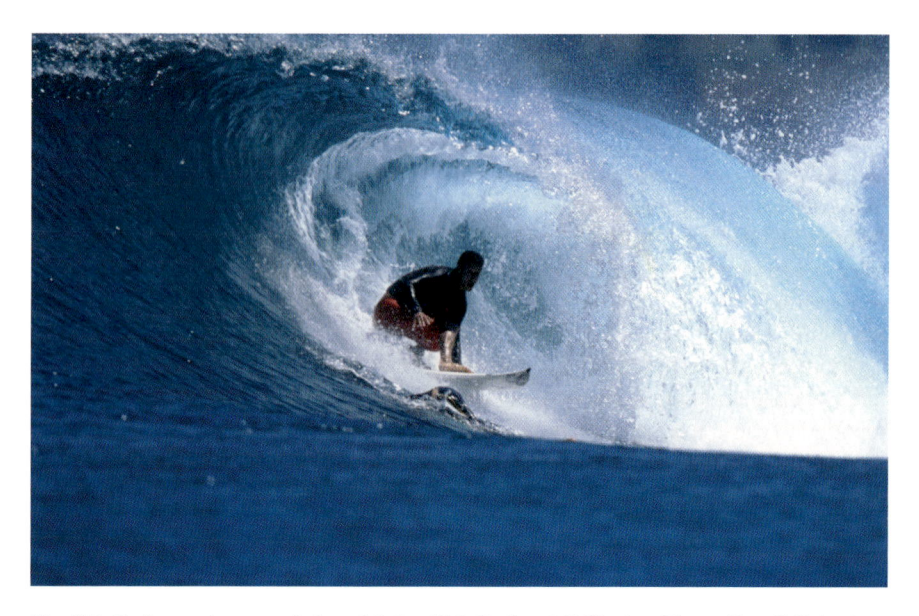

Fig. 7.5 Surfer coming out of a barrel (tube ride). Surfer: Adi Gluska, (Photo: Jhon Callahan)

to the cervical spine [22]. Though some surfers take a casual approach when surfing over a sandy bottom, packed wet sand can be very unforgiving, and headfirst falls onto sand bottoms have resulted in a number of well-publicized and tragic cases of quadriplegia among young surfers [23].

Because bodyboarders and bodysurfers ride headfirst in a prone position, often in near-shore plunging waves, they are at particularly high risk for injuries to the cervical spine. Cheng described a series of 14 cervical spine injuries among bodyboarders and concluded that many of these injuries appeared to be associated with spinal stenosis and cervical spine osteophytes [24]. Chang et al. analyzed 77 patients who suffered wave-related spinal cord injuries in Hawaii. The typical victim was a male tourist of large build in his 40s, with little previous experience in wave-riding activities [25].

Any surfer seen floating on the surface or complaining of severe neck pain after a wipeout should be presumed to have suffered from an unstable cervical spine fracture until proven otherwise. A surfboard and rolled towels on each side of the head can be used to make an improvised backboard and provide spinal immobilization to transport such patients (Fig. 7.6).

Other potential hazards involving the seabed are underwater rock or coral overhangs and obstructions such as kelp or crab traps, which can snag a surfer's leash, tethering them underwater. There are a number of instances in which surfers have had their leashes snagged underwater, were unable to rapidly disengage from the leash's ankle strap, and subsequently drown. Other leash-related injuries occur when an extremity is caught in a loop of leash during a wipeout and the leash is subsequently tugged taught by the force of a wave on the surfboard. Most common

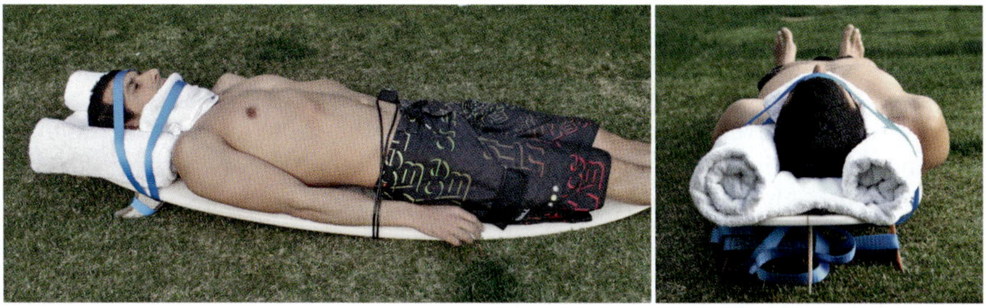

Fig. 7.6 Improvised cervical immobilization. A board, towels, surfboard leash, and roof straps can be used to maintain spinal immobilization in a surfer with a presumed cervical spine injury (Photo: Yaron Weinstein)

among these are fractures and dislocations of the interphalangeal joints, but finger amputations via this mechanism have also occurred.

Wave-Force Injuries

The energy of a breaking wave is considerable. It has been estimated that a 1-m-wide slice of a 3-m-high wave has the equivalent of 73 hp, and because a wave's power increases as a square of its height, a 6-m wave is four times as powerful [21]. Most of a wave's kinetic energy is dissipated in its cascading lip, but not all waves are created equal. Chang et al. describe a four-level grading system that categorizes beaches by the power of the surf, with gentle spilling waves (grade 1) produced in areas with gently sloping bottoms being the least dangerous type and hollow plunging waves (grade 4) found in areas with a steeply inclined bottom being the most dangerous. In his Hawaii-based study of wave-related accidents resulting in cervical spine injuries, 96 % occurred at grade 3 or grade 4 beaches [25].

Surprisingly, traumatic injuries caused solely by the hydraulic forces of a wave (i.e., not involving surfboard or seafloor) are rare, even in very large surf. Most susceptible to wave-force injury is the tympanic membrane (TM). TM rupture can occur when a surfer is hit by the lip of a large wave or when the ear slaps into the water after a high-speed wipeout. Most ruptures involve the pars tensa, below the umbo and malleolus, and heal spontaneously in 4–6 weeks. Immediate symptoms involve conductive hearing loss, ear pain, and the ability to blow air outward through the ear with a pinched nose. There may also be a bloody discharge from the ear [26]. In order to prevent infections of the middle ear, surfers should be advised to keep the ear dry (no surfing, ear covered in the shower) for 4–6 weeks. Rare instances of nonhealing should be referred to an ENT for tympanoplasty. Dizziness or vertigo implies a concomitant rupture of the oval or round windows; these too usually heal spontaneously.

Long bone fractures, shoulder dislocations, and other significant injuries have been attributed to getting hit by enormous waves, but such injuries are unusual unless a surfer hits bottom or is struck by a surfboard.

A much greater danger in large surf is the risk of being held forcefully underwater by a breaking wave's turbulence. Though underwater hold-downs almost never exceed 30 s, even in huge waves, that may be long enough to test the limits of an already winded surfer [27]. Many tow-in surfers wear flotation vests to improve buoyancy in the highly aerated water that is formed after large waves break and a wetsuit is currently being developed with an air bladder that can be rapidly inflated by means of a CO_2 cartridge [28].

Every big-wave surfer's greatest dread is a two-wave hold-down in which they are unable to surface from one wave before getting washed over by the next. While many of today's most notable big-wave surfers have described near-death experiences from getting held under by multiple waves, the fact is that in the absence of trauma, drowning among experienced surfers is exceedingly rare. The number of big-wave surfers that have drowned over the last three decades is in the single digits, and to this author's knowledge, no one has ever drowned while tow-in surfing, despite the fact that tow-in teams have been chasing the largest rideable swells on the planet for over 15 years.

Strong seaward-flowing currents known as "rip currents" (and improperly known as riptides or undertow) pose another danger to those in the surf zone, primarily to inexperienced surfers who fail to appreciate the complex patterns of water flow generated by breaking waves. Experienced surfers use these currents to advantage when paddling out to a surf break, but surfers attempting to reach shore after having lost their boards may find themselves struggling to swim against an outflowing rip current and can become exhausted and drown. According to the United States Lifesaving Association, over 80 % of lifeguard-assisted rescues on ocean beaches are due to rip currents. Surfers who are poor swimmers, lack aerobic capacity, or are inebriated are at particularly high risk of drowning.

Wave-Riding Injuries

Over the last two decades, surfing has become an ever more acrobatic and dynamic sport, particularly at the elite levels. As such, acute muscle and joint injuries acquired while riding waves are on the rise among today's top surfers. In a 2007 study of injuries occurring during surfing contests, 19 % of all acute injuries were found to be knee sprains and strains, up from 10 % reported in a 1987 study [9, 10].

Aerial maneuvers in which the surfer steers sharply up a wave face, becomes airborne, and then lands back on his board carry a high degree of difficulty and score highly in competition (Fig. 7.7). Successfully landing these maneuvers requires that the surfer land on the moving face of the wave with the board squarely under his feet. Mid-flight control of the board is usually achieved by grabbing a rail of the board from a crouched position, but, when landing, the surfer relies solely on air pressure to maintain foot contact with the board, then must compress to absorb the shock of landing. Aerials in which a surfer lands on his board awkwardly or comes down abruptly have become an increasingly common source of ankle and knee injuries. It is now common to see professional surfers sidelined by ankle

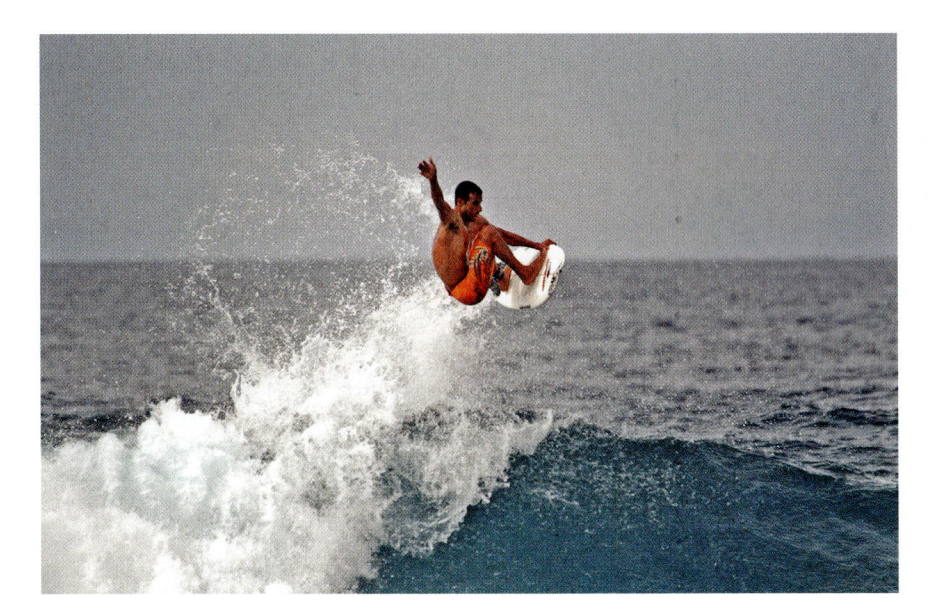

Fig. 7.7 Adi Gluska, airborn. The Maldives Islands (Photo: Shiran Valk)

sprains and fractures as well as ACL rupture and injuries to the meniscus from ill-fated aerials. When wave riding, the knee of the back leg (usually the dominant leg) is in a flexed valgus position, placing high loads on the medial collateral ligament during forceful maneuvers [26].

Radical snaps and laybacks (short-radius turns) requiring highly contorted body positioning are also mandatory for competitive success (Fig. 7.8). These moves demand that the surfer generate power from the relatively unstable surface of their surfboard while riding over the moving and uneven surface of a wave. Poor technique, lack of flexibility, and failure to properly warm up can contribute strains of the hamstrings, neck, and back while executing these aggressive turns.

Overuse Injuries

Given that surfing can only be practiced when there are adequate waves, surfing is an intermittent activity in most areas, even among the sport's most avid participants. High-quality surf is generated by long-period ocean swells originating from distant storms, and these swells typically last anywhere from 2–6 days. When surfing conditions are optimal, surfers may spend upward of 4 h in the water (Mendez), but lack of surf in a given locale may preclude surfing for weeks on end.

Time-motion analysis studies have found that 50 % of a surfer's time is spent paddling and 45 % is spent remaining still, while only 3–5 % is spent actually riding

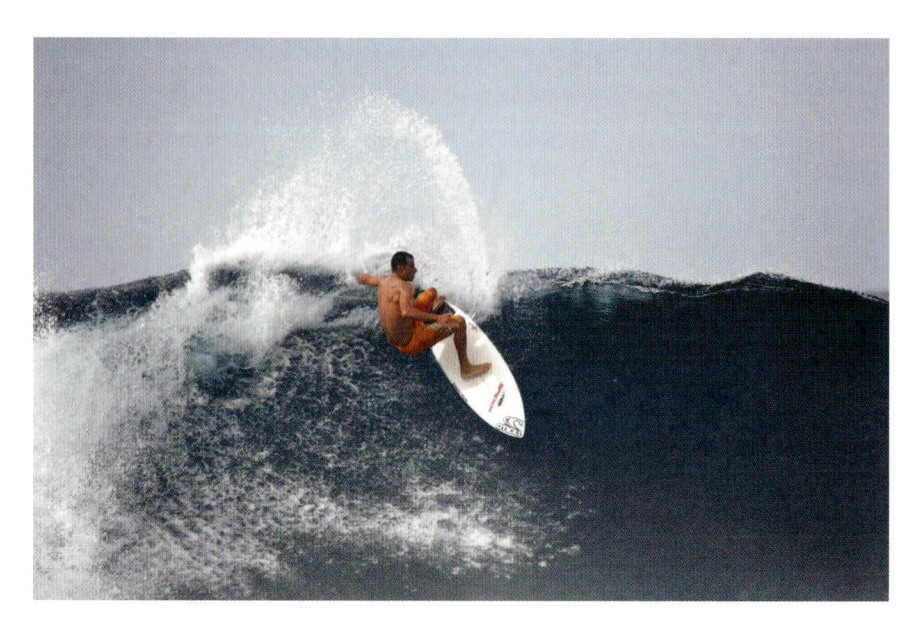

Fig. 7.8 An off-the-lip is one of the core maneuver of modern surfing. The Maldives Islands. Surfer: Adi Gluska, (Photo: Shiran Valk)

waves, so it comes as little surprise that most overuse injuries stem from paddling [29, 30]. Sustained paddling is required to get out to the takeoff zone and maintain one's position in the presence of currents, while short bursts of paddling at maximum effort are needed to successfully catch waves, dodge unfavorable waves, and avoid oncoming surfers.

Lowdon et al. found that among a group of world-class competitive surfers, 29 % of all sprains and strains were related to paddling. In Nathanson et al.'s Internet-based survey, which included 477 surfing-related chronic health problems, overuse injuries to the shoulder (18 %), back (16 %), neck (9 %), and knee (9 %) were most frequently cited [9, 11]. Taylor et al. reported 146 chronic health problems among surfers. He found that pain or stiffness of the neck and back, shoulder, and knee comprised 20% 10% and 8 % of these problems, respectively [8].

Surfers are notorious for not warming up prior to surfing [7, 9]. A fitness program emphasizing flexibility, core strength and balance, as well as a warming up before surfing should be advised as a means of decreasing the incidence overuse injuries.

Neck and Back Pain

Correct prone paddling posture requires extension of the lumbar and thoracic spine so as to raise the upper chest off the deck of the board and allow for an ergonomic paddling stroke. The neck is held in slight extension (Fig. 7.9).

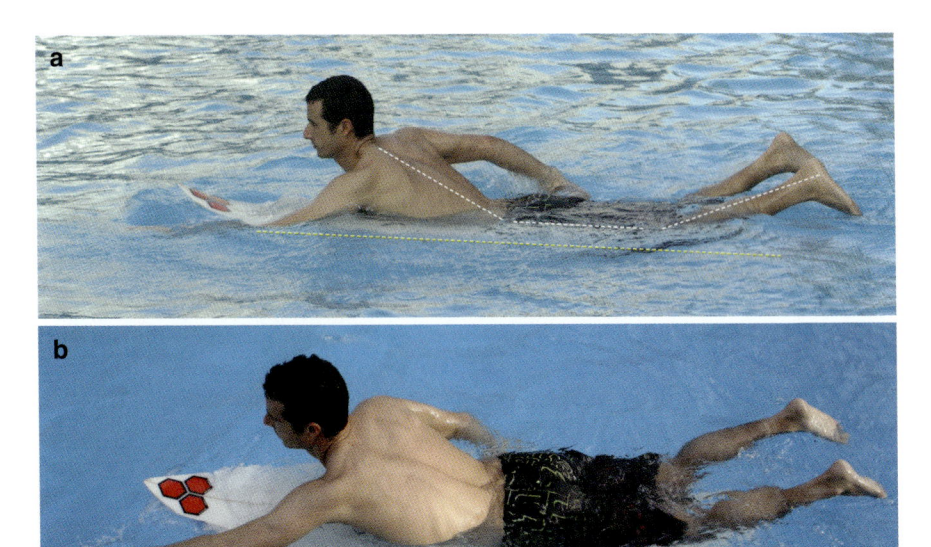

Fig. 7.9 (**a, b**) Surfer paddling. Note chest is raised off board resulting in excessive lordosis (hyperextension of lower back) which by placing the posterior spinal column under continued stress may lead to a stress fracture (spondylolysis) (Photo: Yaron Weinstein)

Strains of the lumbar and cervical paraspinous muscles are common, likely due to sustained isometric contraction of those muscles while paddling. Beginners and those surfing after prolonged periods of inactivity often complain of burning muscular pain in the upper trapezius and rhomboid muscles due to overuse. Neck soreness can be exacerbated by the tendency of some surfers to hyperextend the neck to compensate for inadequate back extension due to fatigue or lack of lumbar and thoracic flexibility [31].

Most neck and back spasms caused by overuse resolve spontaneously, but massage, physical therapy, and chiropractic manipulation can improve acute symptoms. A proper warming up prior to surfing (particularly in cold waters) and routine stretching of the low back, hamstrings, and hip flexors may help prevent this common problem [26]. Actively engaging the core musculature while paddling creates a firm paddling platform, unloading the muscles of the low back. For this reason, land-based exercises aimed at improving core strength among surfers are important. Gillam et al. demonstrated that while surfers had more powerful shoulder flexion and extension than other athletes, they had significantly weaker abdominal strength [6].

Neck pain not resolving after conservative treatment may be due to cervical disk injury, degenerative arthritis in older surfers, or the thoracic outlet syndrome.

Focal low-back pain in adolescent surfers should raise suspicion for spondylolysis, which can be found among other athletes in sports which require low-back extension such as gymnastics and American football. Symptoms are exacerbated by movements that forcefully extend the low back such as duck diving under oncoming waves or popping up (moving from a supine to a standing position) on a surfboard. A one-legged standing extension test reproduces the pain caused by spondylolysis, and a bone scan alongside CT scan and MRI can be obtained to confirm the diagnosis. Stress fractures of the pars interarticularis generally heal with conservative therapy but often require 4–6 months of cessation from sports, though some may require spinal fusion later in life [32].

In 2004, Thompson first described a case series of nine nontraumatic spinal cord injuries among neophyte surfers that he termed "surfer's myelopathy." Afflicted surfers describe feeling low-back pain within an hour of surfing and within the next few hours develop lower extremity weakness, urinary retention, and paralysis [33]. In many cases recovery is complete, but in some instances the victim is left with permanent neurologic deficits including quadriplegia. MRIs of these patients demonstrate findings consistent with thoracic spinal cord ischemia which has been postulated to be caused by kinking or vasospasm of the spinal arteries brought about by the prone hyperextended posture assumed when paddling (Fig. 7.9). Most case series describe this syndrome in first-time surfers who are healthy young adults with normal anatomy and normal coagulation profiles [34, 35]. It remains a mystery why this syndrome only occurs in first-time surfers.

Upper Extremity Pain

Surfing, like swimming, is an overhead sport, and by one estimate, a surfer may take as many as 2,000 paddling stokes in a 2-h session. Shoulder strains and impingement syndromes of the supraspinatus tendon caused by paddling are very common, and intermittent shoulder pain has been found to affect nearly 30 % of amateur surfers [36].

Surfers with scapular instability, muscle imbalance, or poor paddling biomechanics are particularly predisposed to shoulder problems. Those who fail to raise their chests off the deck of their board while paddling require more shoulder flexion during the recovery phase of the paddling stroke, overloading the relatively hypovascular zone of the supraspinatus tendon [31].

Muscle-bound surfers who rely on surfing as their primary means of exercise are prone to shoulder imbalance due to overdevelopment and shortening of the pectoralis and anterior deltoid muscles and relative weakness of the rhomboid muscles, subscapularis, and other scapular stabilizers [36]. This muscular imbalance leads to scapular protraction and movement of the humeral head high into the shoulder socket resulting in compression of the rotator cuff tendons and subacromial bursa, which in turn can cause tendinitis and bursitis [37]. Years of surfing can lead to fraying of the supraspinatus tendon as it courses under the acromion which can progress to a torn rotator cuff.

Shoulder rehabilitation begins with a period of rest, anti-inflammatory medication, and ice. A few days of rest should be followed by gentle stretching of the shoulder using pain as a limiting factor. Early mobilization should include a progressive program of exercises to strengthen the rotator cuff muscles and scapular stabilizers. Each session should begin with isometric muscle contraction and progress to isokinetic exercises. At first, use only the weight of the arm and then advance to light weights or elastic bands, using pain as a rate-limiting factor. A return to surfing should only occur upon restoration of a painless full range of motion, at first surfing on a relatively buoyant, easy gliding board to reduce the paddling burden. Shoulder rehabilitation should last a minimum of 6–12 weeks and may take up to a year.

The repetitive stresses of paddling, duck diving, and popping up may cause lateral epicondylitis or triceps tendinitis. Treatment initially involves cessation of surfing, anti-inflammatory medications, and icing, followed by physical therapy [38]. After a period of conservative treatment, the athlete should return to surfing on a board with efficient paddling characteristics as above. Cho-Pat strapping and various injectables (steroids, PRP, autologous blood) may help alleviate chronic lateral epicondylitis.

Environmental Injuries

The surf zone can be a hostile environment with unremitting exposure to solar radiation, prolonged immersion in salt water, and potential threat from hazardous marine life.

Skin, Eyes, and Ears

Incident and reflected sunlight can take a toll on a surfer's skin and eyes. A small study conducted at a surfing contest in Texas (USA) found that surfers have a higher rate of basal cell carcinoma than their age-matched non-surfing counterparts [39]. It is likely that due to their (often unprotected) prolonged exposure to harmful ultraviolet radiation, surfers are also at increased risk for squamous cell carcinoma and malignant melanoma.

Physical barriers such as wetsuits, rash guards, and hats are the most effective and reliable way for surfers to protect themselves from the sun. In warm climates, long-sleeved, hooded rash guards with SPF >50 should be worn. In smaller surf, hats with chinstraps and sunglasses or goggles with retention straps can be worn. Broad-spectrum (UVA and UVB), water-resistant sunscreen with SPF >15 should be applied to the face and other uncovered skin 30 min prior to entering the water, using approximately 30 ml for an unclothed adult male. Despite manufacturer claims, most sunscreens do not last for more than 2–3 h in the surf and need to be reapplied. While there is good evidence that sunscreen provides protection against squamous cell carcinoma, there is only fair evidence that it protects against basal cell carcinoma and virtually no evidence that it protects against malignant melanoma [40]. Heavily sun-exposed, fair-skinned, and older surfers should be examined at least annually by a dermatologist to screen for skin cancer.

Repeated exposure to bright sunlight, wind, dust, and salt spray can lead to triangular yellow growths over the nasal aspect of the conjunctiva, known as pterygia. Often seen among those surfing in sunny climes, these benign fibrovascular growths can cause eye irritation and may affect vision if they extend over the cornea. Use of sunglasses or goggles on and off the water can prevent the formation and growth of pterygia. Pterygia affecting vision should be referred to a corneal specialist and may be amenable to surgical removal.

External auditory canal exostosis (EAE) or "surfer's ear" is remarkably common among surfers. These painless bony growths of the external auditory canal are benign but can cause water and other debris to get trapped in the ear canal leading to recurrent bouts of otitis externa. Severe exostosis, blocking greater than 66 % of the ear canal, may also cause some degree of hearing loss.

Wong et al. examined the ears of 307 surfers at the US Open of Surfing and found that the overall prevalence of EAE was 73.5 %. In the group that had surfed for over 20 years, 91 % had evidence of EAE, with 16 % of that group having severe exostosis [41]. Kroon et al. showed that those who surfed predominantly in colder waters were at significantly increased risk of EAE (odds ratio 5.8), and that the number of years surfed increased one's risk of developing exostosis by 12 % per year [42].

Broad-spectrum antibiotic drops containing a steroid and an analgesic (e.g., Cortisporin otic suspension) should be prescribed to surfers with otitis externa. Among surfers who frequently suffer from otitis externa (both with and without exostosis), drying the ear canals with isopropyl alcohol after surfing is recommended. The use of Q-tips or other objects in the ear canal should be highly discouraged as this often leads to otitis externa.

Though never proven, the consensus among otolaryngologists is that earplugs can prevent the formation of bony exostosis. Large exostoses causing a decrease in hearing or leading to recurrent episodes of otitis externa should be removed using a transcanal approach by an otolaryngologist experienced in this procedure. After the procedure, surfers are usually "dry-docked" for 4–6 weeks. Unfortunately EAE often regrow after surgery.

Hazardous Marine Life

Despite the widely held perception that dangerous marine animals, most notably sharks, pose a significant risk to surfers, less than 3 % of all surfing injuries are caused by marine life, and the majority of them are due to jellyfish and sea urchins (Table 7.3). Annually there are approximately 30 shark attacks on surfers worldwide with a fatality rate of less than 8 %. The prevention and treatment of marine bites and stings are beyond the scope of this chapter, but a summary of recommendations can be found in Table 7.4.

7 Surfing Injuries

Table 7.4 Treatment of bites and stings from hazardous marine animals

Animal	Habitat/range	Injury/symptoms	Treatment	Prevention
Sea urchin	Rock/reef bottom	Puncture wounds with retained spines. Venomous species	Surgically remove spines in fingers or joints. Other spines best left in place. Envenomation: soak in hot water (45°C) for 15–30 min	Booties. Avoid stepping on seafloor
Stingray	Sandy bottom	Jagged wound and envenomation. Radiating pain nausea and vomiting	Soak in hot water (45°C) for 15–30 min. Remove retained spine and sheath. Prophylactic abx's. Leave wound open versus loose closure	Shuffle feet to scare away animals
Shark	Near steep drop-offs, seal breeding colonies, river mouths	Deep lacerations, hemorrhage, avulsion	Apply direct pressure or tourniquet. In OR, repair damaged structures loose closure. Prophylactic abx's	Avoid surfing at dawn, at dusk, in murky water, or alone. If shark of >2 m is seen, slowly exit water
Jellyfish	Warm waters worldwide	Painful sting, whiplike rash on exposed skin. Allergic reactions	Flush skin with seawater. Topical steroid crème for dermatitis. Portuguese man-of-war: hot water. Australian box: vinegar, antivenom. Hawaiian box: hot water. Allergic rxn: standard treatment	Rash guard or wetsuit Safe Sea® lotion on exposed skin
Sea bather's eruption	Warm waters, summer (jellyfish larvae)	Extremely pruritic papular rash on *clothed* skin surfaces	Topical steroid crème. Oral diphenhydramine	Remove wetsuit or bathing suit before exiting water
Stonefish	Indo-Pacific, rock or reef bottom	Painful sting, severe edema of foot	Soak in hot water (45°C) for 15–30 min. Remove retained spine if presented. Elevate extremity	Avoid stepping on seafloor

Wound Care

Lacerations, abrasions, and puncture wounds are a major reason for surfers to seek medical care. Several factors should be considered when treating these injuries.

The sea is home to a variety of human pathogens such as *Vibrio, Mycobacterium, Pseudomonas*, and other gram-negative organisms, many of which are not sensitive to antibiotics commonly used to treat soft tissue skin infections. When treating a wound infection acquired in the marine environment or providing prophylactic antibiotics, consider adding an antibiotic such as doxycycline or ciprofloxacin to cover marine flora. Most marine organisms are halophilic (salt loving) and will not grow in standard culture media, so when obtaining a wound culture, alert the laboratory to the need for specialized culture media [43]. *V. vulnificus* and *V. damsela* have been reported to cause severe wound infections among surfers. Because of their propensity to cause necrotizing fasciitis, severe infections from these organisms are best treated with intravenous imipenem [44].

Like other extreme athletes, surfers tend to be a hardy breed, and if wave conditions are good, they will return to the water after wound repair, despite advice to the contrary. Nonabsorbable sutures and staples hold up best in the marine environment, whereas surgical adhesives and wound closure strips tend to slough off. For those insistent on surfing, a waterproof wound dressing that will hold up to the rigors of the surf zone can be made as follows: After a wound has been closed, apply a thin layer of an antibiotic ointment to the wound, cover it with a flexible adhesive bio-occlusive dressing, and cover that with a sturdy reinforced tape such as duct tape. If feasible, a wetsuit or wetsuit bootie should be worn over the injured area for further protection. Upon return to shore, the dressing should be removed, the wound rinsed with clean fresh water, and another layer of antibiotic should be applied to the wound which is then covered by a standard gauze dressing.

Coral abrasions require scrubbing and copious irrigation to remove any retained coral fragments and minimize the risk of infection. After these wounds have been thoroughly cleansed, they should be coated with antibiotic ointment and then covered with a nonadherent dressing.

Plantar puncture wounds acquired in the marine environment warrant a high index of suspicion to rule out the presence of retained organic material including sea urchin spines, coral reef, and shell fragments. Most of these foreign bodies contain calcium and are well visualized with x-ray or ultrasound. Due to the high incidence of infection associated with puncture wounds to the foot, prophylactic antibiotics which include coverage for marine organisms are indicated.

Painful ulcers, termed "sea ulcers," commonly form on the hands, feet, and legs of surfers who have prolonged daily exposure to salt water. These ulcers typically begin as small nicks and abrasions caused by coral reef or rocks but fail to heal and gradually enlarge because repeated soaking in the ocean prevents a protective scab from forming. Without a scab, the delicate collagen matrix essential for the initial stage of the healing process gets washed away each surf session, eroding underlying tissue. Constant friction between a surfer's skin and board, especially at the tops of the feet and knees, can further compound the problem.

While often moist at the base, sea ulcers are typically sterile and generally heal within a few weeks of cessation of surfing. To promote healing, ulcers should be covered with dry gauze to prevent soiling but at bedtime should be left uncovered so they can dry. Particulate matter such as sand, which often gets trapped in sea ulcers of the lower extremity, should be removed. For those who continue to surf, a waterproof dressing as described above can be used when surfing [26].

Injury Prevention

Basic Safety Recommendations

- All surfers should be strong swimmers who can swim 1 km in less than 20 min and are comfortable swimming alone in the ocean [45].
- Each surf break is unique and has different characteristics depending on wave height, tide, and wind. When surfing in a new locale, surfers should familiarize themselves with safe entry and exit points, currents, and underwater hazards. This is best done by talking to local surfers and observing the surf break for a minimum of 10 min prior to entering the water.
- Surfing is a skill sport that takes many, many years to master. Surfers should respect their own limits and gradually work their way up the ladder in terms of wave size and difficulty.
- Surfing to exhaustion, particularly in large surf, is foolhardy. Wise surfers pace themselves so that at any given moment they are able to hold their breath for at least 20 s in preparation for an unexpected hold-down. Fatigued surfers should paddle to shore or rest outside of the takeoff zone.
- Breath-hold training may induce syncope and should only be practiced on land in a safe, supervised environment.

Equipment

Collisions with surfboards are the leading source of surfing injuries with 60–70 % of those injuries inflicted by the board's sharp fins, nose, or tail (Fig. 7.2). Minor modifications in surfboard design, described below, are unlikely to significantly alter performance characteristics and would likely go a long way toward reducing injury rates.
- The Surfrider Foundation Australia suggests that sharp surfboard noses and tails should be rounded off to a minimum radius of 37 mm. At the very least, the sharp nose of a surfboard should be covered with a shock-absorbing rubber tip.
- Trailing edges of surfboard fins should be dulled to a minimum width of 2 mm with fine-grit sandpaper. Rubber-edged fins are commercially available and are highly recommended. Fins should be designed to break away on impact.

- Beginners should use boards made entirely of shock-absorbing closed-cell foam and equipped with flexible rubber fins. These boards provide an extra measure of safety for neophytes who have minimal board control or familiarity with the surf and are at high risk of being struck by their own boards. These boards also reduce the risk of injuring near by surfers
- In all but small, uncrowded surf, a leash should be used. Leashes keep the surfer's board close at hand, and the board can be used as a flotation device should a surfer become exhausted or injured. Leashes also reduce the risk of a loose board injuring another surfer [46]. All leashes should be equipped with a single-pull quick-release mechanism should the surfer need to rapidly disengage from the leash (e.g., leash snagged on seafloor). In large surf, a stronger, longer leash is less likely to break and will keep a surfer farther away from his or her board.

Personal Protective Gear

- Temperature-appropriate wetsuits should be worn because they protect against hypothermia, provide a modicum of flotation, provide abrasion resistance, and block harmful UVA and UVB solar radiation. In warmer waters, a long-sleeved rash guard should be worn to provide protection from the sun as well as from jellyfish stings.
- Studies have shown that 26–49 % of surfing injuries involve the head and occasionally result in loss of consciousness and drowning, so it makes sense for surfers to wear helmets. Although surfing-specific helmets are commercially available, studies have shown that few use them. Many surfers perceive helmets as restrictive, feel they restrict hearing and sense of balance, and are concerned that the additional surface area will interfere with duck diving [11, 46]. Surfers should use a helmet when surfing in large hollow waves over a shallow reef, in crowded conditions, or if they are learning how to surf using a traditional fiberglass/epoxy surfboard.
- Booties should be considered to prevent foot injuries when surfing over coral reef.
- Earplugs and/or a neoprene cap should be considered to prevent surfer's ear.

References

1. Warshaw M. The history of surfing. San Francisco: Chronicle Books; 2010.
2. ASP World Tour. http://www.aspworldtour.com/schedule/asp-world-tour-schedule/. Accessed 10 Aug 2011.
3. Warshaw M. Surfline.com who knows. http://www.surfline.com/community/whoknows/who-knows.cfm?id=1012. Accessed 1 Sept 2011.
4. The Outdoor Foundation. Outdoor recreation participation report. 2010. outdoorfoundation.org/pdf/ResearchParticipation2010/pdf. Accessed 22 July 2011.
5. Board Track.net. http://board-trac.com/images/2009_Surf_Fact_Sheet.pdf. Accessed 29 Aug 2011.

6. Renneker M. Surfing: the sport and the life-style. Phys Sport Med. 1987;15(10):157–62.
7. Lowdon B, Pateman N, Pitman A. Surfboard-riding Injuries. Med J Aust. 1983;2:613–6.
8. Taylor D, Bennett D, Carter M, Garewal D, Finch C. Acute injury and chronic disability resulting from surfboard riding. J Sci Med Sport. 2004;7(4):429–37.
9. Lowdon B, Pateman N, Pitman A, Kenneth R. Injuries to international competitive surfboard riders. J Sports Med. 1987;27:57–63.
10. Nathanson A, Bird S, Dao L, Tam-Sing K. Competitive surfing injuries: a prospective study of surfing-related injuries among contest surfers. Am J Sports Med. 2007;35(1):113–7.
11. Nathanson A, Haynes P, Galanis D. Surfing injuries. Am J Emerg Med. 2002;20:155–60.
12. Galanis D. Drownings in Honolulu County 1993–2000: medical and toxicological factors. aloha.com/~lifeguards/drownings93_97.html. Accessed 11 June 2011.
13. Allen R, Eiseman B, Strackly C, Orloff B. Surfing injuries at Waikiki. JAMA. 1977;237:668–70.
14. Chang L, McDanal C. Boardsurfing and bodysurfing injuries requiring hospitalization in Honolulu. Hawaii Med. 1980;39:117.
15. Taniguchi RM, Blattau J, Hammon W. Surfing. In: Schneider RC, editor. Sports injuries: mechanisms, prevention and treatment. New York: Williams and Wilkins; 1985. p. 278–89.
16. Hay C, Barton S, Sulkin T. Recreational surfing injuries in Cornwall, United Kingdom. Wilderness Environ Med. 2009;20:335–8.
17. Lopez G. In: Nathanson AT, Everline C, Renneker M, editors. Surf survival: the surfer's health handbook. New York: Skyhorse Publishing; 2011. p. xi.
18. Kim J, McDonald H, Rubsamen P, Luttrall J, Drouilhet J, Frambach D, et al. Surfing-related ocular injuries. Retina. 1998;18(5):424–9
19. Zoumalan C, Blumenkranz M, McCulley T, Moshfeghi D. Severe surfing-related ocular injuries: the Stanford Northern Californian experience. Br J Sports Med. 2008;42:855–7.
20. Choo K, Hansen J, Bailey D. Beware the boogie board: blunt abdominal trauma from bodyboarding. Med J Aust. 2002;176:326–7.
21. Anthoni J. Oceanography: waves theory and principles of waves, how they work and what causes them. http://www.seafriends.org.nz/oceano/waves.htm. Accessed 7 July 2011.
22. Scher AT. Bodysurfing injuries of the spinal cord. S Afr Med J. 1995;85:1022–4.
23. Billauer J. They will surf again. http://www.liferollson.org. Accessed 10 May 2011.
24. Cheng CL, Wolf L, Mirvis S, Robinson L. Bodysurfing accidents resulting in cervical spine injuries. Spine. 1992;17:257–60.
25. Chang S, Tominaga G, Wong J, Weldon E, Kaan K. Risk factors for water sports-related cervical spine injuries. J Trauma. 2006;60:1041–6.
26. Sunshine S. Surfing injuries. Curr Sports Med Rep. 2003;2(3):136–41.
27. Renneker M. Surviving big surf. In: Nathanson AT, Everline C, Renneker M, editors. Surf Survival: the surfer's health handbook. New York: Skyhorse Publishing; 2011. p. 239–40. Chap 12.
28. Koteen C. Flotation innovation. *Transworld Surf Magazine*. Summer issue: 86; 2011.
29. Mendes-Villanueva A. Bishop, David: physiological aspects of surfboarding riding performance. Sports Med. 2005;35(1):55–70.
30. Meir R, Lowdon R, Davie A. Estimated energy expenditure during recreational surfing. Aust J Sci Med Sport. 1991;23(4):70–4.
31. Fyfe S. Surfing injuries, surfing training. Sports injury bulletin.com. Sportsinjurybulletin.com/archive/surfing-injuries.html. Accessed 22 May 2011.
32. Moeller J, Rifat S. Spondylolysis in active adolescents. Phys Sport Med. 2001;29:27–32.
33. Thompson T, Pearce J, et al. Surfer's myelopathy. Spine. 2004;29:353–6.
34. Aviles-Hernandez I, Garcia-Zozaya I, DeVillasante J. Nontraumatic myelopathy associated with surfing. J Spinal Cord Med. 2007;30:288–93.
35. Chung Y, Sun F, Wang L, Lai H, Hwang W. Non-traumatic anterior spinal cord infarction in a novice surfer: a case report. J Neurol Sci. 2011;302:118–20.
36. Steinman J. Shoulder problems. In: Steinman J, editor. Surfing and health. Maidenhead: Meyer and Meyer Sport; 2009. p. 129–51.

37. Everline C. Chronic surfing injuries: avoidance and rehabilitation. In: Nathanson AT, Everline C, Renneker M, editors. Surf survival: the surfer's health handbook. New York: Skyhorse Publishing; 2011. p. 239–40. Chap 5.
38. McDanal C, Anderson B. Surfer's elbow. Hawaii Med J. 1977;36:108–9.
39. Dozier S, Wagner Jr RF, Black SA, Terracina J. Beachfront screening for skin cancer in Texas Gulf coast surfers. South Med J. 1997;90:55–8.
40. Burnett M, Wang S. Current sunscreen controversies: a critical review. Photodermatol Photoimmunol Photomed. 2011;27:58–67.
41. Wong B, Cervantes W, Doyle K, Karamzadeh A, Boys P, Brauel G, Mushtaq E. Prevalence of external auditory canal exostoses in surfers. Arch Otolaryngol Head Neck Surg. 1999;125:969–72.
42. Kroon D, Lawson M, Derkay C, Hoffmann K, McCook J. Surfer's ear: external auditory exostoses are more prevalent in cold water surfers. Otolaryngol Head Neck Surg. 2002;126:499–504.
43. Auerbach P, Burgess G. Injuries from non-venomous aquatic animals. In: Auerbach P, editor. Wilderness medicine. 5th ed. Philadelphia: Mosby Elsevier; 2007. p. 1691–749. Chap 72.
44. Dryden M, Legarde M, Gottlieb T, Brady L. Vibrio damsela wound infections in Australia. Med J Aust. 1989;151:540.
45. Renneker M. Surfing: medical aspects of surfing. Phys Sportsmed. 1987;15(12):96–105.
46. Taylor D, Bennett D, Carter M, Garewal D, Finch C. Perceptions of surfboard riders regarding the need for protective headgear. Wilderness Environ Med. 2005;16(2):75–80.

Chapter 8
Kite Surfing and Snow Kiting

Mark Tauber and Philipp Moroder

Contents

The Origin of the Sport and Its Development to the Current Stage	173
The Equipment Used: Essential and Safety Requirements	177
Kite Surfing	177
Snow Kiting	180
Injury and Fatality Rates and Specific Types of Injury Related to Each Sport	180
Kite Surfing	180
Snow Kiting	182
Common Treatments for Each Sport and Relevant Rehabilitation	183
Proposed Prevention Measures	185
References	187

The Origin of the Sport and Its Development to the Current Stage

Kite surfing and snow kiting are two of the newest and trendiest disciplines in outdoor sports and gained enormous popularity in recent years. It is estimated by experts and the industry that actually more than 500,000 people are practicing these extreme sports. Unfortunately, detailed demographic data about these popular sports are actually lacking.

M. Tauber, M.D., Ph.D. (✉)
Shoulder and Elbow Service, ATOS Clinic Munich,
Munich, Effnerstrasse 38, 81925, Germany
e-mail: tauber@atos-muenchen.de

P. Moroder, M.D.
Department of Traumatology and Sports Injuries,
Paracelsus Medical University Salzburg,
Salzburg, Austria

O. Mei-Dan, M.R. Carmont (eds.), *Adventure and Extreme Sports Injuries*,
DOI 10.1007/978-1-4471-4363-5_8, © Springer-Verlag London 2013

The origins of this sport cannot exactly be traced back since there is a lack of documentation. From a historic point, the concept of kite surfing was already in Eastern cultures a long time ago. In the twelfth century, Indonesian and Polynesian fishermen used kite to help propel their fishing boats. By the thirteenth and fourteenth centuries, in China and Polynesia, kite sailing was an established form of transportation in the Pacific Rim.

In the 1800s, kites of increased size have been used by George Pocock to propel carts and ships using a four-line control system. Main reason for this invention was the need for an alternative power system to horsepower, partly to avoid the horse tax levied at that time. In 1903, the British aviation pioneer Samuel Franklin Cody developed a "man-lifting kite" and crossed successfully the English Channel in a small collapsible canvas boat powered by a kite.

However, one of the pioneers in engineering modern kites was Dieter Strasilla from Berchtesgaden, Germany, who in the 1960s and 1970s developed early prototypes with the help of his brother Udo, who at that time worked for the NASA in the USA. In 1979, he patented an inflatable kite design for kite surfing. Contemporaneously, the Legaignoux brothers in France developed and patented an inflatable kite for kite surfing in 1984. They evolved their kite designs and succeeded with the "WIPIKA" (wind-powered inflatable kite aircraft) design in 1997, which facilitated water relaunch due to its bow kite design with preformed inflatable tubes and a simple bridle system to the wingtips.

In the USA, development of modern kite surfing was pushed by Bill Roeseler, a Boeing aerodynamicist, and his son Cory in the early 1990s. They patented the "KiteSki" system, which consisted in water skis propelled by a two-line delta-style kite with a bar for kite controlling. The "KiteSki" system became commercially available in 1994, and after a few years, the ski was replaced by a single board.

In 1996, kite surfing was presented as a new sport at the Hawaiian coast of Maui by the windsurfers Laird Hamilton and Manu Bertin, and since then, kite surfing has progressed as a discipline of its own right.

Board designing has been influenced decisively by the French pair of Raphaël Salles and Laurent Ness. Until 2001, the single-direction boards dominated the kite surfing scene and have then been increasingly relieved by twin-tip bidirectional boards similar to wakeboards.

The first competition was held in September 1998 in Maui and was won by the US-American Flash Austin.

Increasingly, special kite surfing schools and associations were founded. The British Kite surfing Association (BKSA) was one of the earliest, formed in 1999. In the same year, already the first association for winter practice of this sport was founded in Austria (Austrian Snowkiting Association). As attempt to provide an international platform to kite surfing sports people, in April 2008, the International Kite boarding Association (IKA) was founded, after the International Sailing Federation (ISAF) had included the principle of surfers being propelled by a kite in the "ISAF Equipment Rules of Sailing." Kite boarding was then adopted in November 2008 as an ISAF international sailing class. Currently, campaigns are running to establish kite surfing as Olympic discipline at the Olympic Games 2016 in Rio de Janeiro (BRA).

8 Kite Surfing and Snow Kiting

Fig. 8.1 (**a**) Kite surfing allows for high velocity converting the propelling force of the kite into high speed on water. The kite forces are transferred to the kiter through the central lines and the belt harness. Spectacular jumps are possible, transforming the wind power into vertical lift power. (**b**) wave kite surfing. The surfer uses both the wind (kite) and the wave to increase performance (Courtesy of Ronen Topelberg)

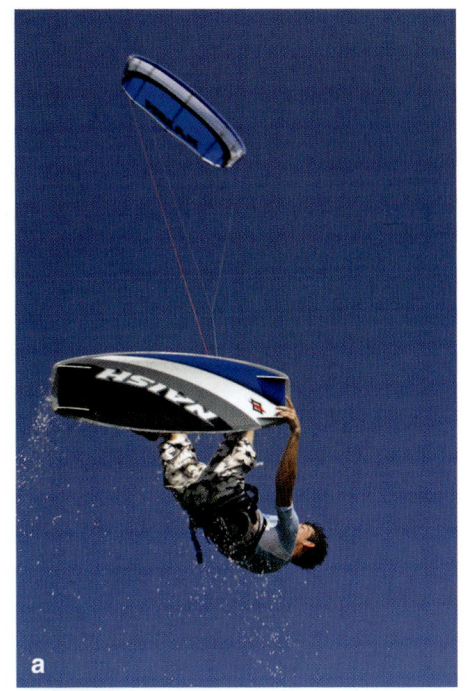

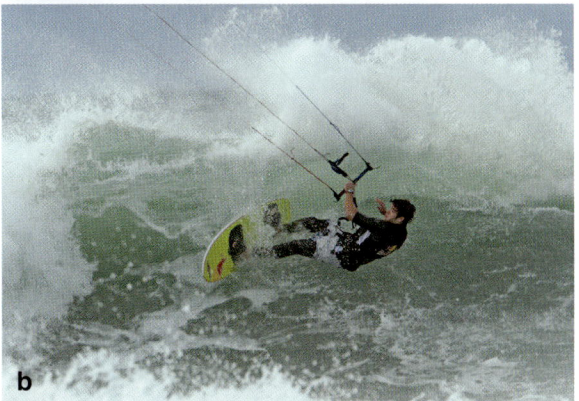

In the last decade, kite surfing (Fig. 8.1) became very popular, and nowadays at nearly every beach with favorable wind conditions, kite surfers can be admired doing spectacular jumps with flips and rotations. It almost looks like kite surfing passed windsurfing as the former dominant action-water sport in windy areas.

The idea of practicing kite surfing during the winter season in areas with sufficient snowfall and favorable wind conditions seemed to be a natural progression. Making use of the same principle of transforming the wind energy into a propelling force, snow kiters are able to reach high velocities (Fig. 8.2a, b), go uphill, and perform spectacular jumps (Fig. 8.3) because of the vertical lift created by the kite. The most

Fig. 8.2 (**a**) Snow kiting works according to the same principles as kite surfing. The skis used are freestyle skis with bidirectionality. The official high-speed world record for snow kiting is 111.2 km/h held by Hardy Brandstoetter. (**b**) Snow kiting is performed using snowboards, as well. The propelling force generated by the kite is transformed over the harness to the kiter (Courtesy of Hardy Brandstoetter)

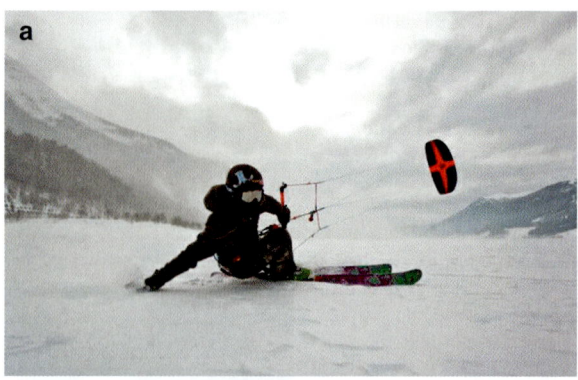

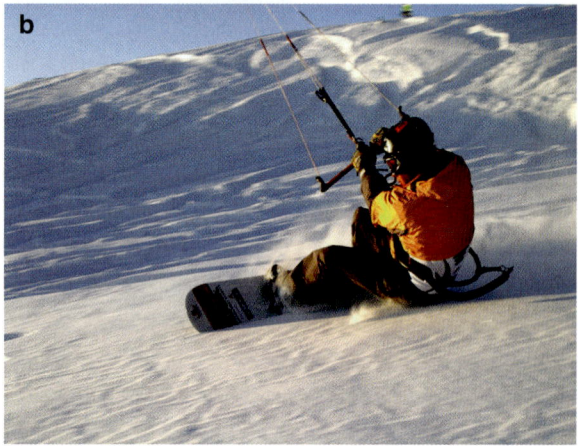

Fig. 8.3 Snow kiting using boards is similar to kite surfing. The freestyle design of the board allows for bidirectionality. The enormous wind forces allow the snow kiter to reach high-speed velocity (Courtesy of Hardy Brandstoetter)

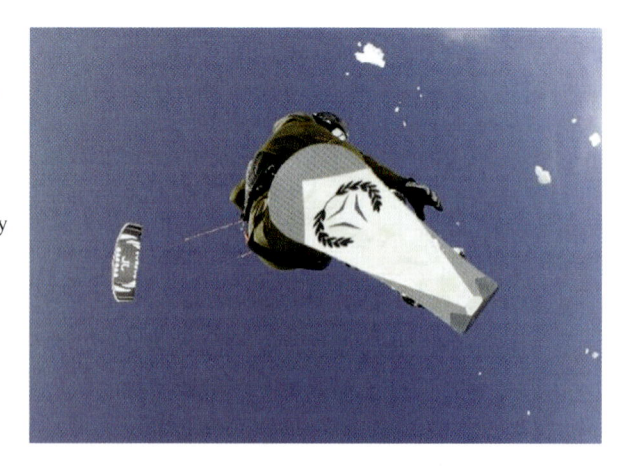

evident differences are the skis or snowboard they use to move on the snow and design of the kite. In contrast to kite surfers, who use tube kites with inflatable air chambers, snow kiters prefer foil kites with air cells to provide it with lift and a fixed bridle to maintain the C shape of the kite. Snow kiting is practiced all around the world, wherever you can find snow and enough wind. Many people practicing Kite surfing during the summer successfully started trying to snow kiting on snow-covered planes or frozen lakes by just combining the kite that they use for kite surfing with a snowboard or skis. Obviously, as the number of snow kiters grew, it did not take too long that special snow kite equipment was developed.

The Equipment Used: Essential and Safety Requirements

Kite Surfing

To practice kite surfing, a kite, board, harness, and other basic equipment are needed. The equipment has to be adjusted to the rider's weight, his skill level, and to water and wind conditions.

Board

Three different types of kite boards have to be distinguished: "twin tips," mutant boards, and directional surf-style boards. In contrast to conventional surfboards, all three types do not have any significant buoyancy, which develops hydrodynamically during the ride. In dependence on skill level, wind force, body weight, and kite size, the board dimensions have a length between 120 and 165 cm and a width ranging from 26 cm up to 45 cm. Twin-tip boards are similar to wakeboards showing bidirectionality. They are easy to learn and meanwhile became the most popular boards under both beginners and experts. They are symmetric regarding outline, shape, and order of the foot straps, allowing for maintenance of the foot position when changing the direction of surfing. Mutants represent a hybrid form between twin tips and directionals. Basically, it is designed for directional riding, but due to two fins at the bow, bidirectional surfing is possible. Finally, the directional board represents the mother of the kite surfing boards. It was taken from surfing and can be ridden only in one direction because of lacking fins at the bow and the spired shape. To change the direction, the foot position has to be changed as well.

Kite

Two major forms of power kites are available at the market. Leading edge inflatable (LEI) kites (known also as inflatables or C-kites) are produced from ripstop polyester with an inflatable main plastic tube at the front edge and separate smaller tubes (struts) perpendicular to the main bladder to form the chord of the kite. The air chambers are inflated before starting with a pressure of 0.4 to 0.6 bar. The air tubes save the shape of the kite and prevent sinking of the kite once dropped in the water.

This type of kite is favored by most of the kiters due to its quick and direct response to the rider's inputs, easy relaunchability, and stability. The next generation of LEI development was the flat LEI or bow kite. The C-shape profile was lower, and the main front tube had bowed ends, which gave the name to this type of kite. The most obvious advantage is the possibility to change the kite's angle of attack and to depower it completely, which represents a decisive key safety feature rendering it suitable for beginners. Hybrid or SLE (supported leading edge) kites are characterized by several lines fixing the front tube, achieving a high depower efficiency associated with improved cruising characteristics due to direct kite control. In 2007, delta-shape kites were introduced into the market. They are similar to bow kites and have four to five lines. The depower efficiency is extremely high, and the easy relaunchability makes them attractive for beginners.

In contrast to LEI kites, foil kites are similar to a paraglider and are suitable mostly on land, that is, for snow kiting. Foil kites with closed cells can be used also on the water, keeping the air inflated for longer time due to an inlet valve mechanism making relaunching the kite much easier. Usually, three lines are sufficient to control the kite; however, some have four.

The size of the kite depends on the wind force and on the weight of the rider. Usually, kite sizes range from 9 to 12 m^2. It always has to be kept in mind that doubling of the wind speed results into a fourfold increase of the kite power.

Lines and Bar

A typical kite has four lines with a length of 24–30 m. The lines that originate from the center part of the kite run medially through the handlebar and are connected to the kite surfer's harness through the so-called chicken loop. They provide the necessary propelling force to put the kite surfer into motion. The two lines, each originating from one edge of the kite, are firmly attached to the edges of the handlebar (Fig. 8.4). They enable the kite surfer to control and guide the kite by pulling on one end of the bar and pushing the other. A safety system comes as standard with most kites nowadays and represents an absolute essential. In case of an accident, the kite surfer can detach her or his harness from the chicken loop by activating the so-called quick-release system. When activating this system, the "chicken loop" releases the hook of the harness and the kite surfer only remains attached to the kite by a so-called kite leash which completely depowers the kite and does not produce any pull. The "depower" system reduces the kite's angle of attack to the wind, thereby catching less wind and reducing its propelling power. The safety leash enables the kite surfer to disconnect himself completely from the kite in exceptional situations.

Other Equipment

Aside from the board and kite, there is an armory of equipment that athletes need to have before getting out on the water, independently from the place where they ride.

Fig. 8.4 The handlebar allows the kiter to control and depower the kite. The central lines transfer the kite power to the kiter, who is attached by the so-called chicken loop to the harness. The two main safety tools are the quick-release system for immediate disengaging of the chicken loop from the harness in case of emergency and the kite leash, which in case of activation of the quick-release system, completely depowers the kite and does not produce any pull (Courtesy of Hardy Brandstoetter)

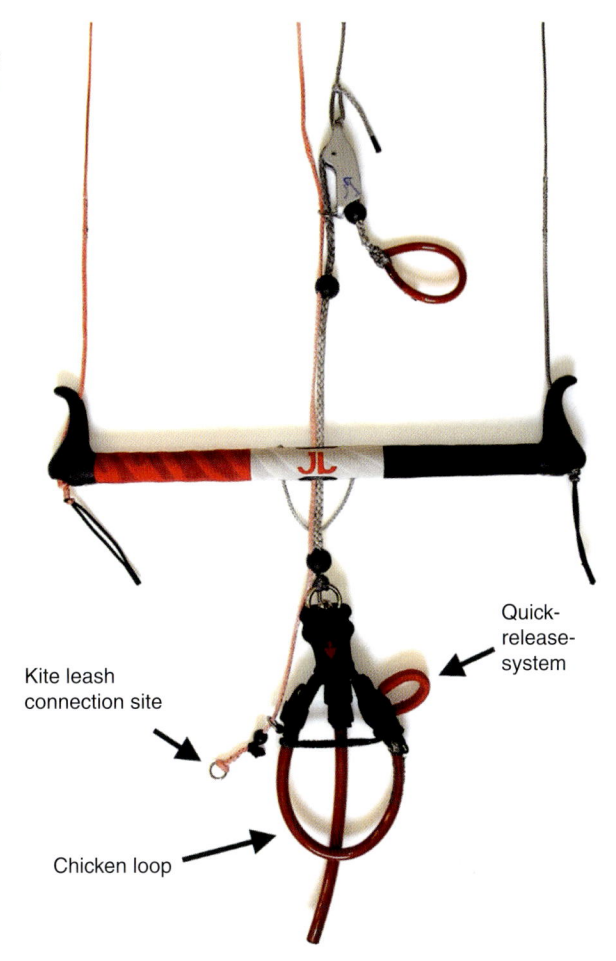

A harness is absolutely essential. It is generally available in two styles. The belt harness fits around the waist, and the seat harness is a full crotch fit. The seat version reduces the center of balance and pull, making boarding more stable. A further absolutely equipment essential is the wetsuit, available in thicknesses from 3 to 7 mm, depending on how cold it is likely to be. They come in different leg and arm lengths with a shorty suit in 3 mm for warm-water riding. Even in tropical waters, wetsuits can protect the kite surfer from crash landings and hypothermia. Flotation or buoyancy is mandatory with some belt-style harnesses now incorporating buoyancy. Another essential requirement is a helmet. There is no excuse for not wearing one since the risk for sustaining a head injury amounts to 15 % for these extreme sports. Furthermore, the use of a board leash is recommended. It attaches the board to the surfer's ankle or rear of the harness via a Velcro strap fastening and an approximately 3-m-long vinyl cord in order to avoid board loosening. A clear disadvantage is the increased risk of getting injured by the fixed board.

Prior to start, wind conditions should be analyzed. The wind strength influences the kite size and/or line length. In order to get adequate information, other kite surfers can be asked for the wind and sea conditions. However, an anemometer for self-measurement of the wind power should make part of the equipment.

As with any sports equipment, material failures may occur, and the kite surfer should be prepared for those cases. A puncture repair kit for the inflatable tubes represents an essential part of the equipment, as well as spare flying lines, a spare control bar, spare fins for the board, spare straps or bindings, and a spare harness.

Snow Kiting

Typically, snow kiters use regular freestyle snowboards and skis to practice snow kiting. Both, skis and boards, enable the snow kiter to run bidirectionally and to perform quick direction turns. Regarding the kite, however, special designs for use on snow are available. Kite surfers use so-called tube kites, which are kept in shape by an inflatable air chamber that prevents the kite from sinking in case it hits the water. Snow kiters, in contrast, tend to use the cheaper foil kites, which occupy less space when stored in a backpack and are easier to start and land. The kite sizes vary from 2 to 20 m^2, and the length of the lines ranges from 20 to 30 m. Lines, handlebar, and safety system including quick-release system and kite leash are the same as for kite surfing.

Further safety equipment often used are helmets (92 %) and spine protectors (51 %), while shoulder, hip, wrist, elbow, and knee protectors are more scarcely used.

Injury and Fatality Rates and Specific Types of Injury Related to Each Sport

Kite Surfing

The conversion of wind energy into speed and vertical lift power enables the kite surfer to perform fast runs and high jumps. The actual speed record is about 55.6 knots (102 km/h) held by the US-American Rob Douglas in 2010, reached at the Lüderitz Speed Challenge in Namibia. The highest documented jump reached 10 m (unofficially 48 m) and the longest, 250 m. In July 2007, Jessie Richman performed a 22-s jump in the Golden Gate, Bay of San Francisco, which is the longest jump documented to date. Enormous, often unpredictable natural forces expose the kite surfers to an increased risk for injuries and render kite surfing and snow kiting extreme sports.

The first report in the literature regarding injury types and rates among kite surfers was published in 2001 by Kristen and Kröner [1]. They reported retrospectively about the World Cup competition on the largest continental lake in Austria. The most severe injury in this series was a cervical spine fracture with a tetraparesis. However, most of the injuries were minor.

Similar injury rates and patterns have been reported by Petersen et al. in a more comprehensive survey study [2]. Retrospectively, 72 kite surfers have been analyzed during the 2001 season using a questionnaire. Injuries have been classified as severe in terms of polytrauma; moderate, requiring medical assistance; and minor, without the need for medical assistance. Thirty-one injuries have been registered, 5 moderate and 26 minor injuries resulting in an incidence of moderate kite injuries of 1 per 1,000 h and 5 per 1,000 h for minor injuries, respectively. In addition, kite injuries have been registered from surrounding trauma centers resulting in one polytrauma and three further moderate injuries. Most of the moderate injuries have been fractures involving the radius, fifth metacarpal, ankle, patella, or ribs. The most frequent mechanism leading to injury was a direct trauma against objects such as stones and boats lying on the beach. The most common reason for injury was lost of control over the kite on or close to the beach due to technical mistakes of the kite surfer, oversized kites, or the unfavorable wind conditions as onshore wind or gusts.

In the following year 2002, a prospective study including 235 kite surfers in northern Germany with an average age of 27.2 years was carried out by the same study group [3]. During a 6-month observational period, 124 injuries have been recorded resulting in a self-reported injury rate of 7.0 per 1,000 h of practice. One fatality and 11 severe injuries occurred during the study period. The most common injury types and regions interested are shown in Tables 8.1 and 8.2. Fifty-six percent of the injuries were attributed to the inability to detach the kite from the harness in a situation involving loss of control over the kite. A tendency was observed for athletes using a quick-release system to sustain fewer injuries than athletes without such a release system.

In 2005, Exadaktylos et al. [5] presented a prospectively observational study analyzing kite surfing-related air rescue missions in Cape Town, South Africa. During a 6-month period from 2003 to 2004, 30 kite surfing-related air rescue missions have been collected with 25 in support of the National Sea Rescue Institute (NSRI) and five based on primary rescue calls. Twenty-five accidents (83 %) were attrib-

Table 8.1 Affected body sites in cases of injury in kite surfing [3] and snow kiting [4]

Region	Kite surfing (%)	Snow kiting (%)
Head	13.7	15.2
Trunk	16.1	21.7
Shoulder/arm	1.6	15.2
Elbow	4	6.5
Forearm/wrist	11.3	4.3
Hip/thigh	2.4	6.5
Knee	12.9	17.4
Calf	5.6	4.3
Ankle/foot	28.2	4.3
Others	4.2	4.6

Table 8.2 Types of injury in kite surfing [3] and snow kiting [4]

Injury	Kite surfing (%)	Snow kiting (%)
Contusion	33.8	32.7
Joint sprain	9.7	15.2
Abrasion	27.4	13
Muscle strain	n.a.	8.7
Fracture	3.2	4.3
Shoulder dislocation	n.a.	4.3
Ligament rupture	1.6	4.3
Concussion	0.8	4.3
Laceration	19.9	4.3
Others	3.6	8.9

uted to the inability to detach the kite from the harness in a situation with loss of control over the kite. These were pure search missions supporting the NSRI. Five rescue missions (17 %) have been injury related. All five injured individuals were male. Two kite surfers were hit by their board and suffered fractures of the ankle, ribs, and humerus. Two other kite surfers were dragged into the open sea due to inability to detach the kite and suffered from hypothermia, and one patient experienced severe exhaustion and lacerations and contusions in the head and neck region. All individuals were rescued successfully with no fatal accidents.

In 2007, Spanjersberg and Schipper [6] from the Netherlands reported about a case series of severe kite surfing injuries with need for helicopter emergency medical service over a 3-year period. They distinguished four main types of trauma mechanism: (1) cuts and bruises owing to sharp edges and ropes or rocks, (2) high-energy trauma owing to frontal collision, (3) high-energy trauma owing to falls from height, that is, vertical deceleration trauma, and (4) drowning. Five patients have been included, with an Injury Severity Score (ISS) ranging from 3 to 75. The injury patterns varied from extremity fractures, spine fractures, bilateral dissection of the internal carotid arteries with left frontal lobe ischemia, and shoulder dislocation, and one patient suffered a fatal head injury. Main injury mechanism has been collision of the surfer with an object. The reason for these collisions was a loss of control, most likely owing to wind conditions.

In a recently published study, the risk of injury was highest for kite surfing compared to personal watercraft and towed water sports among recreational water users in Australia with an overall reported rate of 22.3 injuries per 100 h [7].

Snow Kiting

Due to the vertical lift of the kite, snow kiters are able to perform huge jumps. Sometimes, it even occurs that a snow kiter "takes off" involuntarily due to a strong wind gust and is not able to depower her or his kite in time using the quick-release system. Therefore, snow kiting conveys a great risk of injury, especially when considering the often hard surface the sport is performed on (e.g., frozen lakes). In a recent study performed at the authors' institution, 80 snow kiters from Austria, Germany, Italy, and Switzerland were surveyed over the course of one winter season to determine the injury rate, cause, and patterns [4]. The calculated injury rate was 8.4 injuries per 1,000 h of snow kiting, which is slightly higher than what was reported for kite surfers. No significant difference in injury rates was found between practice (8.5 injuries per 1,000 h of exposure) and competition (7.5 injuries per 1,000 h of exposure). The most commonly injured body part while snow kiting is the back, followed by the knee, shoulder, and head. Most snow kiting incidents result in contusions, abrasions, and joint sprains (Table 8.2).

When the snow kiters begin to perform at a higher level, for example, practicing high jump, rotations, and flips, injuries tend to become more severe. When compared with experts (5.1 injuries per 1,000 h of exposure), beginners had a significantly increased risk of getting injured (20.8 injuries per 1,000 h per exposure). When looking at the injury severity, beginners accounted for 10.4 mild injuries per 1,000 h of exposure, whereas experts sustained no mild injuries at all. Conversely, no severe injuries occurred in the beginner group, while expert snow kiters accounted for 4.1 severe injuries per 1,000 h of exposure. Interestingly, athletes using snowboards for snow kiting sustained three times more injuries than athletes using skis (11.7 vs. 4.1 injuries per 1,000 h of exposure, respectively). As a matter of fact, most snow kiting accidents occur while performing a jump. The same pattern can be observed in many extreme sports. The main causes of injury in snow kiting are riding errors caused by the athletes themselves, sudden wind gusts unexpectedly lifting the riders in the air, and poor snow conditions.

Common Treatments for Each Sport and Relevant Rehabilitation

Most injuries in kite surfing and snow kiting are minor or moderate. In the largest prospectively observed series reported in the literature regarding kite surfing injuries, only 10 % were severe injuries with one fatality due to polytrauma [3]. The relationship between moderate to minor injuries in this sport is 1:5. The distribution of injury severity is similar in snow kiting with a certain increased amount of severe and moderate injuries. The prospective study of snow kiting injuries published by the authors showed 61 % of injuries to be mild, 21 % to be moderate, and 18 % to be severe.

The treatment of injuries follows general treatment guidelines of trauma care and sports medicine. Mild injuries interest mainly skin abrasions or lacerations and can be handled by outpatient treatment with adequate wound care management. Obviously, kite surfers suffer more frequently from skin lesions, and wounds are often soiled in contrast to lacerations during snow kiting. Thus, adequate, quick primary wound care management with cleaning and disinfection represents an

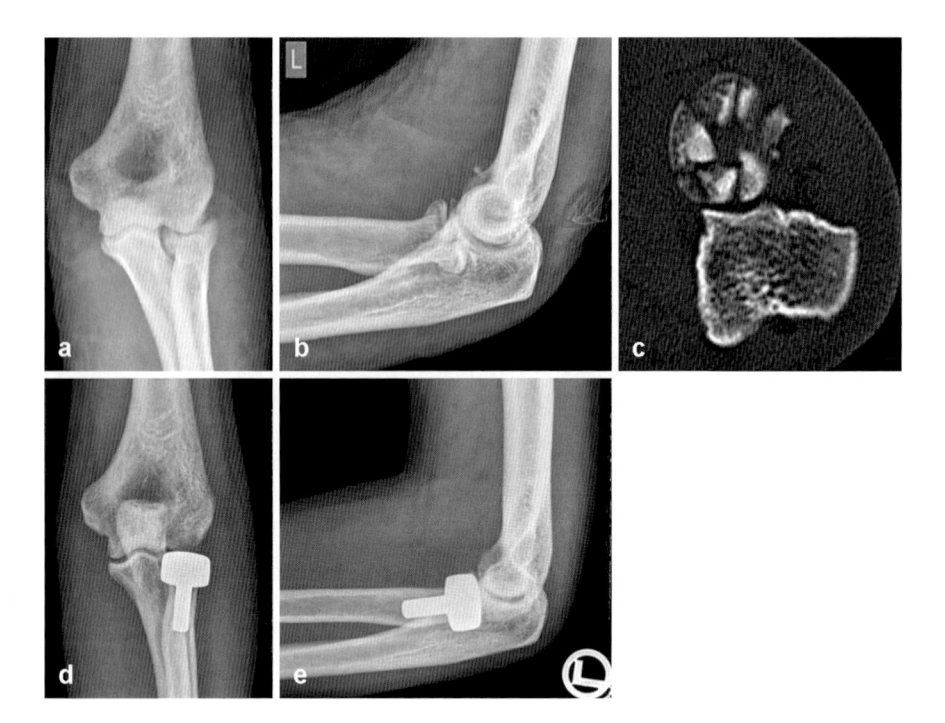

Fig. 8.5 Radiographs showing the left elbow of a 40-year-old male patient with a comminuted dislocation fracture of the radial head and concomitant rupture of the ulnar collateral ligament during kite surfing. Preoperative standard plain radiographs (**a** and **b**) were completed by a CT scan (**c**), which shows the real extent of radial head comminution. Surgical treatment addressed fixation of the ulnar collateral ligament avulsion and radial head replacement using a monopolar prosthetic design (**d** and **e**) (With permission from the American Journal of Sports Medicine [4])

important aspect already as first-aid measurement at the shore. Joint sprains, muscle sprains, and ligament injuries are treated conservatively as well, with functional treatment using splints or special joint orthoses.

Fractures represent the main part of moderate injuries. The decision on surgical or nonsurgical treatment depends on several factors and must be taken by the trauma surgeon individually (Fig. 8.5).

Head injuries are very frequent in kite surfing (13.7 %) and snow kiting (17.4 %). A gross neurological evaluation should be performed with assessment of the Glasgow Coma Scale. Signs of concussion have to be taken seriously with admission of the patient to the neurology ward for observation even in young patients.

Rehabilitation times are injury dependent and have to be assessed individually by the treating physician. An important aspect after long injury-related abstinence from sports represents the general physical condition and fitness. Recent physiological studies on kite surfing have shown that at light and mid-wind conditions (12–15 knots and 15–22 knots, respectively), up to 85 % of maximal heart rate and 80 % of maximal oxygen uptake are achieved, showing that a high-energy and physical demand is required for practice of this extreme sport [8, 9]. Thus, not only injury-specific rehabilitation measures should be taken to gain full convalescence, but general fitness and physical training programs are also recommended.

Proposed Prevention Measures

Kite surfing and snow kiting are extreme sports and are therefore potentially dangerous to both the kiters and others. These sports should not be attempted by beginners without appropriate instruction. Basically, kite flying skills, basic water and snow skills, and basic boarding skills are recommended as minimum competence levels before practicing. This includes all aspects of safe handling of kites on land and water, the ability to launch and land unaided on a specific spot on land, bodysurfing with kite along and back to shore, water launching onto board, getting on a board and traveling a distance under kite power, emergency stop in every situation stopping with the kite aloft, and returning to base on land either by kite boarding, paddling, or bodysurfing home.

All kite surfers and snow kiters are required to respect general safety guidelines, as staying clear of power lines and overhead obstructions or avoiding dangerous weather conditions such as thunderstorms. Kites hitting the water may look like planes crashing, which can be misinterpreted by the uninitiated and lead to false alarming of the coast guard or the beach warden. If kiting off shore or off the piste, an accompanying kiter should be present.

An often underestimated risk factor is the power of the wind. To assess the adequate wind power, the kiter should be able to walk backward when the kite is flying overhead with a minimum power. If this is not the case, the kite is too big or the wind too strong. A wind meter should be in every kiter's bag to get a realistic idea regarding the wind conditions, which never should be underestimated.

The use of an open quick-release harness system is of crucial importance for safe practice for both extreme sports, kite surfing and snow kiting. A sportsman tethered to the kite with a close system has no chance to disconnect himself from the wind power, which can be fatal in unexpected situations on water/snow or gusts. Further factors regarding the equipment should be taken into consideration. Every product has its limitations, which are depictured by the manufacturer's instructions and safety guidelines and have to be followed. A regular check and maintenance of the equipment are necessary to warrant its safety.

A list of prevention measurements and the associated preventions for kite surfing are shown in Table 8.3.

Certain prevention measures should be considered when snow kiting. Beginners should be introduced to this sport by a professional instructor or more advanced rider in order to be informed about the correct technique, favorable wind and snow conditions, adequate equipment, and potential hazards to be aware of. It is also recommendable to first learn how to snowboard/ski and how to guide a kite separately, before combining the two sports in terms of snow kiting. For every snow kiter, it is of great importance to know the local wind and weather conditions very well. An

Table 8.3 Prevention measures and preventions

	Measures	Prevention
1	Use of a "quick-release system"	Collision trauma after loss of control over the kite
2	Use of adequate kite sizes	Loss of control over the kite
3	Accurate weather observation	Loss of control over the kite
4	Avoid storm conditions (Beaufort >8)	Collision trauma
		Loss of control over the kite
5	Performance of tricks and jumps with a safe distance to the shore or other obstacles	Collision trauma
6	Learning under professional instruction	Technical errors due to theoretical lacks
7	*Wearing a helmet if a board leash is used*	Head injuries
8	Use of a kite leash	Collisions, injuries of other water users or people on the beach
9	Delimitation of kite areas	Collisions, injuries of other water users or people on the beach
10	Kite surfing lee sided to other water users	Collisions, injuries of other water user
11	Not surfing next to cliffs or dikes in case of onshore wind	Vertical lift due to upcurrent

unexpected weather change and the sudden occurrence of strong wind gusts can bring a snow kiter into great danger when not reacting properly. A snow kiter should also pay attention to choose the right spot to practice snow kiting. Many snow kiters like to perform their sport on frozen lakes. Due to the hard landing on the ice in case of an accident, these spots convey an increased risk of injury. A field covered with sufficient powder snow is certainly safer, especially when performing jumps. Still, in that case, it must be paid close attention that no obstacles, such as fences, are hidden underneath the deep powder snow. Areas where electricity poles or trees are located downwind of the snow kiting spot should be avoided for obvious reasons. Regarding safety equipment, every snow kiter should wear a helmet and also a back protector. Both the spine and the back are at great risk of injury when trying high jumps on a hard surface such as snow or ice. Of course, many other kinds of protectors that are available can be of benefit in case of an accident and should be considered. A safety device that every snow kiter should be equipped with is the quick-release system. In case of emergency, a snow kiter needs to be able to detach her- or himself from the kite as quickly as possible. Unfortunately, even when using a quick-release system, it often occurs that a rider is suddenly lifted in the air by a wind gust, before she or he is able to react properly and activate the system. Similarly, if snow kiters hit their head in an accident and become unconscious, the release system cannot be activated and the kite keeps dragging the injured kiter. The development of more advanced (maybe even automatically activating) devices is admittedly difficult but would increase the safety of the riders significantly, when functioning properly.

Finally, both sports, kite surfing and snow kiting, have to be seen under the light of extreme sports. This means all people practicing these sports should be in excellent physical conditions and in top form. Muscular power, endurance, and mental strength for practice under competition conditions are required for athletes. Thus, a special physical preparation before the season makes sense for untrained athletes. The training should focus on endurance, strength, and balance and flexibility in order to resist physical demands and to reduce the risk of injury.

All in all, it can be said that the upcoming extreme sports kite surfing and snow kiting belong to the most action-packed and fascinating sports available on water and snow. In certain ways, they add a new dimension to surfing and to snowboarding and skiing, allowing for huge jumps and stunning hang time. Of course, as every extreme sport, they convey a certain risk of injury. However, with the right instructions, equipment, and safety precautions, those risks can be limited.

References

1. Kristen K, Kröner A. Kite surfing-Surfen mit Lenkdrachen, Präsentation und Risikoabschätzung einer neuen Trendsportart. Sportorthopädie Sporttraumatologie. 2001;17:6.
2. Petersen W, Hansen U, Zernial O, Nickel C, Prymka M. Mechanisms and prevention of Kite surfing injuries. Sportverletz Sportschaden. 2002;16(3):115–21.
3. Nickel C, Zernial O, Musahl V, Hansen U, Zantop T, Petersen W. A prospective study of Kite surfing injuries. Am J Sports Med. 2004;32(4):921–7.
4. Moroder P, Runer A, Hoffelner T, Frick N, Resch H, Tauber M. A prospective study of snowkiting injuries. Am J Sports Med. 2011;39(7):1534–40.
5. Exadaktylos AK, Sclabas GM, Blake I, Swemmer K, McCormick G, Erasmus P. The kick with the kite: an analysis of kite surfing related off shore rescue missions in Cape Town, South Africa. Br J Sports Med. 2005;39(5):e26.
6. Spanjersberg WR, Schipper IB. Kite surfing: when fun turns to trauma-the dangers of a new extreme sport. J Trauma. 2007;63(3):E76–80.
7. Pikora TJ, Braham R, Hill C, Mills C. Wet and wild: results from a pilot study assessing injuries among recreational water users in Western Australia. Int J Inj Contr Saf Promot. 2011;18(2):119–26.
8. Camps A, Vercruyssen F, Brisswalter J. Variation in heart rate and blood lactate concentration in freestyle kytesurfing. J Sports Med Phys Fitness. 2011;51(2):313–21.
9. Vercruyssen F, Blin N, L'Huillier D, Brisswalter J. Assessment of physiological demand in Kite surfing. Eur J Appl Physiol. 2009;105(1):103–9.

Chapter 9
Windsurfing

Daryl A. Rosenbaum and Bree Simmons

Contents

Origins and Development of the Sport	189
Equipment and Basic Technique	192
Injuries	192
Incidence	192
Lower Extremities	194
Upper Extremities	197
Back Pain	198
Brain and Spinal Cord Injury	199
Common Skin Problems	199
Infectious Diseases	200
Injury Prevention	200
Summary	201
References	202

Origins and Development of the Sport

People have practiced using a flat platform and an attached sail for movement across water for millennia. Centuries ago, Polynesians were known to use these sailed boards for day trips across the open seas [1].

D.A. Rosenbaum, M.D. (✉)
Department of Family and Community Medicine,
Wake Forest University School of Medicine,
1920 W 1st Street, Suite #3, Winston Salem, NC, 27104, USA
e-mail: drosenba@wakehealth.edu

B. Simmons, M.D.
Sports Medicine, St. Vincent Health,
Joshua Max Simon Primary Care Center,
8414 Naab Rd, Suite 160, Indianapolis, IN 46260, USA
e-mail: bsimm002@stvincent.org

In 1948, Newman Darby of Pennsylvania designed the first small catamaran with a handheld sail and rig mounted on a universal joint [2]; however, other sources recognize British inventor Peter Chilvers as the originator of windsurfing. In 1958, at the age of 12, he also attached a sail on an upright pole to a board by a free-moving universal joint [3]. But it was Californians Jim Drake and Hoyle Schweitzer who finally patented the "windsurfer" in 1970. They credited Darby's and Chilvers' ideas as major influences on their final construction [2].

Though windsurfing may be considered a minimalistic version of sailing, its athletes enjoy skills and tricks well beyond the scope of any other sailing craft design [4]. Windsurfers, also called sailors or board heads, can perform jumps, inverted loops, spinning maneuvers, and other "freestyle" moves. They were the first to ride the world's largest waves, such as Jaws off the island of Maui [4].

Drake and Hoyle marketed their product well, and its popularity boomed in the late 1970s, leading to windsurfing becoming an Olympic sport in 1984. There are now eight recognized disciplines: Olympic Windsurfing Class, Formula Windsurfing Class, Raceboard Class, Slalom, Super X, Speed Racing, Freestyle and Wavesailing.

Olympic windsurfing is a racing event in which all competitors use the same windsurf equipment. These "One Design" boards allow for performance in a range of sailing conditions. The 2012 Olympic Games in London will use the RS:X, a 9-ft, 5-in.-longboard weighing 15.5 kg with a daggerboard (retractable keel) and a sail based on the Neil Pryde formula windsurfing sail RS4 [5].

Formula windsurfing was developed in the mid-1990s. The boards in this class of windsurfing are regulated by the International Sailing Federation and have a maximum width of 1 m and a maximum single fin length of 70 cm. They have large sails up to 12.5 m^2 in size to facilitate high performance in light and moderate winds. Within these parameters, the equipment can be modified to suit the preferences of the sailor and maximize his or her speed. The racecourse is usually a box shape with longer downwind and upwind legs, and events are usually held on "flat water" as opposed to coastal surf. Formula windsurfing represents one of the fastest course-racing sailing crafts on the water.

Raceboarding uses longer windsurf boards with a daggerboard and movable mast rail. Sailors typically race in an Olympic triangle course.

Slalom involves high-speed racing on one of two types of courses: a figure-of-eight course or a downwind course. Boards are small and narrow and require high winds between 9 and 35 knots.

The super X class is a cross between freestyle and slalom, requiring sailors to race a short downwind slalom course and perform tricks along the way.

Under the ISAF, the International Speed Windsurfing Class organizes speedsurfing competitions. These events are made up of heats sailed on a 500-m course, and the average of a sailor's two fastest times is used to determine a winner.

Freestyle windsurfing is a judged event. Sailors perform tricks, and the winner usually has the greatest repertoire or completes the most stunts. Performing stunts on both the port and starboard areas of the board and performing them while fully planing score the sailor higher marks.

Wavesailing is the most "extreme" discipline within windsurfing and includes both wave riding and wave jumping (Fig. 9.1a, b). Wave jumping involves similar

9 Windsurfing

Fig. 9.1 Wave jumping and wave riding (Photos: Ronen Topelberg)

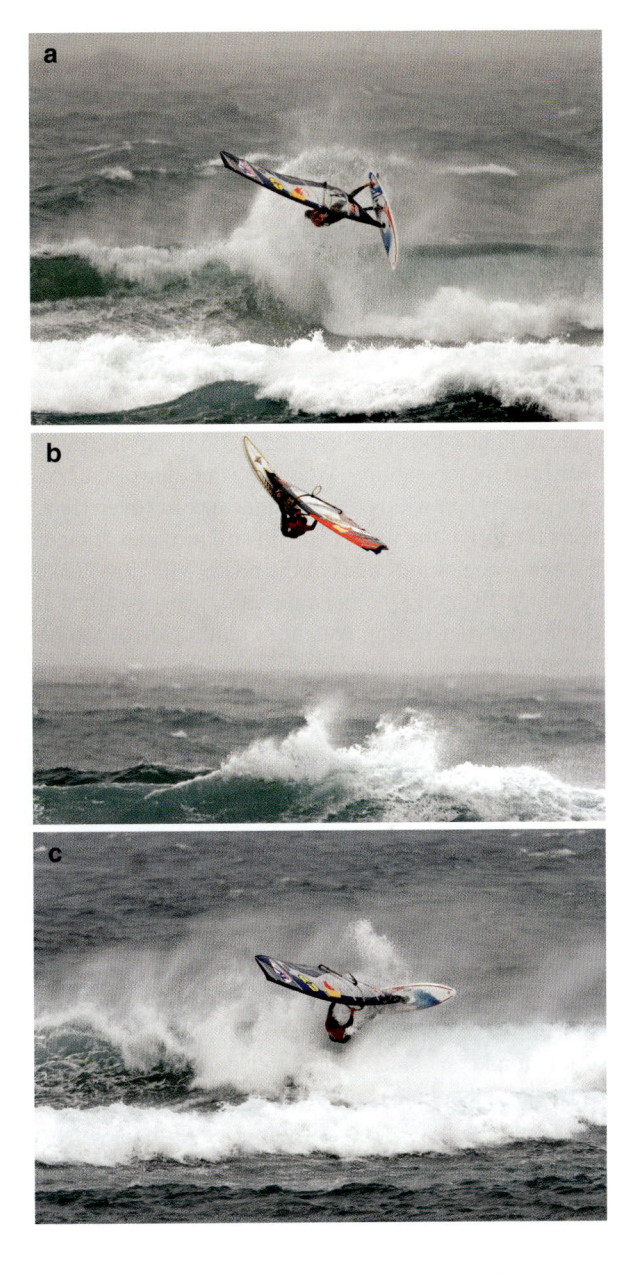

stunts as performed in freestyle but uses the peak of an unbroken wave like a ramp. The stunts therefore are more aerial in nature and allow the competitor to complete single and double rotations in the air. Wave riding is very similar to surfing and involves some turning and cutbacks while the sailor rides an unbroken wave to shore. Since this type of windsurfing requires very specific conditions of large waves and strong winds, it is difficult to organize competitions in advance. Most world-class wavesailing occurs in freeriding sessions.

Equipment and Basic Technique

The main piece of equipment is an 8- to 12-ft-long plastic or fiberglass-covered board with fins on the underside of the stern. Synthetic sails of varying sizes can be attached to a free-pivoting mast that rises from the center of the board. The windsurfer holds on to a chest-high boom. An optional harness attached to the boom supports the waist, allows the body weight to counteract the pull of the wind, and relieves pressure on the arms and lower back. The feet can be inserted under straps at the rear of the board for improved stability and steering in high winds. Additional equipment includes a wet or dry suit, footwear, helmet, and personal flotation device; however, there are no specific laws or guidelines dictating their use.

A sailboard will move by either sailing or hydroplaning (planing). Sailing takes place in light winds and involves the hull moving through the water using a centerboard and fin for stability. Weighting one side of the board or sinking the tail changes direction. When winds reach higher speeds (over 10–15 knots), the board begins to plane the top of the water. The fin still provides some lateral resistance for stability. Engaging one of the edges of the board will "jibe" or "carve" or turn the board over the water. Bringing the mast forward or backward will help steer the board during sailing, but transferring weight to either side of the board is the primary means of controlling the board during planing.

Injuries

Incidence

Despite routinely reaching speeds of 30 mph and jumps of 10–15 ft, windsurfing is a relatively safe sport. One retrospective study found approximately 1 injury per 1,000 sailing days [6]. A retrospective study comparing injury epidemiology in competitive raceboarders, competitive wave/slalom boarders, and recreational windsurfers found an annual injury incidence of just 1.0, 2.0, and 1.2, respectively [7].

Due to the unique equipment used and the often extreme conditions of wind and water, serious injuries do occur. A study performed in Greece in 2002 found 22 cases of severe accidents sustained during windsurfing in the Aegean Sea during a 12-month period. Prolonged hospitalizations, severe disability, and two deaths occurred as a consequence of the injuries. The types of accidents included drowning and near-drowning, spine fracture, concussion, facial fracture, shoulder dislocation and fracture, lower limb fracture, and large or deep lacerations [8].

The most common types of injuries include sprains (26.3 %), lacerations (21.2 %), contusions (16.2 %), and fractures (14.2 %) [6]. One more recent study found muscle/tendon strains to account for as much as a third of all injuries [7] (Chart 9.1). Less common occurrences include dislocations, disk herniations, jellyfish stings, hypothermia, near drowning, and concussions [6].

The most frequently affected body areas of windsurfers are the lower extremities (44.6 % of acute injuries), the upper extremities (18.5 %), the head and neck (17.8 %), and the trunk (16 %) [6] (Chart 9.2).

Injuries can be specific to the skill level of the athlete and surfing discipline. In general, wave/slalom windsurfers have more new and recurrent injuries compared to raceboarders and recreational windsurfers [7].

The longer, heavier boards used in raceboarding can lend to more chronic tendinopathies and muscle strains compared to the other disciplines. A British study in 2006 found that muscle and tendon strains made up over half of all injuries in raceboarders [7].

For wave/slalom windsurfers, collision with equipment in powerful winds and high waves are a major contributory factor to injury occurrence [7].

Ligament sprains in the ankle and foot are more common in recreational windsurfers, while ligamental injuries of the knee are more common in the wave/slalom athletes [7].

The prevalence of back strain is significant in all groups. Uphauling the sail out of the water seems to be a particularly risky maneuver for lumbar muscular strain in longboard sailors [7] (Fig. 9.2). The risk of acute injuries is greater in high winds, while chronic lower back pain occurs predominately during lighter wind conditions, likely due to prolonged maintenance of a lordotic posture [9].

During strong wind conditions, women have nearly twice the incidence of injury of men [9]. This is the only reported gender difference in injury epidemiology to date.

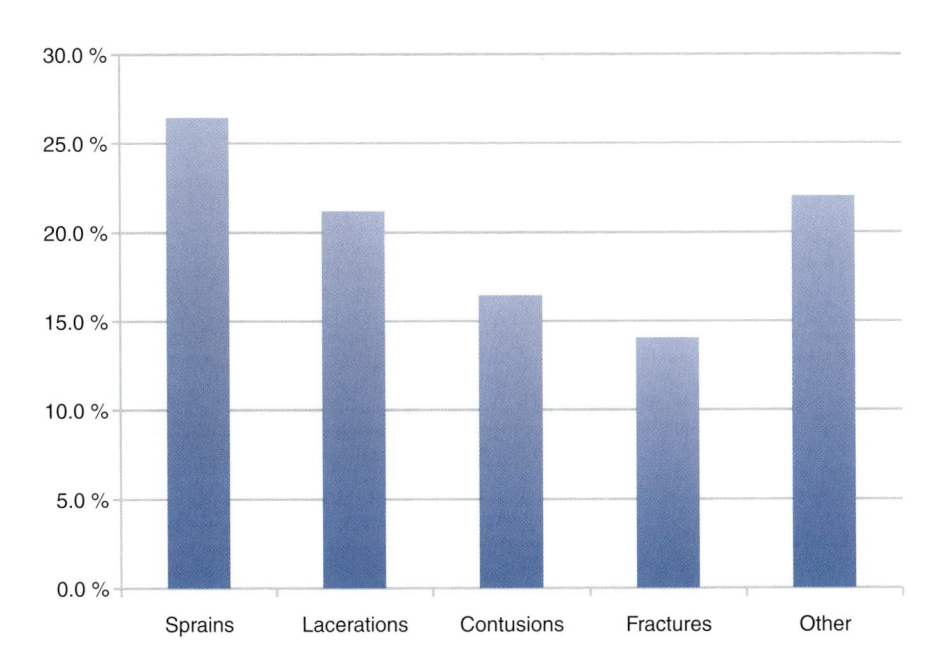

Chart 9.1 Windsurfing injuries by type

Injury distribution

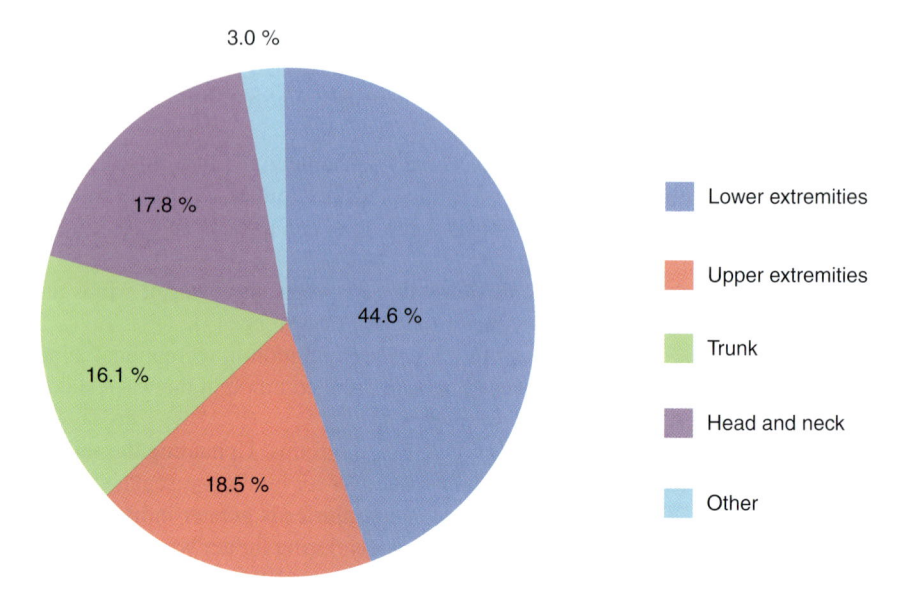

Chart 9.2 Windsurfing injuries by body area affected

Fig. 9.2 Uphauling a sail on a longboard

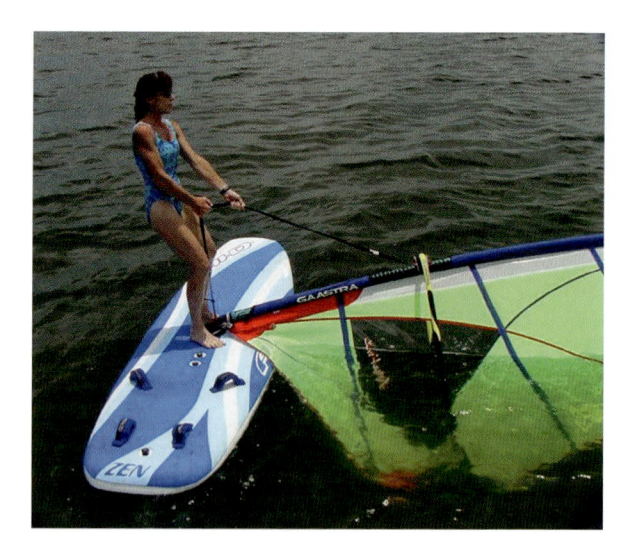

Lower Extremities

Injuries to the ankles and feet can be quite severe, and nearly half are fractures or ligament damage [6]. About 75 % of fractures and ligament injuries result from falling while the foot is engaged in the strap [6]. Being thrown off the sailboard with the strap still across the dorsum of the foot can apply significant counteractive forces across the ankle and foot.

Lisfranc Dislocation or Fracture

The common traumatic mechanism of the foot strap mandates high suspicion for a Lisfranc dislocation or fracture in any windsurfer with midfoot pain, especially if the pain is reproduced by passive pronation and abduction of the forefoot while the hindfoot is fixed. Weight-bearing radiographs in the anteroposterior and lateral planes plus a 30° oblique view should be obtained to look for the characteristic findings.

The x-ray findings for Lisfranc fracture can be subtle and are missed in as many as 20 % of cases [10] (Fig. 9.3 – collage). Comparison views of the other foot can help the clinician distinguish between subtle and normal x-ray findings. If initial radiographs appear negative, vigilance is still required because this injury may not always be evident on plain films. Continued midfoot pain and swelling and difficulty bearing weight 3–5 days post-injury demand further imaging, such as a computed tomography scan [11].

Some minor tarsometatarsal sprains may be treated nonsurgically with casts, but Lisfranc injuries usually require referral to an orthopedic surgeon. Most authors feel that surgical fixation is necessary to achieve precise anatomic reduction [10–13]. Early and accurate diagnosis is the best way to prevent long-term morbidity.

Knee and Leg Injuries

There are two case reports of injury to the lower leg due to foot fixation. A 27-year-old man fractured his lower leg, and an 18-year-old man sustained an ACL and MCL rupture during windsurfing. In both cases, the patients reported a twisting force on their legs and their feet being fixed in foot straps [14].

Chronic Injuries

Foot straps have also been blamed for two cases of extensor digitorum longus tendonitis published in the windsurfing literature. The persistent loading that foot straps create across the midfoot during planing was the proposed mechanism [15]. In both cases, the surfers were positioning their straps across the metatarsophalangeal joints as opposed to the midfoot. Treatments with rest, nonsteroidal anti-inflammatory drugs, physiotherapy, and repositioning the feet with the straps across the midfoot were successful. The surfers returned to full activity.

Thus, there is some controversy regarding foot straps from an injury prevention perspective. Certainly, a quick release mechanism is desirable to prevent the described fracture and ligament injuries. However, ideal placement of the straps is

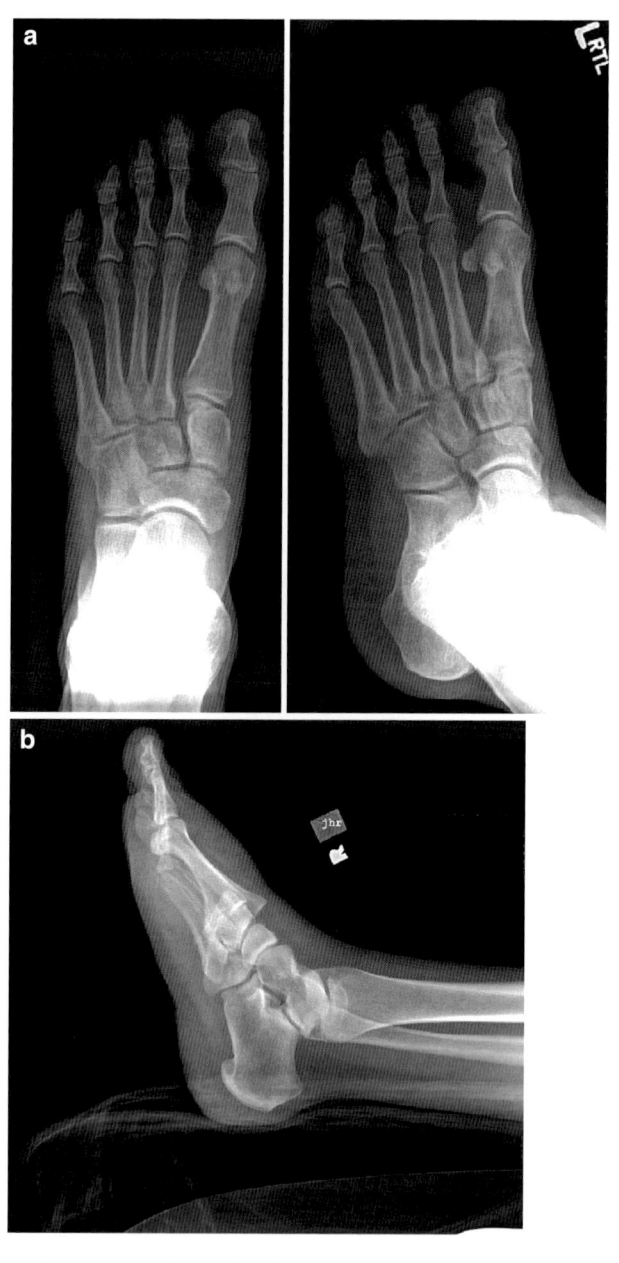

Fig. 9.3 *Lisfranc joint injury radiographs*: AP view (*left*), notice subtle widening between base of first and second metatarsals and lack of congruence between the medial edges of the second metatarsal and second cuneiform. A positive "fleck sign", not present in this example, would be a small avulsion fragment off the base of the second metatarsal found in this same space. Oblique view (*right*): look for lack of alignment between the medial edges of the third metatarsal and third cuneiform (not found in this example). Lateral view, look for a step off deformity when tracing a line along the superior aspect of the second metatarsal to the tarsals

less clear. Though any position comes with its inherent risks, it seems that placing the foot so that the strap crosses the metatarsophalangeal joint avoids a more severe acute injury such as the Lisfranc fracture while risking the development of a less severe condition such as extensor digitorum tendonitis.

Upper Extremities

Shoulder Dislocation

The classic windsurfing injury of the upper extremity is a shoulder dislocation. The usual mechanism involves hanging on to the boom during a fall, which can anteriorly dislocate the humeral head. We have not seen a posterior shoulder dislocation from windsurfing.

On the scene, an attempt at reduction can be made before muscle spasm sets in but only if the care provider is experienced with shoulder injuries. It is important to perform a complete neurovascular exam of the injured limb, including an assessment of deltoid contraction, before reduction is attempted to determine if an associated axillary nerve injury is present. If reduction is not attempted, the arm should be immobilized in the adducted position before transporting the patient to emergency care.

Nerve Injuries

Peripheral nerve injuries due to blunt trauma, acute stretch, and exertional compression have been reported in the literature.

In one case study, a 21-year-old male experienced a sharp daggerlike pain in his shoulder while uphauling. He later developed posterior shoulder muscle atrophy and weakness consistent with a suprascapular neuropathy. EMG study results at that time were not made available, but following 6 months of conservative therapy and rest, the patient was asymptomatic and returned to windsurfing without limitation [3].

A 3-year study by Ciniglio et al. identified 23 windsurfers with exertional upper extremity pain, paresthesia, and weakness compatible with transient compression of the posterior interosseus nerve during windsurfing. All athletes complained of exertional weakness of the wrist extensor muscles. Symptoms were relieved by elbow flexion, wrist flexion, supination, and support with the contralateral hand. A retrospective analysis of the 23 athletes' windsurfing positions noted that 19 held the boom with their forearms in pronation. All athletes were treated with 2 weeks of rest, given physiotherapy, massage, and ultrasound therapy. They were coached to hold the boom with the forearm in supination. The majority of the athletes reported complete alleviation. Symptoms eventually returned in only five athletes, and they were treated with casting of the elbow at 90° with the forearm supinated and wrist in neutral position for 10 days. One of the casted athletes had recurrent symptoms, and surgical exploration of his posterior interosseus nerve revealed fibrosis in the arcade of Frohse where it contacts the nerve [3].

Even in supination, a windsurfer can be at risk for nerve entrapment. Prolonged contraction of the biceps in a flexed arm holding the boom can compress the lateral antebrachial cutaneous nerve (LAC) as it passes under the biceps aponeurosis. A 19-year-old woman presented 3 weeks after developing pain and paresthesia in the right forearm following a long day of windsurfing. Her exam showed that the pain in the radial aspect of her forearm was reproduced by extension at the elbow. She also had a well-defined area of hypersensitivity to touch and decreased sensitivity to pin stimuli in the distribution of the LAC. Tinel's sign was absent, but she had tenderness to palpation and percussion just lateral to the biceps tendon at the elbow. EMG confirmed the diagnosis of LAC neuropathy, and she was treated with methylprednisolone. This relieved the pain but left a numb sensation. She was able to return to windsurfing, but the decreased sensation was still present at 1-year follow-up [3].

Back Pain

Low-back pain is one of the most common chronic conditions that affect windsurfing athletes. More common in longboard sailors [6], it seems to be aggravated by increased sailing duration in light winds [16], suggesting that maintaining a static posture of lumbar lordosis for prolonged periods may fatigue and strain low-back muscles. Especially with a longboard, repetitive uphauling may place flexion overload on the lower back if done with poor technique (Fig. 9.2). Theoretically, this flexion load could lead to a strain of the lumbar extensors or even disk disruption or herniation. Preventive measures include using a waist harness (when conditions and experience allow) or doing a pelvic tilt to relieve some of the continuous burden on the back and strengthening the trunk muscles with exercises, such as prone leg extension.

Shortboard, high-wind sailors are not immune to low-back injury. In fact, Locke and Allen [16] found an increased incidence of disk protrusions and pars interarticularis defects in a small group of elite windsurfers compared to the general population. They theorized that gusting winds and higher waves or twisted posture and fatigue put enough stress on the spine to produce pathologic changes. Prolonged hyperextension of the lumbar spine from leaning back too far in the harness could also explain the increased incidence of pars fractures.

If a pars defect is suspected based on history and physical exam, then AP, lateral, and oblique view plain radiographs of the lumbar spine should be obtained. If suspicion is high but radiographs are normal, then advanced imaging is recommended using single-photon emission computed tomographic (SPECT) scan followed by computed tomographic (CT) imaging or magnetic resonance imaging (MRI). Once the diagnosis is made, most patients do well with conservative care. This can include relative rest, lumbar corset bracing for 3–6 weeks, and extension-limiting bracing for 3–6 months depending on the athlete. Osseous healing is not necessary for full return to activity, though it is desirable [17].

Brain and Spinal Cord Injury

A fall from the board or a strike from the board or boom can cause skull fractures, concussions, spine fracture dislocations, burst fractures, wedge compression fractures, and spinal cord injuries [3]. Patel et al. published a report of two windsurfers with transient thoracic spinal cord pathology that may have been ischemic in origin. In one case, a 19-year-old demonstrated bilateral brisk reflexes, flexor weakness of the lower extremities, and a left-sided sensory level at T10 after windsurfing in rough weather. In the other case, a 30-year-old presented after windsurfing in similar conditions with a sensory deficit to pain and temperature at the level of T7 on the right and increased tone with ankle clonus in the left lower extremity. Both had only thoracic spine degeneration on CT myelography and had normal CSF and evoked potential studies. Both made full recoveries with only conservative therapy [3].

Common Skin Problems

Other than sprains, the most common injury suffered by windsurfers is a laceration, usually to the head or lower extremity [5, 18]. The usual cause is from contact with the fins or other parts of the equipment, but lacerations can also result from hitting rocks, coral, shells, and other underwater objects. To avoid infection, athletes should avoid exposing wounds to salt water for at least 48 h after repair to allow time for a waterproof and bacteria-resistant epithelial bridge to form [19].

Jellyfish pose another hazard. Of the 73 athletes who responded to a questionnaire, 26% had been stung by jellyfish while windsurfing [17]. Jellyfish stings should be immediately rinsed with seawater. Avoid using fresh water or rubbing the affected area; both may cause remaining nematocysts to discharge venom. Follow with a vinegar rinse to interrupt envenomation, and then apply a cool compress and a topical preparation such as hydrocortisone cream to soothe the area [20].

Like other water sports, enthusiastic windsurfers are at risk for two classic causes of a pruritic red papular rash [21]. Seabather's eruption or "sea lice" occurs in areas of high friction and those covered by swimwear after exposure to ocean water. It is caused by the venom of *Linuche unguiculata* or "thimble jellyfish" larvae that are found in the ocean waters of the southern United States, Caribbean, and South America. Treatment is symptomatic with topical corticosteroids and oral antihistamines. Prevention involves removing swimwear and showering as soon as possible after exiting the water.

Cercarial dermatitis or "swimmer's itch" is caused by the burrowing larval trematodes of *Schistosoma* and *Trichobilharzia* that can be found in freshwater. As the parasites die upon entering human skin, treatment is also symptomatic with oral antihistamines. Applying either a niclosamide plus water-resistant sunscreen formulation or Safe Sea™, a cream originally designed to prevent jellyfish stings, before entering the water [22] or brisk toweling after exiting can decrease risk.

Infectious Diseases

Windsurfing is often tolerated on waters judged unsafe for swimming because of pollution [23]. Significant health hazards can result from exposure to contaminated water. The 1984 Windsurfer Western Hemisphere Championships were held in Quebec City on the St. Lawrence River in the Baie de Beauport, an area contaminated by sewage. A team of physicians conducted a prospective study measuring the incidence of gastroenteritis, otitis, conjunctivitis, and skin infections in competitors compared to staff controls. They found a relative risk of 5.5 for gastrointestinal symptoms and an average relative risk of 2.1 for all skin symptoms, otitis, and conjunctivitis. Competitors were more likely to complain of symptoms if they fell into the water more than 30 times in the 9-day competition.

In 2004, Ulusarac and Carter published an article reviewing a case of Vibrio vulnificus infection in a windsurfer [24]. A 27-year-old male was struck by lightning while windsurfing off the coast of Pensacola, Fla. He was found pulseless in the water and was resuscitated and intubated by emergency medical personnel and transported to a nearby hospital. During his hospital course, he was found to have compartment syndrome in all four extremities and underwent emergency fasciotomies. Blood cultures grew *V. vulnificus* and *Enterobacter aerogenes*. Despite developing ARDS and requiring repeat fasciotomies of all four extremities, the patient did eventually recover and was discharged from the hospital in stable condition.

Injury Prevention

The first and most obvious safety tip is to be prepared. In an Internet survey by Peterson et al. analyzing acute injuries in 327 German windsurfers, the athletes underestimated wind conditions for 7.3 % of accidents [25]. Sailors should study local water currents, obstacles, wind patterns, weather, and boat traffic and choose an area that matches their ability. A windsurfing board is considered a sailing vessel, so the athlete must follow the usual rules of sailing and respect others in the same area. Sailing with a buddy can ensure that help is available in case of injury or equipment failure.

Protective gear is another important part of windsurfing safety. Helmets help avoid lacerations, concussions, and other head trauma. Helmets designed and certified for water sports (e.g., windsurfing, waterskiing, wakeboarding) have a light, impact-resistant plastic shell with a padded liner that drains water and provides adequate peripheral vision and hearing. Beginners should always wear helmets when sailing because of the risk of being struck if the mast is released during a fall. More experienced windsurfers should wear a helmet when sailing in crowded areas or when performing high-speed or aerial maneuvers. A personal flotation device is also highly recommended.

The skin should also be protected from sun damage by applying a waterproof sunscreen with a sun protective factor of at least 30 an hour before exposure and every 2 h thereafter. In addition to protecting the eyes from trauma, shatterproof sunglasses can also prevent problems from long-term sun exposure. A wet or dry suit and protective footwear such as neoprene booties or slippers can prevent many lacerations, and gloves can decrease abrasions and blisters on the hands.

Informed coaching of sailors on correct technique and appropriate progression of physical and technical development can also be important parts of injury prevention [8]. Specific strength training can increase the resilience of body regions at high risk of injury [8]. Neville and Folland recommend that strengthening exercises for windsurfers at all levels should involve synergist and joint stabilizing muscles. They point out rotator cuff, scapular and glenohumeral stabilizing exercises, ankle and knee proprioceptive training, and transversus abdominis and multifidus activation exercises as specific examples for injury prevention strategies. Flexibility exercises for the anterior chest and shoulders of windsurfers can also help maintain healthy muscle balance [8].

Achieving adequate overall fitness can help to limit both acute and cumulative injuries caused by fatigue-induced technique or performance errors. The introduction of a new Olympic class windsurf board in the late 1990s prompted sailors to develop a new technique of sail "pumping" (rhythmically pulling the sail so that it acts as a wing) [26]. A French study examining the physiologic demands of this technique found that the mean distance sailed was shorter and the board speed greater with this technique. Though the new technique was sustained at a significantly higher fraction of VO_2 max compared to the old technique, total energy expenditure and blood lactate concentration 3 min into recovery were not different [26].

Equipment ergonomics can also be an important factor in preventing injury. Current literature focuses on two pieces of equipment: the foot straps and the boom. As discussed earlier, foot straps that do not allow quick release of the foot have been blamed for significant and possibly preventable injuries such as Lisfranc fractures and ligamental injuries in the ankle and knee. The caliber or diameter of the boom may be important in improving grip and overall control.

Summary

Physicians are likely to see more windsurfing injuries as the popularity of the sport increases. The clinician's awareness of common windsurfing injuries can lead to prompt and accurate diagnosis and treatment. Physicians can help reduce injuries by prompting safe sailing habits and protective equipment use.

References

1. http://www.worldofwindsurfing.net/en/press-lounge/basics/legends-of-the-sport/jim-drake.html. Accessed 20 Oct 2011.
2. http://www.surfertoday.com/windsurfing/2323-windsurfing-was-invented-60-years-ago-by-newman-darby. Accessed 20 Oct 2011.
3. Jablecki C, Garner S. Neurological complications of windsurfing (sailboarding). Semin Neurol. 2000;20(2):219–23.
4. http://en.wikipedia.org/wiki/Windsurfing. Accessed 20 Oct 2011.
5. http://www.sailing.org/olympic_about_rules_regs_class_rules_.php<http://www.sailing.org/olympic_about_rules_regs_class_rules_.php>. Accessed 20 Oct 2011.
6. Nathanson AT, Reinart SE. Windsurfing injuries: results of a paper- and internet-based survey. Wilderness Environ Med. 1999;10(4):218–25.
7. Dyson R, Buchanon M, Hale T. Incidence of sports injuries in elite competitive and recreational windsurfers. Br J Sports Med. 2006;40:346–50.
8. Kalogeromitros A, Tsangaris H, Bilalis D, Karabinis A. Severe accidents due to windsurfing in the Aegean Sea. Eur J Emerg Med. 2002;9:149–54.
9. Neville V, Folland J. The epidemiology and aetiology of injuries in sailing. Sports Med. 2009;39(2):129–45.
10. Goossens M, De Stoop N. Lisfranc's fracture-dislocations: etiology, radiology, and results of treatment. A review of 20 cases. Clin Orthop. 1983;176:154–62.
11. Lu J, Ebrahim NA, Skie M, et al. Radiographic and CT evaluation of lisfranc dislocation: a cadaver study. Foot Ankle Int. 1997;18(6):351–5.
12. Arntz CT, Hansen Jr ST. Dislocations and fracture-dislocation of the tarsometatarsal joints. Orthop Clin North Am. 1987;18(1):105–14.
13. Myerson M. The diagnosis and treatment of injuries to the lisfranc joint complex. Orthop Clin North Am. 1989;20(4):655–64.
14. Witt J, Paaske BP, Jorgensen U. Injuries in windsurfing due to foot fixation. Scand J Med Sci Sports. 1995;5(5):311–2.
15. Hestroni I, Mann G, Ayalon M, Frankl U, Nyska M. Extensor digitorum longus tendonitis in windsurfing due to footstrap fixation. Clin J Sport Med. 2006;16:74–5.
16. Locke S, Allen GD. Etiology of low back pain in elite boardsailors. Med Sci Sports Exerc. 1992;24(9):964–6.
17. Standaert CJ, Herring SA. Spondylolysis: a critical review. Br J Sports Med. 2000;34:415–22.
18. McCormick DP, Davis AL. Injuries in sailboard enthusiasts. Br J Sports Med. 1988;22(3):95–7.
19. Roberts JR, Hedges JR. Clinical procedures emergency medicine. 3rd ed. Philadelphia: WB Saunders; 1998. p. 533, 553.
20. Auerbach PS. Wilderness medicine: management of wilderness and environmental emergencies. 3rd ed. St. Louis: Mosby-Year Book; 1995. p. 1335.
21. Monckton R, Fagan B, Frayne DJ, Colvin GF. Pruritic erythematous maculopapular rash. J Fam Pract. 2011;60(10):613–5.
22. Wulff C, Haeberlein S, Haas W. Cream formulations protecting against cercarial dermatitis by Trichobilharzia. Parasitol Res. 2007;101(1):91–7.
23. Dewailly E, Poirier C, Meyer F. Health hazards associated with windsurfing on polluted water. Am J Public Health. 1986;76(6):690–1.
24. Ulusarac O, Carter E. Varied clinical presentations of vibrio vulnificus infections: a report of four unusual cases and review of the literature. South Med J. 2004;97(2):163–8.
25. Petersen W, Rau J, Hansen U, Zantop T, Stein V. Mechanisms and prevention of windsurfing injuries (German). Sportverletz Sportschaden. 2003;17(3):118–22.
26. Castagna O, Brisswalter J, Lacour JR, Vogiatzis I. Physiological demands of different sailing techniques of the New Olympic windsurfing class. Eur J Appl Physiol. 2008;104:1061–7.

Chapter 10
Sailing and Yachting

Michael R. Carmont

Contents

Background	203
Dinghy Sailing	205
Yacht Sailing	209
Injury Incidence and Mechanisms	210
Injuries Characteristics with Dinghy Racing	210
Injury Characteristics of Yachting	213
Specific Injuries	218
Back Pain	218
Knee Pain	218
Elbow Pain	218
Fitness Training	218
Injury Prevention and Return to Play	220
Summary	221
References	221

Background

Sailing today encompasses many disciplines but is defined as the propulsion of a vehicle and control of its movement with sails, rigging, and a rudder. The first references to sailing have been estimated to originate from Kuwait in 5,000 years BC. Other references have been found in Arabian, Chinese, Indian, and European ancient literature.

M.R. Carmont, FRCS (Tr&Orth)
The Department of Orthopaedic Surgery,
Princess Royal Hospital, Shrewsbury and Telford NHS Trust,
Telford, UK

The Department of Orthopaedic Surgery, The Northern General Hospital
Sheffield Teaching Hospitals NHS Foundation Trust,
Sheffield, UK
e-mail: mcarmont@hotmail.com

Wind power allowed long-distance nautical travel compared to rowing, and during the thirteenth and fourteenth centuries permitted long-distance exploration with the principal aim of acquiring land and wealth. It was the Portuguese sailor Ferdinand Magellan who is accredited with having completed the first circumnavigation. In a voyage funded by the King of Spain to search for the "spice islands," he set sail westward to the far Pacific. Here he unfortunately met his demise at the hands of a local king in the islands now known as the Philippines due to persistent attempts to convert the inhabitants to Christianity. He had reached a similar area on a previous easterly voyage and so it credited with the first circumnavigation.

The propulsion of the craft by the use of sails occurs due to two principles. When sailing downwind, the wind catches within the sails and the craft moves forward. Sailing vessels can also travel into the wind by performing a series of tacks or turns across the wind. Based on the obliquity of the tack, the sail hanging behind the mast directs the winds toward the rear of the boat. This increases the relative air pressure at the stern and decreases the pressure at the bow, and so the boat moves in a forward direction. The presence of a keel or centerboard effectively deepens the hull within the water. This prevents sideways drift due to the wind or tides. These may be raised and lowered as required.

Although long-distance water travel was primarily sustained by sail power, now the use of motors and engines has superseded sail for commercial water travel. The use of sailing power remains for recreational activities and competitive racing. The Dutch were the first to take up sailing as a pastime in the seventeenth century sailing on small vessels called "jaghts," hence the development of the word yacht. Sailing for recreation or sport may be divided into dinghy sailing and cruising or yachting depending upon the size of the vessel.

International competitive sailing began in the mid-nineteenth century when members of the New York Yacht Club raced British competitors around the Isle of Wight. Cowes in Hampshire may be considered to be home of yacht racing after the first regatta was held there in 1812 organized by the Royal Yacht Club. Since the founding of the Royal Yacht Squadron in 1815, the Cowes Regatta has been held every year since 1826.

The world governing body for sailing was formed in Paris in 1907; this was initially known as the International Yacht Racing Union but was changed to the International Sailing Federation in 1996. The rules of different sailing competitions were uniformed at the Yachting Congress at the Royal Victoria Yacht Club in June 1868, and these complex documents are currently listed on the International Sailing Federation website together with medical guidelines 2009–2012 [1]. The ISAF World Championships have been held every 4 years since 2003.

Yachting was first contested at the Olympic Games in 1900 and subsequently at every game since 1908. The initial races were for yachts with crews of between 10 and 12 sailors; however, since the 1950s, the emphasis has changed to much smaller boats. At the 2000 Olympic Games in Sydney, the name of the event was changed from yachting to sailing.

Racing is divided into numerous different categories and subclasses as follows:

Olympic: 8 classes
Centerboard: 40 classes
Keelboat: 29 classes
Multihull: 1 class
Yachting: 10 classes
Radio-controlled

From the initial form of exploration, long-distance yachting is considered as a form of adventure with considerable challenges involved. Joshua Slocum from the United States is the first person to sail around the world solo in 1898 on a voyage completed in an 11-m sloop "Spray." It was however over 50 years later, in 1966, when Francis Chichester completed the first solo circumnavigation on Gipsy Moth IV. Chay Blyth completed a solo nonstop circumnavigation passing from east to west aboard the ketch British Steel in 1972. This voyage is considered to be much more arduous as in this direction the winds are less favorable.

There are numerous sailing records ratified by the World Sailing Speed Record Council, and it would be beyond the scope of this chapter to list all of these; many are listed in the accompanying table (Table 10.1). There are in addition notable speed challenges. In small boats, dinghies, etc., the record for the nautical mile is currently held by Alain Thebault who attained a speed of 50.17 kts sailing a Hydroptere at Hyree in France. When measured over a 500-m distance, Rob Douglas from the USA achieved a speed of 55.65 kts at Luderitz in Namibia.

In offshore sailing, the 24-h distance record was set in 2009 by Pascal Bidegorry sailing a 131″ trimaran Banque Populaire 5, covering a distance of 908.2 nm corresponding to a speed of 37.84 kts [2].

Dinghy Sailing

Dinghy sailing may be performed on lakes, landlocked areas of water, or close inshore. Dinghies are small boats with one or two sails and a center or dagger board with a rudder. The centerboard or dagger board may be raised or lowered depending on the side-to-side balance of the boat. Boats are typically crewed by one or two people. The positioning of the crew within the boat and the strength and direction of the wind determine the speed and direction of the boat.

The crew may sit leaning over the side of the boat with their feet held in straps. This is termed hiking and allows the crews' weight to generate righting moments to counteract the heeling forces of the boat. A heeling force is generated by wind across the sails causing the boat to tip away from the direction of the wind [3].

The use of a trapeze allows the crew to hang outside the boat on a harness; thus, their weight can be taken further from the midline of the craft (Fig. 10.1). When using a trapeze, the crew person sits in a harness and is suspended from the mast by halyards.

Table 10.1 Speed records

	Distance (m)	Date	Skipper	Yacht	Duration	Speed
Transatlantic W > E Ambrose Light to Lizard Point	2,880	2009	Pascal Bidegorry	Banque Populaire	3 day 15 h 25 min	32.94 kts
Transatlantic W > E Ambrose Light to Lizard Point (single handed)	2,880	2008	Thomas Coville	Sodebo	5 day 19 h 30 min	20.87 kts
Round-the-World Nonstop Crewed (any type)	21,760	Jan–Mar 2010	Franck Cammas	Groupama 3	48 day 7 h 44 min	18.76 kts
Round-the-World Female Nonstop (single handed)	21,760	Nov 2004–Feb 2005	Dame Ellen MacArthur	B&Q	71 day 14 h 18 min	12.66 kts

10 Sailing and Yachting

Fig. 10.1 The use of a trapeze to allow crew to position their weight over the side of the catamaran (Photo: Omer Mei-Dan)

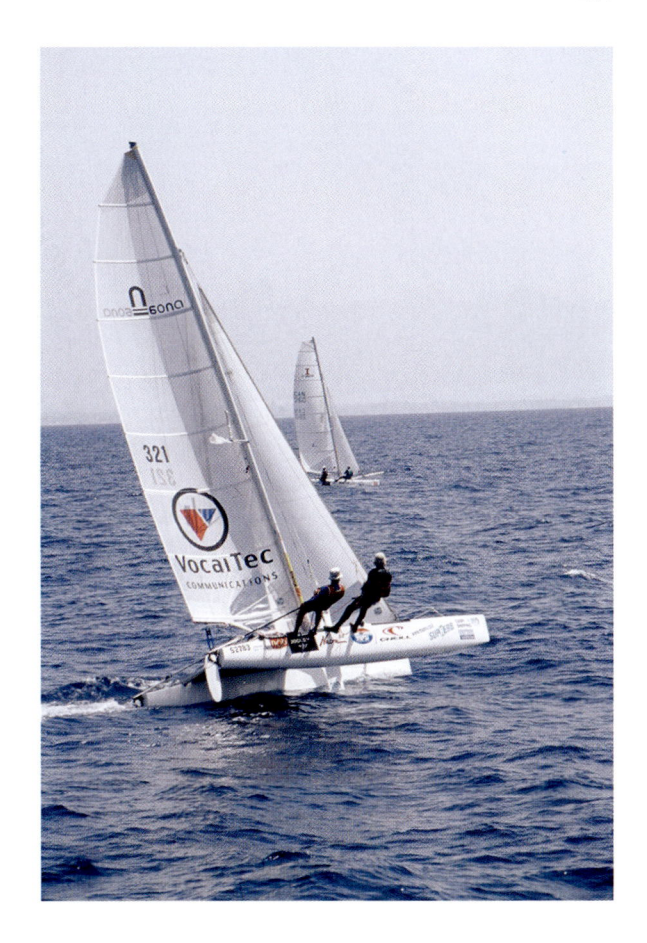

The speed of the boat also depends on the design of the hull. Narrow-hulled vessels may be supported by additional hulls or outriggers. Two-hulled craft are called catamarans (Fig. 10.2) and three hulls a trimaran. Advanced hull shapes allow lighter boats to plane and rise out of the water on their own bow wave and skim across the surface. Further advances include the placement of battens in the mainsail and aerodynamic rotating masts.

The traditional Olympic triangle course consists of an equilateral triangle, three equal sides and angles of 60°, and a ratio of windward to reaching legs of 1:1 (Fig. 10.3). From the start, sailors beat or work to windward from the starting line to the top weather or windward mark, with a first reaching leg to the wing mark, also known as the jibe mark; a second reaching leg from the wing mark to the bottom or leeward mark, called a hot dog; a beat to the top mark with a square run back to the bottom mark; another lap; and then a beat to the finish line. The finish line may be at the top mark or may be set beyond the top mark.

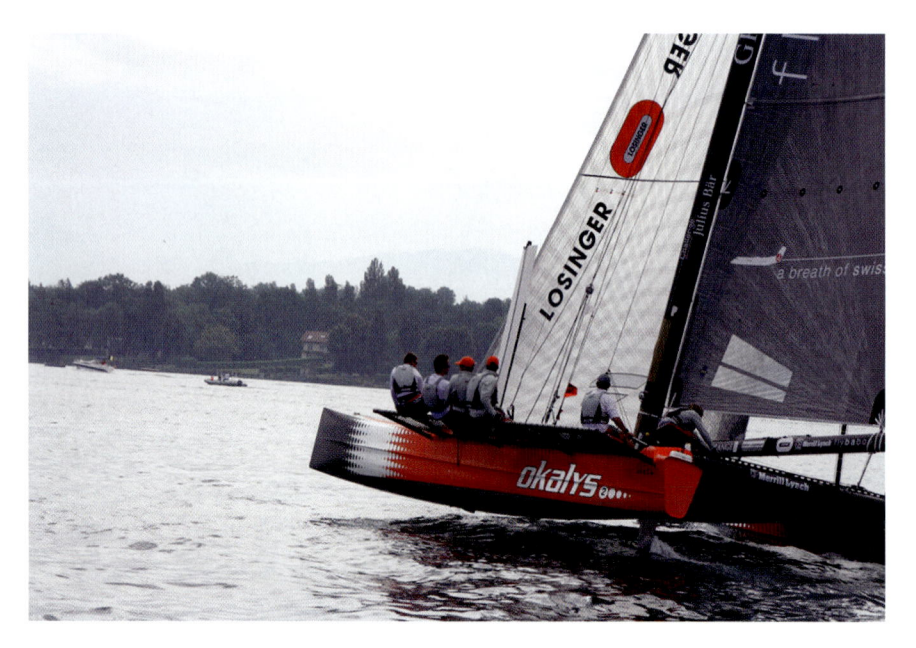

Fig. 10.2 A catamaran with one hull lifted high from the water (David Carlier/www.bivouac44.com)

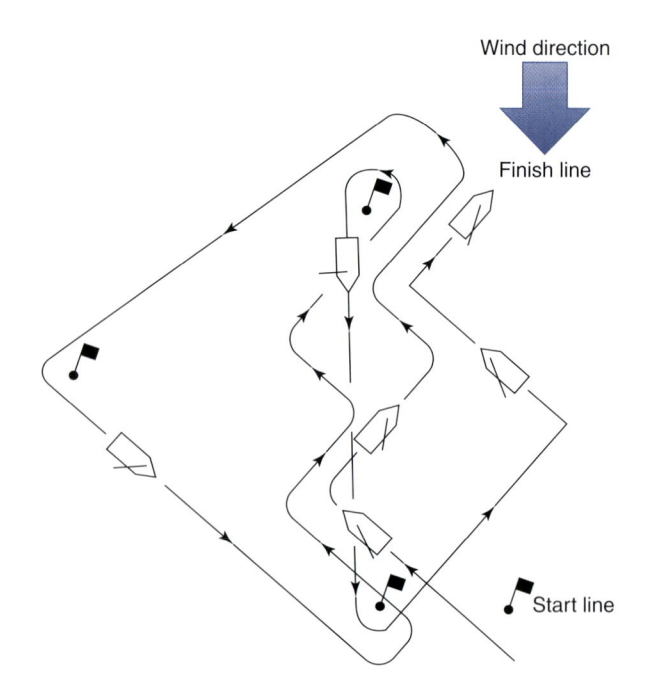

Fig. 10.3 The Olympic sailing course

Yacht Sailing

Yachting tends to be the recreational or competitive sailing of a large vessel specifically designed for this purpose. These are typically specifically built racing monohull or multihull vessels. Yacht races may consist of short races of several hours duration around a specific course up to long-distance round-the-world voyages either nonstop or with multiple stop-off points. Given the cost of these boats, it is not surprising that racing tends to occur at a professional corporate level with full-time crews preparing with extensive training programs.

The oldest of these races may be considered to be the America's Cup (Fig. 10.4). This competition was established following a challenge to the American yacht racing club in New York in 1851. This trophy has been held by New York Yacht Club until 1983 when they were finally beaten by Australia II from the Perth Yacht Club [4].

The first round-the-world yacht race took place in 1973. Originally sponsored by Whitbread, it is now known as the Volvo Ocean Race and incorporates a distance of 39,000 miles with yachts passing through the most treacherous seas on the planet. There are around five stop-off points at which yachts may be repaired and supplies replenished. This race is undertaken by professional crews and skippers and takes place every 4 years.

The amateur version is called the Clipper Round the World Yacht Race and passes through much smoother waters. Sailors pay the organizers to compete and are formed into crews led by a professional skipper and race identical yachts.

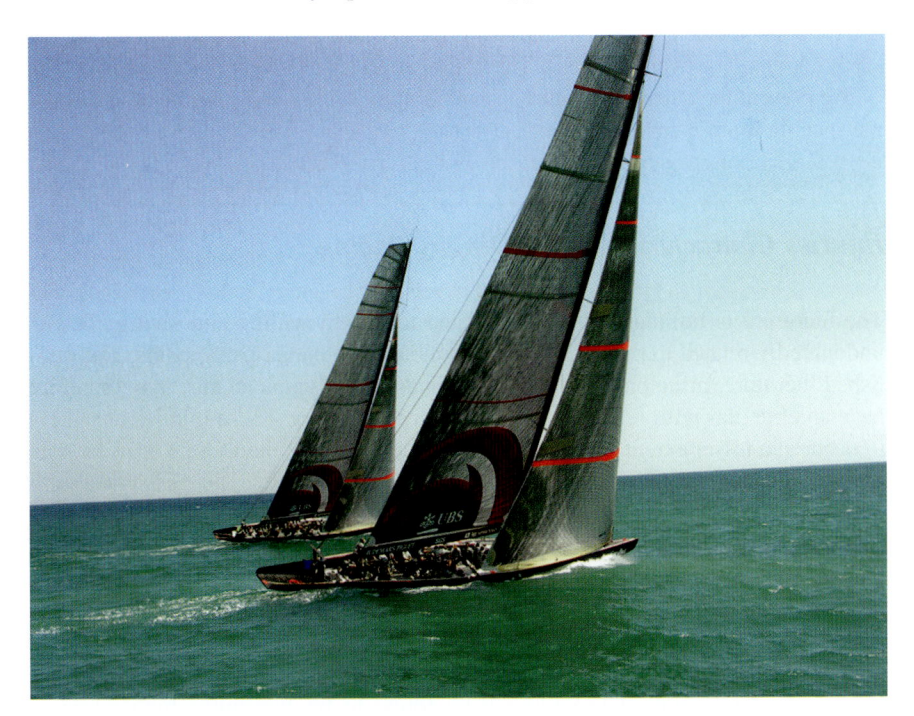

Fig. 10.4 America's Cup yacht racing. Valencia (David Carlier/www.bivouac44.com)

The Vendee Globe single-handed nonstop race was founded by Philippe Jeantot in 1989 and also takes place every 4 years. In this race, sailors compete in monohulls and pass through electronic waypoints according to global positioning systems, starting and finishing in Sables-d'Olonne in France.

Shorter but also challenging races include the Single-Handed Transatlantic Race (STAR) or the Rolex Sydney to Hobart Yacht Race.

Injury Incidence and Mechanisms

The activity characteristics of those sailors competing on dinghies and yachts are similar in some respects however different in others. Both involve physical strength with sudden bouts of anaerobic activity in cramped confined conditions. Both have significant differences related to on-deck activity.

Given the large number of recreational participants in both dinghy sailing and yachting, it is virtually impossible to determine injury rates in this aspect of the sport. Questionnaire surveys may gain some insight but these are subject to recall bias.

Organized regattas, competitions, and races allow a degree of data collection and epidemiological study. The relatively large infrastructure and financial resources of yacht racing have meant that much of the published literature has come from this aspect of the sport. The epidemiological studies of America's Cup racing have yielded useful information. This event consists of a series of match races of two boats at a time. Each race lasts 2–3 h, and teams may compete in up to 50 races during the event taking place over 22 weeks. The competition is held every 3–4 years [4].

We present the current literature in both dinghy sailing and yachting and discuss the specific injuries involved.

Injuries Characteristics with Dinghy Racing

The literature is limited for injuries related to dinghy sailing and racing. This is undoubtedly related to the considerable numbers of amateur participants. The published literature, principally on national squads and Olympic teams, may therefore have an elite bias with regard to certain patterns of injury. These injuries are likely to occur at a lesser extent in the recreational sailor and are therefore worthy of note to medical personnel providing healthcare for these athletes.

Incidence

In elite Olympic class sailing, the incidence of injury is approximately 0.2 injuries/athlete/year with the lumbar and thoracic spine and knee most commonly injured. Injuries in Paralympic class sailing were found to be at a much higher rate of approximately 100 injuries/1,000 days of sailing in 1999. This is a considerable discrepancy, which was thought to be due to more difficult sailing conditions. The majority of injuries were chronic in nature, predominantly sprains and strains of the upper extremity [5]. This may have been due to the level of disability of the competitors.

Nathanson has reported an online survey of recreationally competitive sailors performed during 2006 looking at the relative frequency, patterns, and mechanisms of sailing-related injuries in dinghies and keelboats [6]. A total of 1,715 injuries were reported from 1,188 respondents. The rates of injury and severe injury were 4.6/1,000 and 0.57/1,000 days of sailing, respectively.

A retrospective review of injuries at the Kiel Regatta from 1984 to 1987 showed that sailing injuries requiring hospital care were three times more common in male competitors and twice as likely from sailing dinghies than keelboats [7]. Another series reporting from a similar event revealed that there was a higher risk of injury for the helmsman than for the fore deckhand but injuries were equally distributed among the sexes [8].

Region

When we compare the anatomical regions where injury was reported, there appears to be a distinction between those injuries reported by elite competitors and recreationally competitive sailors versus beginners.

A review of the 2002 Brazilian Olympic team revealed that the most common painful areas were the lower back (52.9 %) and the knees (25–32 %). In Legg's series, 57 % of New Zealand Olympic sailors' injuries were reported in the preceding 3 years, with lower back (45 %), knee (22 %), shoulder (18 %), and arm (15 %) reported [9]. The most common injuries in the Kiel Week regatta were again back (44 %) and knee pain (30 %) [10].

By comparison, when participants of beginner dinghy sailing courses were reviewed, the distribution of injuries was as follows: upper limbs 39.5 %, head 32.4 %, lower extremities 39.5 %, and the neck or the trunk 1.6 % [8]. This distinction may well be due to the reporting of injuries and the exertion involved. Beginner sailors when questioned may well report all minor knocks, scrapes, and aches, whereas experienced sailors may discount these minor injuries and only report only significantly injured areas. Similarly inexperienced sailors may be in the boats sailing but not necessarily applying the same exertion in the process of sailing the boat.

Type

Contusions were the most common injury (55 %), followed by grazes (17 %), cuts or tears (14.3 %), bruises (6.3 %), tender spots or blisters or callus (4.6 %), lacerations (1.7 %), pulled muscles (0.4 %), and fractures (0.4 %) in sailing at the Kiel Regatta [8].

Scholne also reports on the same regatta but a different cohort of patients with a similar pattern of findings. Injuries reported featured as open wounds (31.3 %), hand injuries (31.3 %), head injuries (22.1 %), contusions (19.7 %), and various fractures (15.1 %) [7].

In Nathanson's survey reporting on 70 severe injuries, 25 % were fractures, and 16 % were torn tendons or cartilage. The most frequent injuries for keelboat sailors were leg contusions (11 %), hand lacerations (8 %), and arm contusions (6 %) showing a predilection for upper limb injuries. Injuries sustained in dinghies were leg contusions (11 %), knee contusions (6 %), and leg lacerations (6 %) [11]. Like all surveys, the accuracy of these findings may be subject to a degree of recall bias, with respondents being more likely to remember severe injuries but forget bruises and contusions.

Causalgia

The causes of injuries can be considered to be either accidental acute trauma or overuse activity. Collision with the boom was the most common accidental injury mechanism (31.1 %), followed by putting the rigging up and down (13 %), capsizing (10.5 %), docking and casting off (9.7 %), the handling of sheets (9.2 %), conditions of the harbor (8.8 %), and slipping while on board (6.8 %). Notably stronger and offshore winds made the sailor more accident prone [8]. Injuries in novice and recreational sailing are predominantly acute in nature with contusions and abrasions typically occurring as a result of collisions with the boom or other equipment during maneuvers. The common mechanisms of injury were trip/fall, being hit by object, and being caught in lines. The common factors contributing to injury are tacking heavy weather and jibing.

By comparison, competitive sailing is a physical sport with large forces suddenly applied to muscle groups in order to make the dinghy go faster.

Actions in sailing are sudden sporadic placing muscles at high risk by performing explosive powerful moves. A lack of warming up, stretching, and cooling down surrounding race also increases risk of injury.

Hiking or sitting over the side of the boat with the feet held beneath foot straps places immense strain on the lower back and the knees [12]. In some classes of sailboats, sailors may spend as much as 94 % of the race in the hiking position [13]. Unaccustomed overarching of the back and weak abdominal muscles will lead to excessive loading of the spine. Inadequate leg strength and poor hiking technique are thought to lead to an imbalance between the medial and lateral quadriceps leading to pain [14]. Inadequate fitness training exacerbates muscular imbalances, changing the forces in opposing muscle groups.

When hiking or using a harness to counterbalance the boat with a trapeze, it may be safest to keep the back straight, depending on the hiking style being performed. Using electromyographic analysis to evaluate static hiking, Hall has suggested that body harnesses include rigid padding, shoulder-through-buttock support, and leg strap supports [15].

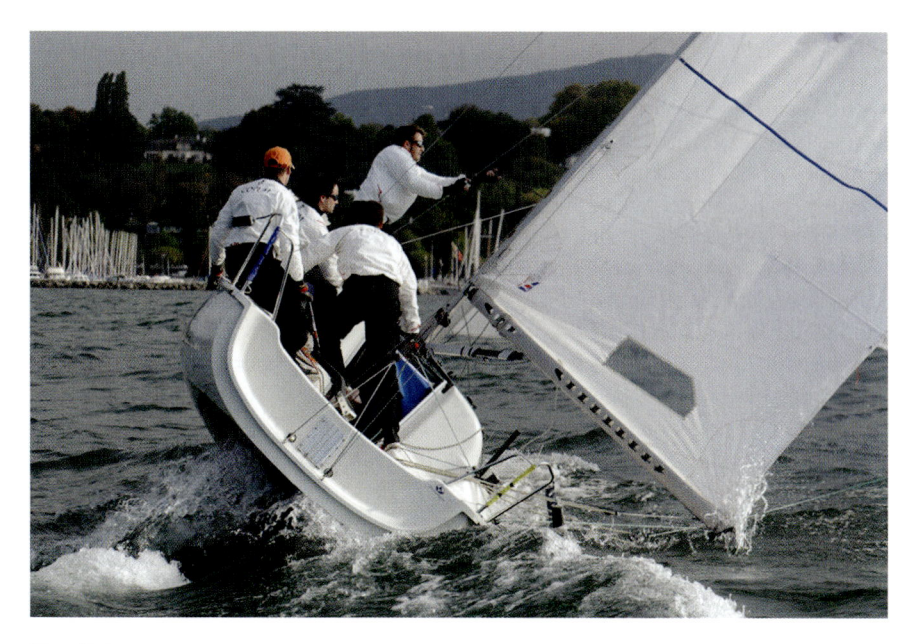

Fig. 10.5 Cramped conditions in dinghy sailing can predispose to injury (David Carlier/www.bivouac44.com)

Maneuvering around the cramped dinghy (Fig. 10.5) and in particular avoiding the boom can be awkward resulting in rotating, hyperextending, locking, or twisting of joints, leading to meniscal or articular cartilage injury principally of the knee.

The handling of the mainsheet against the wind's resistance to increase the dinghy's speed may lead to shoulder and arm injuries particularly sudden eccentric loading.

Injury Characteristics of Yachting

Significant injury epidemiological data has come from large-boat yacht racing. These international corporate events often have the medical infrastructure and financial backing, with some teams having overall budgets in excess of £100 m, to permit data collection and observations to be made.

All maneuvers on board are performed manually placing high physical and psychological demands on the 16-person crew. The intensity and demands depend upon the position and role of the athlete, the weather conditions, the race tactics, and the competitiveness of the opposition. The preparation for the events usually occurs over the 4 years on the buildup to the competition. This introduces the aspect of recording injuries sustained during the training phase of preparation as well as during the period of competition itself.

Incidence

Neville et al. have reported on injuries sustained during training for and competition during the 2003 America's Cup [16]. This prospective study reported an overall incidence of 8.8 incidents/1,000 sailing and training hours. It is interesting to note that there was a higher rate of injury associated with training, 8.6 injuries per 1,000 h of training compared to 2.2 injuries/1,000 h of sailing.

Neville has prospectively studied the injuries sustained by one America's Cup team during the 2003 competition [16]. The exposure time consisted of 74 weeks of sailing and training, and 220 injuries and 119 illnesses were recorded. This allowed the determination of 5.7 injuries per 1,000 training/sailing hours.

Recent studies by Hadala report an overall incidence of 10 injuries per 1,000 h competition during a race series [17].

Given the nature of the event with multiple match races occurring over a short period of time and the professional nature, finance, and prestige associated with the event, caution must be used with the interpretation of some aspects of data collection. Some yachtsmen may not reveal or report injuries to prevent them from being dropped from the racing squad and the event.

Professional yacht racing is such a precise science that yachtsmen have very specific roles on board, and the frequency of injury has been determined for these different activities. A follow-up study completed in 2,000 with contributions from all America's Cup teams determined that bowmen and jib winch grinders were most often injured [18]. Bowmen are considered to have a high risk of injury due to having to perform physical activity in a very confined space, working at the bow or front of the boat, and grinders simply due to the repetitive overuse nature of the grinding action. Grinding is the process of using a winch to raise or lower sails (Fig. 10.6) and is akin to upper limb cycling.

In round-the-world offshore racing, 1.5 injuries/person/round-the-world race (amateur) and 3.2 injuries/person/race (professional) have been reported [19]. Comparison of these two values is difficult in terms of injury definitions and exposure times.

Region

Seventy-six percent of injuries in Allen's series were soft tissue, and common locations were lumbar spine (16 %), shoulder (16 %), knee (10 %), cervical spine (8 %), and hand (7 %) [18]. Allen went on to report a similar location of injures on the all-female yacht of America during the 1995 race that lower back and shoulder injuries were most common and that these were chronic and overuse in nature [20].

In Neville's study on injuries during the 2003 race, the upper limb was the most commonly injured body segment (40 %) followed by neck and spine (30 %) [16].

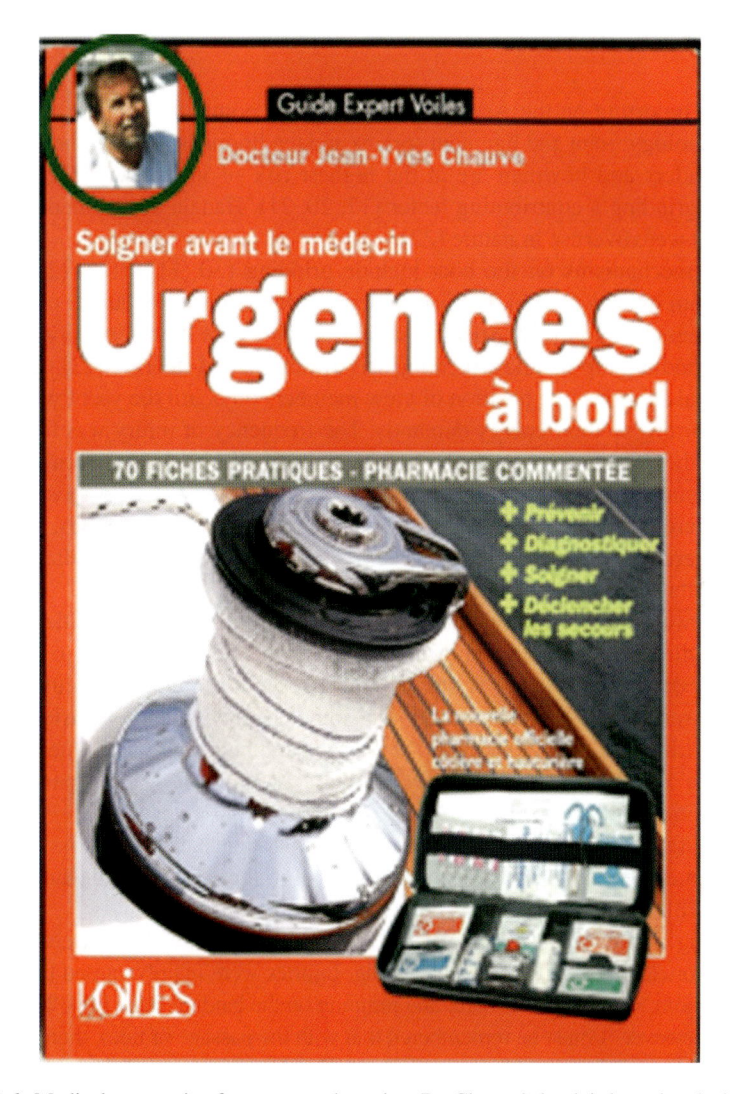

Fig. 10.6 Medical preparation for ocean yacht racing. Dr. Chauve's book is bound to deal with all types of diseases and emergencies in isolated conditions. Algorithms for diagnostic allow to communicate with a distant MD and explain the safe self-treatments

This regional distribution was the same as Hadala's reporting on the following event. In the 2007 race, the most common anatomical location was the upper limb (36.6 %) followed by the upper dorsal and cervical spine (34.4 %) [17].

Over a period of 3 years, 68 sailing injuries were registered at a German clinic at which patients were reviewed during a sailing regatta. The hand (32.3 %) and the head (17.6 %) were the most frequently damaged [7].

Causalgia

All series reporting on the America's Cup report a common theme of nonspecific overuse etiology: joint and ligament sprains and tendinopathies being the most common. Grinders and bowmen are at the highest risk of injury, with the repetitive nature of grinding a contributing factor [17, 20, 21]. Hadala determined that 85 % of injuries were overuse in nature [22].

Injury mechanisms on the boat include grinding (30 %), lifting (24 %), and impact from objects (16 %), but just under a fifth of injuries occurred off the boat during fitness training [20]. Specific sailing activities are high-repetition activities such as grinding, top-handle winching, sail trimming, and steering [23].

In Hadala's series, the position of crew members on board the yacht was categorized according to their energy demands. The frequency of injury was found to be related to the sailor's position on the boat, with most injuries (67 %) occurring in the more demanding activities (grinder, bowman, and mastman). The most common injuries were muscle contractures of the quadratus lumborum, trapezius, and rhomboids. There were 8 cases of elbow epicondylitis, 4 cases of tendinopathy of supraspinatus, and 3 cases of biceps brachii [17].

The forward flexed and rotated position of the spine during the activities of grinding and pulling ropes and trimming sails make yachtsmen susceptible to back pain. Similarly, the cervical spine is susceptible to overuse injuries particularly those related to sustained posture of the cervical spine protraction and extension, characteristic of trimmers while looking up at the sails and helmsmen while steering [24]. Helmsmen are characteristically affected due to steering the yacht, spending long periods of time at the wheel.

During sailing, the bowmen have the highest incidence of injury possibly due to the high intensity of the activities occurring within the very small unstable area of the bow [18].

Bleeding wounds (26.4 %), contusions (22 %), and fractures (17.6 %) were very commonly reported lesions during regatta sailing. Injuries were mainly caused by collision with the boom, stumbling on board, and jumping on the landing stage [25]. This sounds comical; however, it must be remembered that with the passage of tides, there is considerable variation of the height between the water level and the level of the landing stage.

In professional ocean yacht racing, the injury pattern is very different, with a greater proportion of injuries (33 %) occurring below deck as a much greater time is spent below deck and the violent and sudden movements of the yacht. Helmsmen are also at much greater risk of overuse injury due to the arduous demands of steering in heavy weather conditions [23].

Spalding et al. have conducted a prospective investigation of injuries during the 2001–2002 Volvo Ocean Race. Lower back pain, shoulder pain, neck pain, and skin lesions were most problematic. Bowmen (2.9 injuries per leg) and helmsmen (2.6 injuries per leg) were most subject to injury [19]. Similar patterns of injury were reported by Price during the BT Global Challenge Round-the-World Yacht Race 1996–1997 [26].

By comparison, in amateur ocean yacht racing, a much greater proportion of incidents are illness, accounting for 56 % of incidents reported rather than injury, compared to 35 % in the America's Cup series [16, 26]. The majority of injuries are related to impact, e.g., contusions, lacerations, fractures, and sprains. Helmsmen experience mostly upper limb overuse injuries as a result of steering, while mastmen and bowmen are at greater risk of acute injuries. Illnesses and noninjury-related complaints account for a large proportion of the medical conditions of these events.

Further work has looked at the offshore Newport to Bermuda race from 1998 to 2006. At the end of each race, captains were asked to complete a survey (87 % response rate) of injuries sustained by crew members. With an injury/illness rate of 12 per 1,000 h per sailor, most common were injuries of the upper extremity (47 %) and lacerations (45 %). The rates of illness and injury increased in races that took place in heavy weather [11].

Studies highlight that because of the high sailing and training demands, America's Cup crew members are at risk of injury and illness evidenced by the prevalence of crew absent from sailing (6.2 %) and training (15.4 %). Compared to other high-performance team sports, much less resources are allocated to the health and fitness of the athletes but focused on the boats and hardware.

There is clearly a need for effective sports science and sports medicine within the America's Cup. Regular assessments should be performed as well as medical treatment and physiotherapy, both pre-habilitation and rehabilitation, preventative strength and conditioning programs, nutrition and hydration strategies, and monitoring of overall workloads.

Hadala's team also looked into mood profile, metabolic muscle damage, and oxidative stress markers in the America's Cup [27, 28]. Mood was found to be dependent on physical work intensity and related to boat position but not on injury occurrence [27]. Markers of muscle damage, e.g., creatine kinase, were found to be highest in sailors involved in strenuous physical work [28].

Given the physical activity and muscular demands involved in America's Cup racing, it is not surprising that injury prevention strategies have been adopted. These were studied during the 2007 competition. Prior to 2004, the crew did not receive any preventative physiotherapy and acted as a control group. The first phase consisted of stretching exercises before the race and preventative taping. The second phase consisted of the addition of articular mobilization before competition, ice baths following competition, and Kinesio Taping. The final phase consisted of a recovery program with core stability exercises, post-competition stretching, and the wearing of 12 h of compressive clothing. Each phase lasted 1 year. The pre-intervention phase demonstrated 1.66 injured sailors per competition day, which fell to 0.6 in phase three. The number of athletes with more than one injury was significantly reduced from 53 to 6.5 %. Before the program, the mastmen, grinders, and bowmen showed a rate of 2.88 injuries per competition day, which fell to 0.35 injuries by phase 3 [22].

Specific Injuries

Back Pain

Back pain is common to sailors in both dinghy sailing and yachting. As already discussed in dinghy sailing, the main etiology is related to hiking and use of the trapeze. Prevention focuses on back strengthening exercises and the gradual increase in exposure. In yacht racing, back pain is once again posture related due to periods of time spent "grinding" or winching.

Cervical pain typically occurs in grinders and helmsmen spending long periods of time looking up at the sails for wind direction and activity.

Knee Pain

This can also occur in hiking and is related to overuse of the knee extensor mechanism. Knee strengthening programs are beneficial. Unfortunately, it is difficult to reproduce the variability of wind and water on land or gym simulators. Conditioning and preventative exercises are beneficial although progressive exposure may be useful. Adoption of the correct technique will also aid prevention.

Elbow Pain

The elbow is a common site of pain particularly in grinders to the extent that it has been termed grinder's elbow. This is considered to be a combination of tendinitis, fasciitis, and epicondylitis causing local tenderness near the elbow and forearm. There may have been an element of entrapment of the posterior interosseous nerve (PINE) [16]. This has been thought to account for as much as 40 % of elbow injuries reported.

Fitness Training

Generic recommendations are difficult to make given the considerable differing positions during sailing. Sailing dinghies and small keelboats require both aerobic endurance together with muscular strength and endurance.

Hiking relies on muscle groups in the thighs, abdominals, hips, and arms, whereas the sailors principally using the trapeze focus more on upper body strength and endurance together with aerobic endurance and agility.

Larsson found consistently high levels of isometric trunk strength, hiking endurance, and arm endurance on sailors versus non-sailors as one would expect. Superior hiking endurance was felt to reflect high levels of endurance in knee extensors and core musculature [29]. Bojsen-Moller found excellent knee extensor strength of hikers although reduced hamstring to quadriceps strength ratios were worrisome indicators for potential injury [30].

Legg showed that different dinghy classes spend various amounts of time in specific hiking positions, although the time spent in any position rarely exceeded 30 s; however, for other classes, as much as 94 % of the race can be spent in the hiking position [9]. The physical stress of hiking involves contraction of the quadriceps, iliopsoas, and abdominal muscles with body weight loading the patellofemoral joint [31, 32]. Weight loading has been determined to give a maximum quadriceps torque 305–325 Nm during hiking [31]. With fatigue, most sailors tend to isolate vastus lateralis leading to patellofemoral pain; turning out both feet with legs extended increases the workload of vastus medialis. Tight toe straps and plantar flexing the foot may help to straighten the knees, centralize gravity, and reduce the effort required by the quadriceps. Hiking has been described as quasi-isometric contraction of the knee extensor and hip flexor muscles. It is termed quasi-isometric due to small amplitude changes in force production to counteract the changing waves [33]. Strong isometric and eccentric muscle production is required to perform this task, and maximal quadriceps muscle torque values are required to hike successfully [34].

Prolonged isometric contractions are believed to restrict blood supply during contraction, and the resulting ischemia rapidly causes fatigue of the muscles [33]. As yet, there have been no electromyographic studies of hiking, but clinical experience suggests that there is considerable facilitation of vastus medialis.

Fitness training specific to hiking should include muscle strength and endurance of the core and lower extremities, maintaining balanced force and flexibility about each joint. Sailing involves considerable balance training with perturbation. Sailors must perform a full squat to go beneath the swinging boom during turns through the wind, on a wet and continually moving surface.

Training may result in increased tolerance of hiking through decreased lactate production for a given heart rate and VO_2.

The use of a stationary hiking bench can benefit muscular endurance and dynamic repetitions of trunk, and sheeting movements can aid aerobic fitness. In their 1998 study, Aagaard felt that optimal hiking performance may rely on antagonist action of the trunk and hip extensors to stabilize the lower back and spine [34].

Vangelakoudi and Vogiatzis found that elite status of Laser sailors correlated strongly with quadriceps maximal voluntary contraction isometric endurance and tolerance of muscular fatigue [35].

Crew members of all boats involved with sail trimming require highly trained arms, shoulders, and upper back. Grinders and many other big-boat sailors should address aerobic endurance as well as muscular strength, power, and endurance [36].

This fitness work should be developed in the off-season, and reducing heavy training loads before regattas [36] and 4-year preparation programs are established before the America's Cup races.

The training practices of sailors were first published by Legg in 1997 when 28 New Zealand Olympic sailors were surveyed. Sixty-one percent underwent strength/circuit training, 36 % assessed flexibility, 75 % trained aerobically on land, and 86 % performed on water aerobic training [37].

Most sailors reported increased volume and intensity of physical training and aerobic training, together with increased fluid during and a prerace carbohydrate meal consumption on the day of racing. Most sailors felt less prerace anxiety and believed that the adoption of sports science led to increased performance [37].

When surveying 25 Olympic sailors with self-prescribed strength, endurance, and flexibility programs, Legg noted significant changes in body weight, skinfolds, flexibility, aerobic endurance, and strength, but results were inconsistent [13]. In the profiling of Danish Olympic class sailors, Bojsen-Moller reported that the mean weight of Laser sailor was 80.3 kg and that of Finn and Star sailors was 93.5 kg [30].

Injury Prevention and Return to Play

Prevention is best addressed as in all sports through appropriate fitness training and proper care of previous injuries. Effective prevention programs involve a combination of flexibility, hip flexor mobility, and core stability. In addition, ergonomic developments particularly in big-boat design also holds potential for injury prevention.

Returning to the sport depends both upon the nature of the injury and the physical demands of when the athlete is returning to sail. One survey of orthopedic surgeons from the Mayo Clinic reported that many would allow a return to sailing after hip or knee arthroplasty but many said it would depend upon the circumstances [38].

The goals of rehabilitation of an athlete dealing with the conditions unique to sailing include (1) pain-free maximal quadriceps muscle contraction; (2) full resolution of edema; (3) full range of motion of the knees and hips; (4) increased joint stability, balance, and proprioception; (5) maintenance of fitness for sailing; and (6) return to pain-free sailing, especially hiking at the previous competitive level.

A case report published on a Finn class sailor describes the rehabilitation of an Olympic class sailor with a knee medial collateral ligament injury. At day 5 following injury, he was able to flex from 0° to 125° with pain at end of range. He began stationary cycling, closed kinetic chain exercises, and mobility, balance, and flexibility exercises. He was also fitted with a neoprene brace with double upright rigid supports [3].

Sailors of all classes and abilities seem to be at risk of injury particularly from acute impacts with equipment that might be reduced by wearing protective clothing and more ergonomic boat design. High-repetition activities such as hiking, pumping, grinding, and steering are major causes of overuse injury in experienced sailors. Informed coaching of correct technique and appropriate progression of physical and technical developments are required. Competitive sailors should undergo regular health screening with specific strength conditioning of high-risk muscle groups synergists and stabilizers [23].

Summary

Injury incidence rates for different disciplines have been approximately determined:
Elite Olympic class sailing 0.2 injuries/athlete/year

America's Cup	Overall 8.8 incidents/1,000 sailing and training hours
	8.6 injuries per 1,000 h of training
	2.2 injuries/1,000 h of sailing.
Round The World	Amateur 1.5 injuries/person/race
	Professional 3.2 injuries/person/race

Common areas of injury in sailing are the lower back, the knee, the shoulder and the elbow, and the cervical spine. Particular to dinghy sailing included the lumbar spine and knees in racers and traumatic injuries to the hand and upper limb. Those in yacht match racing are overuse injuries to the upper limb and cervical spine. Bowmen, grinders, winchmen, and helmsmen are the positions on the yacht most likely to sustain injury.

Prevention strategies should include core flexibility and strengthening programs for the lumbar spine, quadriceps, and upper limbs.

Sailing is a competitive adventure sport, which may be enjoyed by people of all ages and levels of ability from recreational for beginners to round-the-world competitive challenges. To quote the water rat:

> Believe me, my young friend, there is nothing – absolutely nothing – half so much worth doing as simply messing about in boats.
> Kenneth Grahame, *The Wind in the Willows* [39].

References

1. International Sailing Federation. 2012. http://www.sailing.org/documents.php. Accessed 06 Apr 2012.
2. World Sailing Speed Record Council. 2012. http://www.sailspeedrecords.com/. Accessed 06 Apr 2012.
3. Hunt SE, Herera C, Cicerale S, Moses K, Smiley P. Rehabilitation of an elite class sailor with an MCL injury. N Am J Sports Phys Ther. 2009;4:123–31.
4. Americas Cup. 2012. http://www.americascup.com/. Accessed 06 Apr 2012.
5. Allen JB. Sports injuries in disabled sailing. In: Legg SJ, editor. Human performance in sailing conference proceedings: incorporating the 4th European conference on sailing sports science

and sports medicine and the 3rd Australian sailing science conference. Palmerston North: Massey University; 2003. pp. 58.
6. Nathanson AT, Baird J, Mello M. Sailing injury and illness: results of an online survey. Wilderness Environ Med. 2010;21:291–7.
7. Schonle C. Traumatology of sailing injuries. Aktuelle Traumatol. 1989;19:116–20.
8. Schaefer O. Injuries sustained in dinghy sailing by beginners: an analysis. Sportverletz Sportschaden. 2000;14:25–30.
9. Legg SJ, Miller AB, Slyfield D, et al. Physical performance of elite New Zealand Olympic class sailors. J Sports Med Phys Fitness. 1997;37:41–9.
10. Shephard RJ. Injuries in sailing. In: Renstrom P, editor. Clinical practice of sports injury prevention, vol. 6. Oxford: Blackwell Scientific Publications; 1994. p. 41–54.
11. Nathanson AT, Fischer EG, Mello MJ, Baird J. Injury and illness at the Newport-Bermuda race 1998–2006. Wilderness Environ Med. 2008;19:129–32.
12. Blackburn M. The stayed back: ideas and exercises to avoid problems with the sailing spine. Aust Sailing. 1994;2:43–5.
13. Legg SJ, Mackie HW. Development of knowledge and reported use of sport science by elite New Zealand Olympic Class sailors. J Physiol Anthropol. 1999;18:125–33.
14. Newton F. Dinghy sailing. Practitioner. 1989;233:1032–5.
15. Hall SJ, Kent JA, Dickinson VR. Comparative assessment of novel sailing trapeze harness designs. Int J Sports Biomech. 1989;5:289–96.
16. Neville VJ, Molloy J, Brooks JHM, Speedy DB, Atkinson G. Epidemiology of injuries and illnesses in America's Cup yacht racing. Br J Sports Med. 2006;40:304–12.
17. Hadala M, Barrios C. Sports injuries in an America's Cup Yachting crew: a 4 year epidemiological study covering the 2007 challenge. J Sports Sci. 2009;27:711–7.
18. Allen JB. Sports medicine injuries in the America's Cup 2000. In: Legg SJ, editor. Human performance in sailing conference proceedings: incorporating the 4th European conference on sailing sports science and sports medicine and the 3rd Australian sailing science conference. Palmerston North: Massey University; 2003. pp. 45–6.
19. Spalding T, Malinen T, Allen JB, et al. Analysis of medical problems during the 2001–2002 Volvo Ocean Race. In: Legg SJ, editor. Human performance in sailing conference proceedings: incorporating the 4th European conference on sailing sports science and sports medicine and the 3rd Australian sailing science conference. Palmerston North: Massey University; 2003. pp. 47–50.
20. Allen JB, De Jong MR. Sailing and sports medicine: a literature review. Br J Sports Med. 2006;40:587–93.
21. Neville V, Brooks JH, Allen JB. Sports injuries in an America's Cup yachting crew: a 4 year epidemiological study covering the 2007 challenge- a critical commentary. J Sports Sci. 2010;28:1137–9.
22. Hadala M, Barrios C. Different strategies for sports injury prevention in an America's Cup yachting crew. Med Sci Sports Exerc. 2009;41:1587–96.
23. Neville V, Folland JP. The epidemiology and aetiology of injuries in sailing. Sports Med. 2009;39:129–45.
24. Allen JB. Sports medicine and sailing. Phys Med Rehabil Clin N Am. 1999;10:49–65.
25. Schonle C. Medical aspects of selecting a new high performance Olympic boat. Sportverletz Sportschaden. 1998;12:44–6.
26. Price C, Spalding T, McKenzie C, et al. Patterns of illness and injury encountered in amateur ocean yacht racing; an analysis of the British Telecom Round the World Yacht Race 1996–1997. Br J Sports Med. 2002;36:457–62.
27. Hadala M, Cebolla A, Banos R, Barrios C. Mood profile of an America's Cup team: relationship with muscle damage and injuries. Med Sci Sports Exerc. 2010;42:1408.
28. Barrios C, Hadala M, Almansa I, Bosch-Morell F, Palanca JM, Romero FJ. Muscle damage and oxidative stress markers in an America's Cup Yachting crew. Eur J Appl Physiol. 2011;111:1341–50.

29. Larsson B, Beyer N, Bey P, et al. Exercise performance in elite male and female sailors. Int J Sports Med. 1996;17:504–8.
30. Bojsen-Moller J, Larsson, Magnusson SP, et al. Physiological characteristics of America's Cup Sailors. In: Legg SJ, editor. Human performance in sailing conference proceedings: incorporating the 4th European conference on sailing sports science and sports medicine and the 3rd Australian sailing science conference. Palmerston North: Massey University; 2003. pp. 97–110.
31. Shepherd R. The biology and medicine of sailing. Sports Med. 1990;9:86–99.
32. Cockerill S, Taylor F. No pain: how to develop a hiking style that avoids the knee problems that put many out of the sport. Aust Sailing. 1999:40–2.
33. Tan B, Aziz AR, Spurway NC, et al. Determinants of maximal hiking performance in Laser Sailors. In: Legg SJ, editor. Human performance in sailing conference proceedings: incorporating the 4th European conference on sailing sports science and sports medicine and the 3rd Australian sailing science conference. Palmerston North: Massey University; 2003. pp. 25–50.
34. Aagaard P, Beyer N, Simonsen EB, et al. Isokinetic muscle strength and hiking performance in elite sailors. Scand J Med Sci Sports. 1998;3:138–44.
35. Vangelakoudi A, Vogiatzis I. Anaerobic capacity isometric endurance and performance of Greek Laser class sailors. In: Legg SJ, editor. Human performance in sailing conference proceedings: incorporating the 4th European conference on sailing sports science and sports medicine and the 3rd Australian sailing science conference. Palmerston North: Massey University; 2003. pp. 97–110.
36. Blackburn M. Shapes and sizes: you need to know whether you are a grunter, winger, flapper or grinder to get your body into the best shape. Aust Sailing. 1998:43–4.
37. Legg SJ, Smith P, Slyfield D, et al. Knowledge and reported use of sport science by elite New Zealand Olympic class sailors. J Sports Med Phys Fitness. 1997;32:213–7.
38. McGrory BJ, Stuart MJ, Sim FH. Participation in sports after hip and knee arthroplasty: review of literature and survey of surgeon preferences. Mayo Clin Proc. 1995;70:342–8.
39. Grahame K. The wind in the willows. London: Penguin Classics; 2007.

Chapter 11
Mountain Biking Injuries

Michael R. Carmont

Contents

Background	225
Injury Rates and Demographics	228
Specific Injury Patterns	237
Head and Face	237
Spinal Injuries	239
Upper Limbs	239
Abdominal Viscera	240
Perineum	240
Lower Limbs	240
Adventure Racing	241
Injury Prevention	242
Summary	243
References	243

Background

The origins of mountain biking understandably began as a means of transport rather than recreation during nineteenth-century wartime when "Buffalo" soldiers are reported to have cycled home, cross-country from Missoula, Montana, to Yellowstone. Japanese forces recognized that cycle provided faster travel on some jungle paths during the Second World War.

M.R. Carmont, FRCS (Tr&Orth)
The Department of Orthopaedic Surgery,
Princess Royal Hospital, Shrewsbury and Telford NHS Trust,
Telford, UK

The Department of Orthopaedic Surgery, The Northern General Hospital,
Sheffield Teaching Hospitals NHS Foundation Trust,
Sheffield, UK
e-mail: mcarmont@hotmail.com

Fig. 11.1 Downhill riding has slightly higher risk compared to cross-country (photo: Ronen Topelberg)

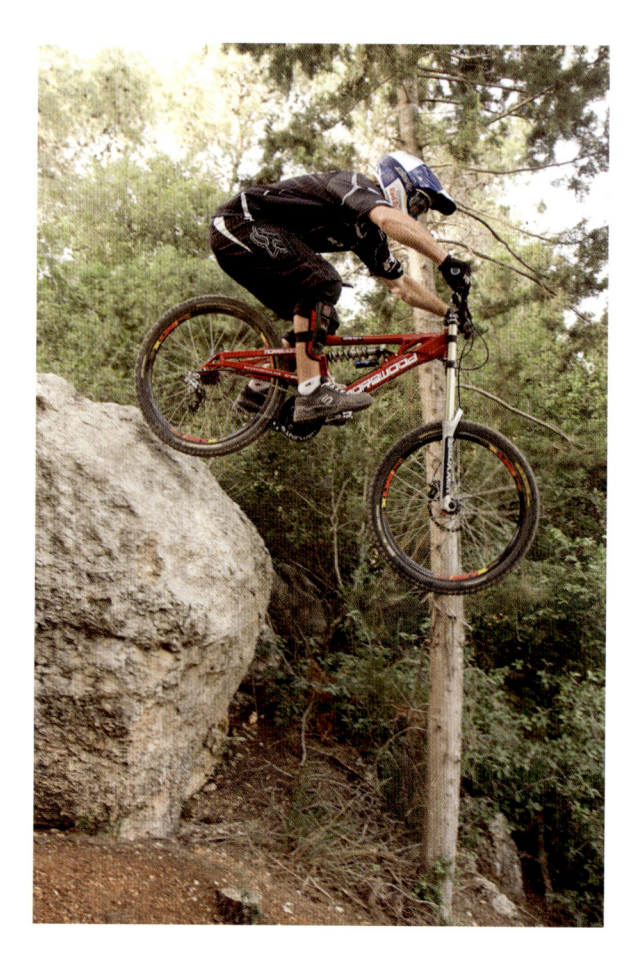

The first recorded development of a bicycle specific for off-road recreational riding was made by John Finley Scott in 1953 with his "Woodsie" bike. Joe Breeze, Otis Guy, and Gary Fisher are attributed to have started mountain bike (MTB) racing in Marin County, California, in the 1970s although riders will have raced against each other recreationally before this date [1]. After inaugural "world championships" were held simultaneously in the United States and Europe, the sport was recognized by the Union Cycliste Internationale (UCI) in 1990. Now, there is an annual World Cup Series and a World Championship, and after demonstration at the Atlanta Olympic Games in 1996, the mountain biking was awarded full Olympic status at the 2000 Games in Sydney [2].

MTB competitions were previously limited to the disciplines of cross-country and downhill, but more recently, dual slalom or four-cross and free or trials riding have developed. Cross-country races require considerable stamina and may last over several hours, whereas downhill events may be over within a couple of intense and stressful minutes. During downhill racing, speeds approaching 70 mph may be obtained over treacherous rocky terrain (Fig. 11.1). At such speeds, the slightest

Fig. 11.2 The higher you jump, the further you fall (photo: Ronen Topelberg)

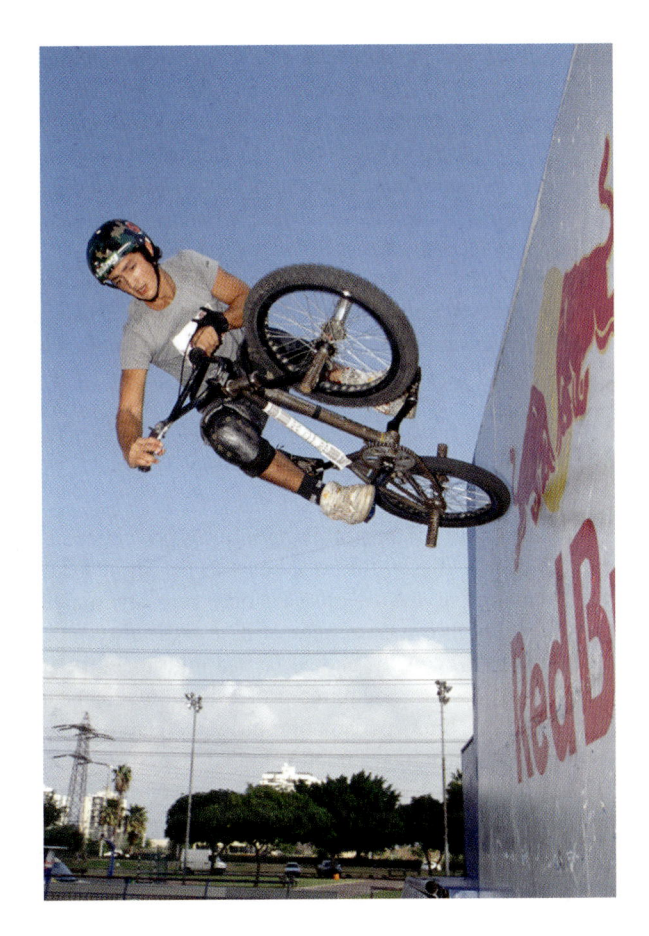

loss of attention can lead to a high-speed crash with obvious consequences of injury. During four-cross and dual slalom races, riders race head-to-head over a prepared artificial course similar to the boarder-cross discipline in snowboarding. Although physical contact is not allowed, riders jostle with each other for the best line and so falls commonly occur. Free or trials riding involves performing stunts and jumps over obstacles. Speeds are relatively low, but the height from where riders may fall is considerable (Fig. 11.2) [3].

The modern downhill racing bike features technology more akin to that of off-road rally driving rather than the vision of the traditional mountain bike. Frames are built from carbon fiber, and both front and rear wheels use suspension systems in an effort to speed descents and increase energy efficiency [4–7]. Suspension systems provide significantly less muscular stress according to Seifert's study [4] and lower power output from MacRae's work [5] although have not shown this to be associated with a significant difference in VO_2 max [5, 6]. Nishii found that over a test course, full suspension leads to an increase in cycling performance with faster cycling but decreased actual pedaling power [7]. The current vogue seems that downhill bikers tend to prefer full suspension systems, whereas there is increased use of hard tail or front suspension only for cross-country riders. The influence of bike weight is clearly a factor. A downhill full suspension bike weighs typically 15–17 kg, whereas cross-country models may weigh almost half this amount. The sport here is analogous to ski racing. Downhill riders use heavier bikes and take ski lifts to the top of their descent runs, whereas cross-country riders have lighter bikes as they will have to race uphill as well as down.

Mountain bike riding is also a popular recreational activity, occurring in both urban and rural surroundings by young and old alike. This chapter focuses on the injury demographics and specific injuries related to mountain bike riding and racing.

Injury Rates and Demographics

The reporting of mountain biking injuries commenced in parallel with sport development principally on the west coast of the United States during the 1990s. Initial questionnaire surveys of off-road bicycling organizations by Chow, Bracker, and Patrick had high response rates of 82.8 %. Eighty-four percent of respondents had been injured previously, and 51 % had injuries in the past year. Most injuries were minor; however, 26 % required professional medical care and 4.4 % required hospital admission. Ninety percent of injuries were abrasions, lacerations, and contusions, whereas 12 % sustained a fracture or dislocation, e.g., clavicle and shoulder. Frequent riding was associated with increased severity of injury, but most (87.6 %) occurred off paved roads. This survey suggested that compared to road cyclists, off-road cyclists had more frequent but not necessarily more severe injuries [8] (Table 11.1).

Pfeiffer surveyed the National Off-Road Bicycling Association (NORBA), a bicycle race series, by questionnaire, and Pro/Elite category in North America, in 1994, allowed further data collection, but response rates were initially poor (40 %), meaning that less firm conclusions can be made from these studies [9]. Wounds and bruises were the commonest type of injury reported, occurring in 58.1 and 68.2 % of males and female riders, respectively. Sprains, fractures, and dislocations occurred much less commonly. In males, the commonest regions injured were the knee (22.6 %) and the lower leg (12.3 %); however, in females, they were the lower back (16.5 %) and the knee (13.2 %). Typically, these are due to the rider falling to the side or putting out the leg in an attempt to slow down (Fig. 11.3). Already the sport was becoming more competitive with racers training for more than 10 h per week on an off-road bicycling. The majority of injuries (56 %) occurred during racing compared to training.

A questionnaire survey of the 1992 cycling season has been reported by Krosnich and Rubin. Injury rates were high with 85.7 % of respondents reporting injuries. Significant injuries were said to have occurred if the cyclist sought medical attention or was unable to ride on the following day. Ninety percent of these injuries were traumatic with fractures being the most common significant injury reported. The shoulder complex was the most commonly involved anatomical region. Loss of

11 Mountain Biking Injuries

Table 11.1 Current literature mountain biking injuries

Ref.	Year of study	Type	Method	Control	Outcome	Additional data
Chow et al. [8]	1993	Cross-sectional study	Questionnaire survey of bicycling club: injuries divided into mild versus moderate/severe	Mild: no hospitalization	MTB more frequent but not more severe injuries	Demographics Injury distribution Ride characteristics
Krosnich and Rubin [10]	1992	Cross-sectional study	Questionnaire survey of 21 bicycling clubs	Injury: sought medical attention or unable ride for 1 day	4× risk injury if competing	Most common: fracture, shoulder Loss control, high-speed descent, and competing main risk factors
Pfeiffer [9]	1992	Cross-sectional survey of competing riders	Comparison of groups surveyed: 1991, 1992, and 1993	No formal control group Injury is defined as one which forces the rider to stop and seek attention before returning to participation	Females more likely to get injured Wounds most common injury Knee most common area injured	Males more likely to sustain an injury during racing
Rajapaske et al. [34]	1992–1994	Cohort study of forearm and wrist fractures in MTB riders	Questionnaire and clinical examination	MTB accidents can result in significant injury, majority do well, with minimum discomfort and no long-term physical and social consequences	Commonest injury undisplaced radial head fracture	

(continued)

Table 11.1 (continued)

Ref.	Year of study	Type	Method	Control	Outcome	Additional data
Krosnich et al. [11]	1994	Cross-sectional study of riders at a single event. Mammoth Mountain, NORBA UCI	Injured riders were asked to complete a questionnaire and examined by a research physician	Injury was significant if occurred during competition and prevented the rider from completing the event. Injuries scored by Injury Severity Score	Injuries more severe when thrown from bicycle. Moderate injuries when thrown over the handlebars, minor injuries when thrown to the side. Most injuries occurred when going DH. Head-to-head events riskier	The small number of riders injured in a single event has limitations for the study
Krosnich et al. [12]	1995	Case control series. Controls were the different groups of injured riders with respect to each condition	Riders sustaining injury at 3 off-road races completed questionnaires and exam	Injury rates 0.49 % for XC and 0.51 % for DH. 0.37 injuries/100-h racing in CC and 4.34/100 h in the DH	Riders falling over the handlebars had significantly higher injury severity scores and more emergency room visits	Risk of being injured in race is similar in both CC and DH. Greater severity of injury when fall forward over the handlebars. Female riders are more likely to fall forward than male riders and more likely to be injured
Krosnich et al. [13]	1994	Cross-sectional study of riders at a single event. Mammoth Mountain	Injured riders completed a questionnaire interview and exam	Overall injury rate 0.40 %, 81.2 % injuries occurred while DH. Abrasions were the most common injury. Head-to-head riding riskier	Injury considered significant if occurred during competition and prevented the rider from completing that event	The small number of injuries that occur in 1 event may not reflect those that occur during a long sports season

Rivara et al. [15]	1992–1994	Cross-sectional study	Questionnaire survey of those injured while riding off road	3.7 % of cyclists injured were sustained cycling off road. Injury is defined as any rider who attends ED with their injury 4 % cyclists had severe injuries (ISS >8)	Upper extremity and lower extremity were most likely to be injured. Abrasion was the most common injury	Majority of injuries minor. Off-road cyclists are less likely to have head injuries than other cyclists? Higher rate of helmet usage (4×)
Gassner et al. [26].	1991–1996	Cross-sectional survey	Notes review and comparison of riders referred to Max. Fax. Dept.	Severe injury profiles of MTB riders compared to road cyclists. 15.2 % Le Fort fractures	Facial rather than jaw fractures	Recommend face guards for MTB riders
Gassner et al. [27]	1991–1996	Cohort studies	Comparison between bicyclists and MTB riders. Review patient records	More severe injury profile with MTB riders	Increased face guard use together with helmets for MTB and bicycle riders	
Grooten et al. [16]	1997	Cross-sectional survey	Mailed self-administered questionnaire survey to riders of Swedish XC World Cup	75 % riders sustain a major or minor injury. 73 % riders sought medical treatment	Minor discomfort while riding, major injury prevents from riding. More training associated fewer injuries	Better-dosed training and the use of better equipment may prevent injuries
Jeys et al. [17]	1999	Cross-sectional study	Notes review from patients seen in orthopedic fracture clinic	23 % required op. treatment, most common injury: clavicle fracture		

(continued)

Table 11.1 (continued)

Ref.	Year of study	Type	Method	Control	Outcome	Additional data
Frauscher et al. [42]		Case control series	Ultrasound comparison of the scrotal contents of MTB riders compared with nonbikers	94 % MTB riders had abnormal scrotal contents. 46 % had Hx of intermittent scrotal discomfort. Commonest: 81 % scrotal calculi, 46 % epididymal cysts	High prevalence of extratesticular and testicular disorders in MTB riders	
Quigley and Boyce [21]	2004	Cross-sectional survey	Questionnaire and notes review of riders attending A&E dept	Peak incidence in June. 8 % were admitted. Low speed, 65 % cases. 69 % XC. 21 % DH		
Gaulrapp et al. [18]		Cross-sectional survey of German magazine readership with >1 year experience off-road riding	Subscribers were randomly selected, subscribers who had not sustained an injury asked not to reply	Overall risk rate of 0.6 %/year and 1 injury/1,000-h riding	75 % injuries were minor (pause in biking for <1 week), 10 % injuries were severe. Commonest site: calf and knee. Commonest fracture: shoulder	Uses the National Athletic Injury Reporting System
Chow and Krosnich [14]	1994–1998	Cross-sectional survey of those injured	Interview and exam of all riders competing at 7 off-road events. Mammoth Mountain 1994–1998, Vail and Mount Spokane in 1995	Most injuries were minor and involved the extremities (70.5 %)	Falling over the handlebars results in injury more frequently than falling to the side, and injuries were more severe (ISS 3.4 vs. 1.7)	Falling over the handlebars produced more head and neck injuries, whereas falling to the side produced more lower limb injuries

Kim et al. [19]	1992–2002	Cross-sectional study	Review of trauma registries entry requirements: presentation within 7 days injury, admission for ≥3 days, ISS >12 and death	3× increase in incidence of MTB injuries over 10-year period	Orthopedic injuries most common (46.5 %). 38 % of injuries and 66 % of patients required surgery	MTB is a growing cause of serious injuries
Nelson and McKenzie [20]	1994–2007	Retrospective case series	Analysis of National Electronic Injury Surveillance System. Presentation with injury related to MTB	Rates of presentation decreased from 23,177 in 1995 to 10,267 in 2007 ($P<0.001$)	The commonest injury: upper extremity 10.6 % and shoulder fractures 8.3 %. Those aged 14–19 more likely TBI	More females were hospitalized 6.1 % compared to males 4.5 %
Aitken et al. [22]	2011	Cross-sectional study	Survey of those visiting a mountain biking area compared to those reporting injuries relating to MTB at surrounding ED	Overall injury rate found 1.54 injuries per 1,000 biker exposure	Males more commonly injured than females, particularly those aged 30–39. Commonest injuries: wounds, skeletal fractures, and soft tissue injuries	
Lareau and McGinnis [50]	?2009	Cross-sectional study	448 participants in cross-country (<6 h), 6–12-h races, and endurance races (>24 h) were surveyed	No increase in injury rate (7.2 %) in cross-country races <6-h duration versus endurance races >6 h (4.7 %) (OR 1.6, 95 % CI)		

Fig. 11.3 Putting the foot down to the side tends to lead to less severe lower limb injuries, but misjudging a sharp turn and accidentally using the foot in order to stop or change directions can result in a major foot and ankle fracture (photo: Ronen Topelberg)

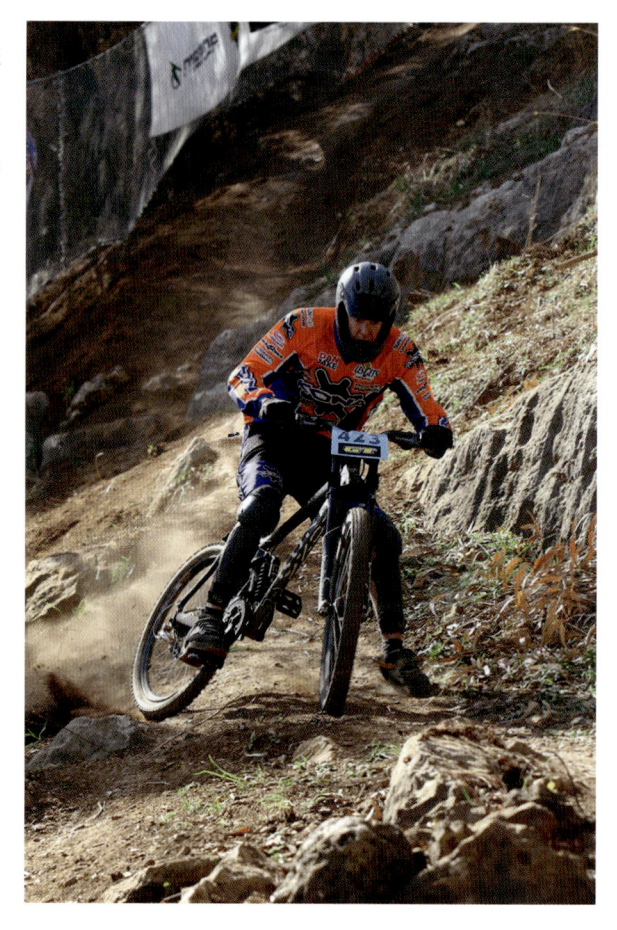

control, high-speed descent, and competitive activity were shown to be variables associated with traumatic injury. In this study, competitive activity level was the only independent risk factor positively associated with traumatic injury, with an adjusted odds ratio of 4.24 [10].

Reports from large mountain bike areas, e.g., Mammoth Mountain Ski Area in the United States, again by Krosnich et al., have revealed injury rates of 60 % for recreational riders; however, the majority of these were superficial injuries (65 %) not requiring medical treatment [11]. Riders that were involved in formal racing had injury rates of 0.39 %, and no differences in the severity of injuries were found between downhill and cross-country riders [11]. Significant injuries are considered to be those in which riders miss a day's cycling, and 26 % of injuries in Krosnich and Rubin's study met these criteria [10]. The commonest of these injuries were fractures, of which 57 % involved the upper extremity compared to 21 % the lower extremity. The acromioclavicular joint was the most commonly injured joint and the clavicle the most common fracture (40 %).

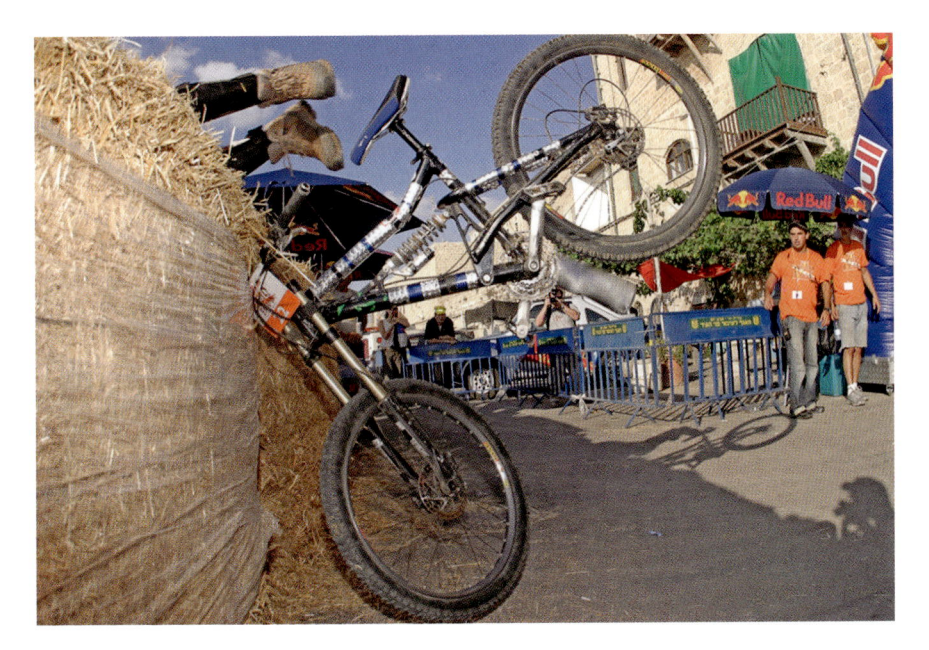

Fig. 11.4 Falling over the handlebars tends to lead to more severe head, neck, and face injuries. Bikers in an urban event (a mountain bike competition within a city) are taking the corner too fast and crash into a thatch block (photo: Ronen Topelberg)

Further studies on the America NORBA series identified injury rates of 0.37 cyclists per 100 h cross-country racing and 4.34 per 100 h of downhill racing [12]. Turning was the commonest reported mechanism of injury, others being loss of control or traction and mechanical problems. Riders who fell forward over the handlebars sustained more severe injuries (Injury Severity Score [12] 3 vs. 1.3) (Fig. 11.4) and required more emergency department visits than those who fell to the side. Also, females were more likely to fall over the handlebars than male riders [12]. This is probably due to female riders being lighter than male. Falling over the handlebars produced more head and neck injuries than falling to the side (56 % vs. 8 %) and generally more severe injuries (with an Injury Severity Score of 3.4 vs. 1.7); conversely, falling to the side generally led to more lower extremity injuries (88 % vs. 57 %) [14]. Thus, female riders could be considered to be more prone to severe injuries.

Other studies consider an injury to have occurred if a rider was unable to complete an event. It must be borne in mind that certainly in downhill events, riders are very "pumped up" and may complete events even with significant injuries, e.g., fractures, if they are mechanically able to ride. Questionnaire surveys may be more accurate than event-side medical care reporting as riders may note abrasions and contusions on a survey of recreational riders, but professional riders may not consider these to be significant enough injuries to trouble event medical support. Surveys may more accurately report a prolonged period of potential exposure compared to the duration of a single or series of events. The American studies tend to involve riders racing on dirt and gravel mountain roads at ski areas. Over other types of terrain, injury patterns may be different.

When injuries sustained during bicycling resulting in attendance at an emergency department were analyzed by Rivara, almost four percent of riders were injured off road. Of these, 73 % were 20–39 years of age and 88 % were males. Injuries were less severe, and riders required less hospitalization than road cyclists [15]. In this questionnaire study at the time of the crash, more off-road riders (80.3 %) wore helmets than other cyclists (49.5 %).

Research into mountain bike accidents has not been totally from the United States. When Swedish racers were surveyed by Grooten, 75 % reported having had an injury, and once again, the knees and lower back were most commonly affected, and 71 % reported minor injuries. Although not statistically significant, riders that trained more and had partaken preseason training sustained fewer injuries [16].

Some studies have reported on the seasonal variation of injuries. Within the United Kingdom, more off-road riders presented to an emergency department during the summer months, most commonly August. In Jey's study, the commonest injury was a clavicle fracture, and alarmingly 23 % of injuries required operative intervention [17].

German questionnaire surveys have revealed an injury rate of one injury per 1,000 h of biking, of which 75 % of injuries were minor and 10 % required hospitalization. Gaulrapp's study revealed comparable injury rates to the North American series [18].

Recent work from Canada has also shown high rates of injury (38 %) requiring surgery [19], and this series has also shown an increasing injury rate with a threefold increase in injuries reported over the last decade [19]. As a result of this increased injury rate, injury prevention has been targeted. It is worthwhile to note that admission to the Canadian trauma registry and an inclusion criteria into the study relied upon presentation within 7 days of injury, a hospital stay of longer than 3 days, and an Injury Severity Score of >12 or expiration in hospital. This means that data from this study cannot be compared directly with other studies, hence the higher operating rate.

A recent review by Nelson of mountain-biking-related injuries treated in emergency departments from 1994 to 2007 has conversely suggested decreasing injury rates falling from 23,177 in 1995 to 10,267 in 2007 (56 %) [20]. The authors commented that reasons for this could be the increase in the use of disc brakes together with suspension. Disc brakes make braking more efficient. They also affirmed that females (6.1 %) were more likely than males (4.5 %) to require hospitalization and that there was an increased risk of traumatic brain injury for those aged 14–19 years (8.4 %). This study reported emergency department data where mountain biking injuries were deemed to have occurred by any person riding an MTB. The results revealed the most common mechanism of injury requiring hospitalization was the rider being commonly struck by motor vehicles termed objects in the series. This study may be more representative of injury patterns of those riding mountain bikes in an urban environment rather than pure off-road riding [20].

Quigley-reviewed mountain-bike-related emergency department presentation to a district general hospital within the United Kingdom has revealed that 74 % (64) of riders were cycling recreationally, 16 % (14) were racing, and 9 % (8) were free riding over man-made/natural obstacles. Seventeen percent of riders were wearing body armor with the majority of these being downhill racers [21].

Another excellent recent study reports on recreational mountain biking from the southeast of Scotland. The number of injuries sustained by bikers was compared to the number of riders visiting a popular mountain biking area. Mechanism and injury data was obtained from questioning riders at the center first aid posts and surrounding hospitals and by follow-up telephone interview (90 %). The overall injury rate was determined to be 1.54 injuries per 1,000 biker exposures. Males were more commonly injured than females with those aged 30–39 being the highest at risk. The commonest types of injury were wounding, skeletal fracture, and musculoskeletal soft tissue injury. Joint dislocations occurred more commonly in older mountain bikers. The limbs were more commonly injured than the axial skeleton. The highest hospital admission rates were observed with head, neck, and torso injuries. Protective body armor, clip-in pedals, and the use of full suspension bikes were thought to confer a protective effect [22].

It must also be remembered that many MTB events occur in small towns in remote mountainous areas. Many riders may sustain significant injury and present over a short-time period. The local hospital's facilities may be rapidly overwhelmed; thus, event organizers may have to warn local hospitals before events so they can arrange extra staffing and equipment [23].

At the Olympic level [24], injury rates in cycling do not form a large component of the injuries sustained at a multisports event. Mountain biking injuries were included within the cycling injuries, and only 30 out of 518 cycling competitors (5.8 %) reported injuries. Two-thirds (20) of these were sustained during competition rather than training (10) [24]. Specifically, only 9 mountain bike riders sustained injuries roughly equally in training (5) and competition (4) (Astrid Junge, personal communication 2011).

Specific Injury Patterns

There are several studies and case reports on specific anatomical areas injured while mountain biking. These include the head and face, the cervical spine, the upper limbs, the abdominal viscera, the perineum, and the lower limbs.

Head and Face

Bicyclists and mountain bikers are prone to facial trauma, and Chow has suggested that conventional bicycle helmets may not provide adequate protection for the face while mountain biking [25]. Gassner from Innsbruck has revealed that mountain bikers have more severe injury profiles than bicyclists for maxillofacial trauma with 55 % having facial bone fractures, 22 % having dentoalveolar injuries, and 23 % having soft tissue injuries. Dentoalveolar injuries were the commonest site of facial

Fig. 11.5 A mountain biker takes a sharp angle turn designed with a berm in order to enable the biker to remain in high speed throughout the turn. The use of a helmet with a face guard may reduce facial injury compared to open face helmets (photo: Ronen Topelberg)

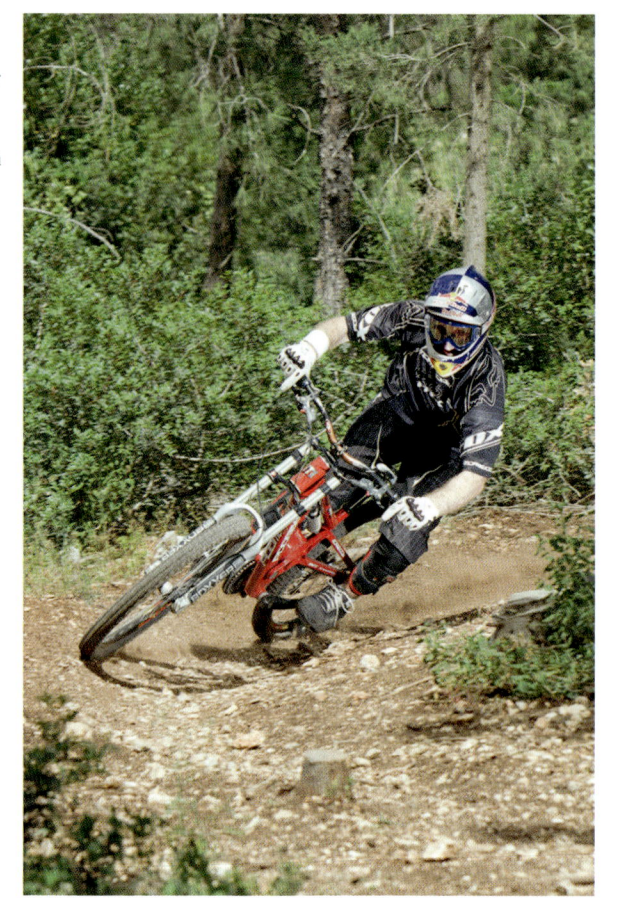

injury in road bicyclists (50.8 %) [26, 27]. Of the facial fractures, 15.2 % were maxillary fractures.

Base of skull fractures may result in injuries to the cranial nerves and bleeding into the middle ear resulting in reduced hearing due to hemotympanum or CSF leak. In one case reported by Saito, a rider sustained a head injury with dislocation of the incus into the external auditory meatus while stunt riding [28].

Kelly reported that 13 % of sports-related head injuries presenting to an emergency department were sustained while cycling [29]. In McDermott's study of 1,710 bicycling injuries, helmet use has reduced the risk of head injuries by 39 % and the risk of facial injury by 28 % [30]. This data on the reduction of the rate of head injury may be extendable to mountain bike riding particularly as we can see from previous papers that it is very difficult to distinguish head injuries sustained by those riding a mountain bike from those partaking in pure off-road MTB riding.

Revuelta has reported on dental injuries including degloving of the mandibular mucosa in children [31]. The high incidence of facial trauma has led to the increased use of helmets with attached face protectors and face guards (Fig. 11.5).

Spinal Injuries

With the speeds involved in downhill racing and the nature of over-the-handlebar injuries, it is surprising that cervical spine injuries do not occur more commonly. A series of paraplegic patients injured while mountain biking have been reported by Aspingi [32]. The three riders in this series had sustained either over-the-handlebar falls or falls directly onto the helmet. The cervical spine is the commonest site of spinal injury, and cord injury was present in 24 % of Kim's series [19].

Dodwell has recently presented a 13-year review of spinal column and spinal cord injuries in mountain bikers. One hundred and seven patients were included. The mean age at injury was 32.7 years, with the majority sustaining cervical injuries (73.8 %) and 40.2 % sustaining a spinal cord injury. Just over 40 % were American Spinal Injury Association grade A and a third improved one ASIA category. This series reports a bleak outcome for those sustaining cervical cord injuries while mountain biking, typically young male recreational riders. The authors of this series recommend that injury prevention should be the primary goal with educational programs, helmets, and other protective equipment awareness [33].

Upper Limbs

The upper limb extremities have already been identified as an area commonly injured. In Rajapaske's series of forearm injuries, the distal radius and scaphoid were commonly injured bones (30 % and 28 %); however, surprisingly, the commonest fracture was the radial head (35 %) [34]. The radial head was either fractured or dislocated due to the energy transmitted down the axis of the forearm from the wrist. This reinforces the importance of examining the elbow in all riders sustaining a wrist injury.

Given the numbers of children riding mountain bikes and the increased popularity of competitions in this age group, it is not surprising that bike use features prominently in childhood and adolescent injuries given that an upper limb fracture is a very common injury in this age group [35].

Prolonged cycle riding of any form has been shown to be associated with nerve compression at the wrist by Patterson, with 23/25 riders reporting sensory or motor, or both, symptoms [36]. When the rough nature of off-road riding is considered, it is no surprise that hypothenar hammer syndrome, i.e., ulnar artery occlusion, has also been reported [37].

During downhill mountain biking, the wrist is held in an extended position and is subjected to repeated forced extension stresses. This has been proposed as the mechanism of injury leading to a case of pisotriquetral instability treated by pisotriquetral arthrodesis using a Barouk screw. The patient returned to professional downhill riding without functional disability although on examination had lost 5° of ulna deviation [38].

Abdominal Viscera

Nehoda has reported a large series of patients with liver hematomata sustained during mountain biking crashes [39]. All of these patients had blunt focal blows to the right abdomen due to the handlebars, and all were using "bar ends" on their handlebars. These bar ends were used to provide additional riding positions and so optimize rider comfort. After a media information program of the implication of bar ends for abdominal injury, bar ends cease to be used in mountain biking. Nehoda's group has noticed an almost complete cessation of liver injury from the sport.

Kim has shown that the spleen was the organ most frequently injured (49 %); the liver (15 %) was injured less commonly. The small bowel was the most frequently injured hollow organ (13 %) [19].

Perineum

Richiuti has shown that perineal numbness due to nerve compression after long periods of sitting on a hard saddle commonly occurs [40]. Modern saddles are molded to reduce pressure on the pudendal nerves in the perineum and aim to alleviate this problem.

The scrotal contents can be subjected to repeated microtraumatization during mountain biking. Work by Frauscher has revealed that 96 % of mountain bikers had pathological abnormalities compared to 16 % of a control group on ultrasound examination [41]. The most common abnormal ultrasound findings were scrotal calculi (81 %), epididymal cysts (46 %), epididymal calcifications (40 %), testicular calcifications (32 %), hydroceles (28 %), and varicoceles (11 %) [42]. Short padding and alteration of the saddle position could help reduce the incidence of these problems.

It is not just the male genitalia which have been shown to suffer from prolonged riding. Female road cyclists have been reported to develop unilateral vulval hypertrophy [43].

Lower Limbs

The shins of bikers are vulnerable to scratches and scrapes when riding through undergrowth, but this can be minimized by wearing long trousers, gaiters, or shin guards. Riders find it essential to have a firm foothold on the pedal to permit stability and pedaling efficiency, and straps or quick-release pedals have been developed for this purpose. These pedals hold the shoe onto the pedal securely allowing improved power transfer [44] but conversely make it more difficult to put the foot down onto the ground when falling off. This delay in foot release means that there is less time to put the foot down for support so it is placed closer to the bike and the sharp teeth of the chain ring. The sharp teeth can result in pretibial lacerations, an area prone to poor healing, and Patel has reported a series, which required debridement under anesthesia and skin grafting [45]. Failure to remove the foot from the pedal can result in the cyclist toppling over onto their side. Although these falls may be perceived as being comical, they can result in significant trauma with the potential for complications. A direct blow to the hip can result in neck-of-femur fractures [46] or acetabulum fractures [47]. Padded shorts are designed to provide protection against this injury. This mechanism also results in more upper limb fracture when the athlete attempts to reduce the impact with his wrist/elbow or shoulder.

In stunt, trials, and downhill events, riders may prefer flat pedals to those with pedal devices or clips for ease of removal and rapid dismount. These pedals, known as "flatties," have a layer of small proud screws on their surface, which give the rider's rubber sole shoe more friction to avoid skidding. These screws are also responsible for major shin laceration when the foot skids backward and the shin meets the rough pedal surface. Putting the foot out in an attempt to slow down may lead to lower tibia spiral fractures or ankle external rotation injuries, but there is no reported literature in this specific area.

Although classically described falling off horses with the foot caught in the stirrup, Lisfranc's dislocation of the midfoot has also been described in a mountain biker. In Callaghan's case, rather than having the foot caught in the toe clip, pain occurred as the rider suffered a forced plantar flexion injury of the midfoot while trying to put his foot on the ground [48].

Adventure Racing

Within the last decade, adventure racing has soared in popularity. These races involve principally mountain biking, mountain running, kayaking, and other disciplines such as caving and rock climbing, and many last for over 24 h. In these events, competitors may ride over forest and mountain trails, and the terrain may be seen to be "softer" than narrow tracks on cross-country or downhill courses. The long duration of these events may well increase injury through falls due to inattention or poor visibility at night; however, lack of experience and reluctance to dismount over difficult terrain have been cited by Greenland as reasons for injury [49].

Lareau and McGinnis have recently suggested that there was no increase in risk of injury in cross-country races, of less than 6-h duration, compared to endurance races of more than 6-h duration (odds ratio 1.6, 95 % CI [0.50, 2.92]) [50]. Data was acquired by surveying the participants in six races: two cross-country (<6 h), two 6–12-h races, and two 24-h races. Endurance races typically involve riding multiple laps of a looped course for a predetermined time period. This means that riders are unlikely to encounter new terrain as they become more tired and as a consequence are more likely to be injured. Riding over MTB terrain at night has added risks, and riders typically use helmet- or handlebar-mounted lights.

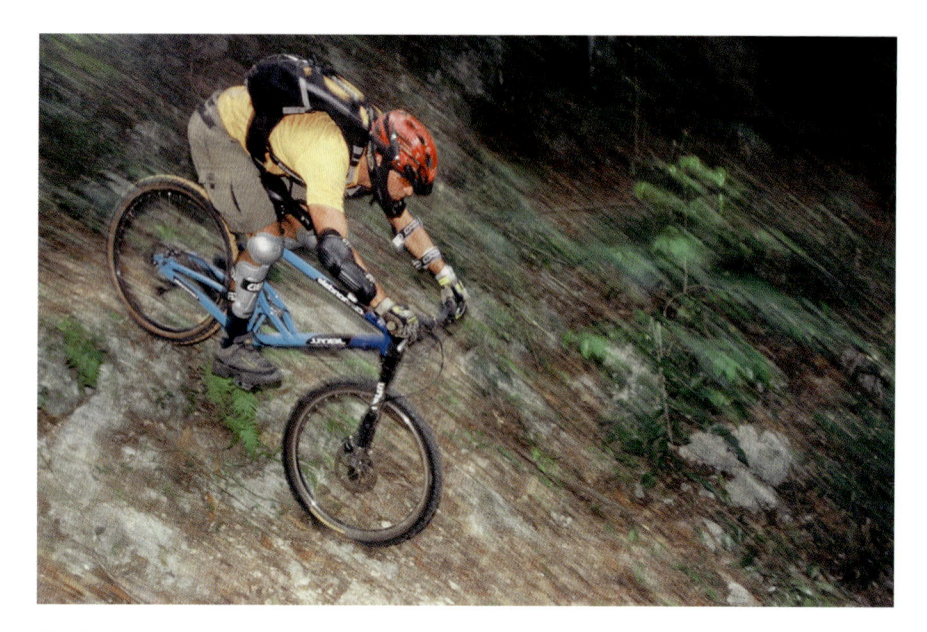

Fig. 11.6 A mountain biker and the common protection used: full face helmet, hard elbow and knee + shin pads, full finger thick gloves, and eye protection. Also, a backpack with water bag and extra cloth is used to pad a potential backward fall/impact, especially if designated spine protection is not used. This use of partial or complete body armor is becoming increasingly common; however, its use may lead to a false sense of security (photo: Yaron Weinstein)

Injury Prevention

A number of methods can be adopted to minimize injury while mountain biking. Riders should be well trained, ride within the level of their capability, learn to dismount safely, and use a well-maintained bike without handlebar ends. Excessive speed, adverse environmental conditions, inadequate conditioning, and rider behavior are factors which contribute to injuries.

Riders are also recommended to wear helmets with facial protection (Fig. 11.5), rather than open face helmets. The use of padded gloves and shorts together with well-cushioned seats and shin protection is recommended.

The use of body armor and leg guards is contentious (Fig. 11.6). It would seem sensible to recommend that all downhill riders use this protective equipment. There is no published literature to support the benefit of its use during mountain biking; however, some research has been done in the sport of off-road motorcycling which may be considered to have similar mechanisms of injury. When off-road motorcyclists were surveyed, 57 % reported that an extremity was most frequently injured; however, the most common type of injury was ligamentous (50 %) and fractures particularly of the foot and ankle (36 %) [51]. Given this predisposition for lower limb ligamentous injury, it is not surprising that the wearing of a prophylactic bracing is associated with reduced rates of both anterior cruciate and medial collateral ligament injuries (ACL 1.515 unbraced vs. 0.701 braced ($P<0.001$) and MCL 0.799 unbraced versus 0.111 braced ($P=0.0274$) injury rates per 1,000 rider hours) [52].

The use of body armor may also lead to a false sense of security for some riders, although its use has been shown to lead to reduced risk of crash-related injury and hospitalization [53]. Unfortunately, motorcycle riders did not, as a rule, learn from their injuries with riders sustaining major injury being less likely to wear protective equipment [54]. This may encourage riders to ride at a level beyond their skill and experience leading to injury. This effect has been shown in the use of helmets in team sports, e.g., schoolboy rugby, encouraging increasingly aggressive play and increased head injury rates as a result [55].

Summary

Mountain biking is a fast, exciting outdoor sport placing riders at risk of injury. A summary of injuries is listed below:

1. Injury rates are 0.37 riders per 100 h cross-country and 4.34 riders per 100 h downhill racing.
2. More serious injuries to the head and neck occur while falling over the handlebars rather than falling off the bike to the side, which tends to result in lower limb injuries. As a consequence of this, female riders, who are lighter and as a result fall over the handlebars easier than male, tend to be more seriously injured than male riders; however, most injuries sustained mountain biking occur to young males aged 20–39 years.
3. Etiological factors for injury are loss of control, high-speed descent, and competitive activity, i.e., riders are most likely to be injured racing downhill rather than training. Turning, loss of traction, and mechanical problems can also lead to injury.
4. The commonest injuries (60–75 %) are soft tissue abrasions, lacerations, and contusions.
5. The commonest fracture is the clavicle, and the dislocation is the acromioclavicular joint.

Mountain biking is a fast adventure sport, which may lead to serious injury; however, the majority of injuries are minor and can be minimized with care and precautions.

References

1. www.mtnbikehalloffame.com/history.cfm. Accessed 26 Nov 2006.
2. International Olympic Committee. The games of the XXXVIII Olympiad mountain bike official results book. Lausanne: International Olympic Committee; 2000.
3. Carmont MR. Mountain biking injuries: a review. Br Med Bulletin. 2008;85:1–12.

4. Seifert JG, Luetkemeier MJ, Spencer MK, et al. The effects of mountain bike suspension systems on energy expenditure, physical exertion and time trial performance during mountain bicycling. Int J Sports Med. 1997;18:197–200.
5. MacRae HSH, Hise KJ, Allen PJ. Effects of front and dual suspension mountain bike systems on uphill cycling performance. Med Sci Sports Exerc. 2000;32:1276–80.
6. Nielens H, Lejeune TM. Energy cost of riding bicycles with shock absorption systems on a flat surface. Int J Sports Med. 2001;22:400–4.
7. Nishii T, Umemura Y, Kitagawa K. Full suspension mountain bike improves off road cycling performance. J Sports Med Phys Fitness. 2004;44:356–60.
8. Chow TK, Bracker MD, Patrick K. Acute injuries from mountain biking. West J Med. 1993;159:145–8.
9. Pfeiffer RP. Off road bicycle racing injuries-the NORBA pro/elite category. Clin Sports Med. 1994;13:207–18.
10. Kronisch RL, Rubin AL. Traumatic injuries in off road bicycling. Clin J Sports Med. 1994;4:240–4.
11. Krosnich RL, Chow TK, Simon LM, et al. Acute injuries in off-road bicycle racing. Am J Sports Med. 1996;24:88–94.
12. Kronisch RL, Pfeiffer RP, Chow TK. Acute injuries in cross country and downhill off road cycle racing. Med Sci Sports Exerc. 1996;28:1351–5.
13. Baker SP, O'Neill B, Haddon N, et al. The injury severity score: a method for describing patients with multiple injuries and evaluating emergency care. J Trauma. 1974;14:187–96.
14. Chow TK, Kronisch RL. Mechanisms of injury in competitive off road bicycling. Wilderness Environ Med. 2002;13:27–30.
15. Rivara FP, Thompson DC, Thompson RS, et al. Injuries involving off road cycling. J Fam Pract. 1997;44:481–5.
16. Grooten WJA, Genberg S, Jonasson L, et al. Injuries among Swedish mountainbike cyclists at an elite level. J Sports Traumatol Rel Res. 1999;21:196–205.
17. Jeys LM, Cribb G, Toms AD, et al. Mountain biking injuries in rural England. Br J Sports Med. 2001;35:197–9.
18. Gaulrapp H, Weber A, Rosemeyer B. Injuries in mountain biking. Knee Surg Sports Traumatol Arthrosc. 2001;9:48–53.
19. Kim PTW, Jangra D, Ritchie AH, et al. Mountain biking injuries requiring trauma centre admission. J Trauma. 2006;60:312–8.
20. Nelson NG, McKenzie LB. Mountain biking related injuries treated in emergency departments in the United States, 1994–2007. Am J Sports Med. 2011;39:404–9.
21. Quigley MA, Boyce SH. Mountain biking injuries in south west Scotland: an analysis of injuries attending A&E. Presented at the British Association of Sport and Exercise Medicine meeting 2005 Edinburgh. Br J Sports Med. 2005;40:90.
22. Aitken SA, Biant LC, Court-Brown CM. Recreational mountain biking injuries. Emerg Med J. 2011;28:274–9.
23. Carmont MR, Daynes R, Sedgwick DM. The impact of an extreme sports event on a district general hospital. Scott Med J. 2005;50:106–8.
24. Junge A, Engebretsen L, Mountjoy ML, Alonso JM, Renstrom PA, Aubry MJ, Dvorak J. Sports injuries during the Summer Olympic Games 2008. Am J Sports Med. 2009;37:2165–72.
25. Chow TK, Corbett SW, Farstad DJ. Do conventional bicycle helmets provide adequate protection in mountain biking? Wilderness Environ Med. 1995;6:385–90.
26. Gassner R, Tuli T, Emshoff R, et al. Mountain biking- a dangerous sport: comparison with bicycling on oral and maxillofacial trauma. Int J Oral Maxillofac Surg. 1999;28:188–91.
27. Gassner RJ, Hackl W, Tuli T, et al. Differential profile of facial injuries among mountain bikers compared with bicyclists. J Trauma. 1999;47:50–4.
28. Saito T, Kono Y, Kukuoka Y, et al. Dislocation of the incus into the external auditory canal after mountain biking accident. ORL. 2001;63:102–5.

29. Kelly KD, Lissel HL, Rowe BH, et al. Sport and recreation-related head injuries treated in the emergency department. Clin J Sports Med. 2001;11:77–81.
30. McDermott FT. The effectiveness of bicyclist's helmets: a study of 1710 casualties. J Trauma. 1993;34:834–45.
31. Revuelta R, Sandor GKB. Degloving injury of the mandibular mucosa following an extreme sport accident: a case report. J Dent Child (Chic). 2005;72:104–6.
32. Aspingi S, Dussa CU, Soni BM. Acute cervical spine injuries in mountain biking. Am J Sports Med. 2006;34:487–9.
33. Dodwell ER, Kwon BK, Hughes B, Koo D, Townson A, Aludino A, Simons RK, Fisher CG, Dvorak MF, Noonan VK. Spinal column and spinal cord injuries in mountain bikers. A 13 year review. Am J Sports Med. 2010;38:1647–52.
34. Rajapaske BN, Horne G, Devane P. Forearm and wrist fractures in mountain bike riders. N Z Med J. 1996;109:147–8.
35. Aleman KB, Meyers MC. Mountain biking injuries in children and adolescents. Sports Med. 2010;40:77–90.
36. Patterson JMM, Jaggars MM, Boyer MI. Ulnar and Median Nerve palsy in long distance cyclists. Am J Sports Med. 2003;31:585–9.
37. Applegate KE, Speigel PK. Ulnar artery occlusion in mountain bikers. J Sports Med Phys Fitness. 1995;35:232–4.
38. Singer G, Eberl R, Hoellwarth ME. Pisotriquetral arthrodesis for pisotriquetral instability. J Hand Surg Am. 2011;36:299–303.
39. Nehoda H, Hochleitner BW, Hourmont K, et al. Central liver haematomas caused by mountain bike crashes. Injury. 2001;32:285–7.
40. Ricchuti VS, Haas CA, Seftel AD, et al. Pudendal nerve injury associated with avid cycling. J Urol. 1999;162:2099–100.
41. Frauscher F, Klauser A, Hobisch A, et al. Subclinical microtraumatisation of the scrotal contents in extreme mountain biking. Lancet. 2000;356:1414.
42. Frauscher F, Klauser A, Stenzl A, et al. US findings in the scrotum of extreme mountain bikers. Radiology. 2001;219:427–31.
43. Humphries D. Unilateral vulval hypertrophy in competitive female cyclists. Br J Sports Med. 2002;36:463–4.
44. Fregly B, Zajac F. A state space analysis of mechanical energy generation, absorption and transfer during pedalling. J Biomech. 1996;29:81–90.
45. Patel ND. Mountain bike injuries and clipless pedals: a review of three cases. Br J Sports Med. 2004;38:340–1.
46. Slootmans FC, Biert J, de Waard JW, et al. Femoral neck fractures in bicyclists due to clipless pedals. Ned Tijdschr Geneeskd. 1995;139:1141–3.
47. Barnett B. More on mountain biking. West J Med. 1993;159(6):708.
48. Callaghan MJ, Jane MJ. Fracture dislocation of the tarsometatarsal (Lisfranc's) joint by a mountain biker. Phys Ther Sport. 2000;1:15–8.
49. Greenland K. Medical support for adventure racing. Emerg Med Australas. 2004;16:465–8.
50. Lareau SA, McGinnis HD. Injuries in mountain bike racing: frequency of injuries in endurance versus cross country mountain bike races. Wilderness Environ Med. 2011;22:222–7.
51. Colburn NT, Meyer RD. Sports injury or trauma? Injuries of the competition off road motorcyclist. Injury. 2003;34:207–14.
52. Sanders MS, Cotes RA, Baker MD, Barber-Westin SD, Gladin WM, Levy MS. Knee injuries and the use of prophylactic knee bracing in off-road motorcycling: results of large epidemiological study. Am J Sports Med. 2011;39:1395–400.
53. de Rome L, Ivers R, Fitzhams M, Du W, Haworth N, Hertlier S, Richardson D. Motorcycle protective clothing: protection from injury or just the weather? Accid Anal Prev. 2011;43:1893–900.
54. Mangus RS, Simons CJ, Jacobson LE, Streib EW, Gomez GA. Current helmet and protective equipment usage among previously injured ATV and motorcycle riders. Inj Prev. 2004;10:56–8.
55. Finch CF, McIntosh AS, McCrory P. What do under 15 years old schoolboy rugby union players think about protective headgear? Br J Sports Med. 2001;35:89–94.

Chapter 12
Paragliding

Lior Laver and Omer Mei-Dan

Contents

Background and Development of the Sport	248
Equipment	249
Control, Maneuvers, and Basic Terms	252
Steering	252
Launching	252
Landing	253
Slope Soaring	254
Thermal Flying	254
Cross-Country Flying	254
Collapse (In-Flight Deflation)	254
Competitive Flying Disciplines	255
Injuries	255
Spinal Injuries and Related Mechanism	257
Lower Extremities Injuries	260
Upper Extremity Injuries	261
Other Associated Injuries	261
Fatality	262
Injury Patterns and Causes	263
Takeoff/Launching Accidents	263
In-Flight Accidents	266
Landing Accidents	266
Main Cause of Accidents	267
Safety Requirements and Prevention	269
Level of Training	270
Summary	270
References	271

L. Laver, M.D. (✉)
Department of Orthopaedics,
Sports Medicine Unit, "Meir" Medical Center, 59 Tschernichovsky st, Kfar-Saba, Israel
e-mail: laver17@gmail.com

O. Mei-Dan, M.D.
Division of Sports Medicine, Department of Orthopaedic Surgery,
University of Colorado School of Medicine, Aurora, CO 80045, USA

CU Sports Medicine, Boulder, Colorado, USA
e-mail: omer@extremegate.com, omer.meidan@ucdenver.org

O. Mei-Dan, M.R. Carmont (eds.), *Adventure and Extreme Sports Injuries*,
DOI 10.1007/978-1-4471-4363-5_12, © Springer-Verlag London 2013

Background and Development of the Sport

Paragliding is a recreational and competitive flying sport. It is defined as a sport using a single seater, nonmotorized, foot-launched flexible aircraft which is steered aerodynamically and able to start from ground level without requiring a free-fall phase. The paraglider, an advanced form of the parachute, consists of an upper and lower sail, with "ribs" dividing it into numerous separate compartments that are stabilized by air pressure. Accurate maneuvers are enabled using two steering lines attached to the rear corners of the parachute. Despite not having an engine, paraglider flights performed by experience pilot can last many hours and cover large distances (up to many hundreds of kilometers). The paraglider pilot also has the ability to gain altitude, using air thermals, often climbing few kilometers over the surrounding countryside/geographic surface.

Being an easily transportable, cheap form of aircraft, paragliders have gained increasing popularity.

Naturally, the evolution of the paraglider began with the normal parachute. American Domina Jalbert, in 1952, advanced governable gliding parachutes with multicells and controls for lateral glide (sideways gliding) [1]. Later, in 1963, he invented and patented the parafoil which had sectioned cells in an aerofoil shape, an open leading edge (known as the "nose") and a closed trailing edge (the "tail"), inflated by passage through the air – which is commonly being referred to as the

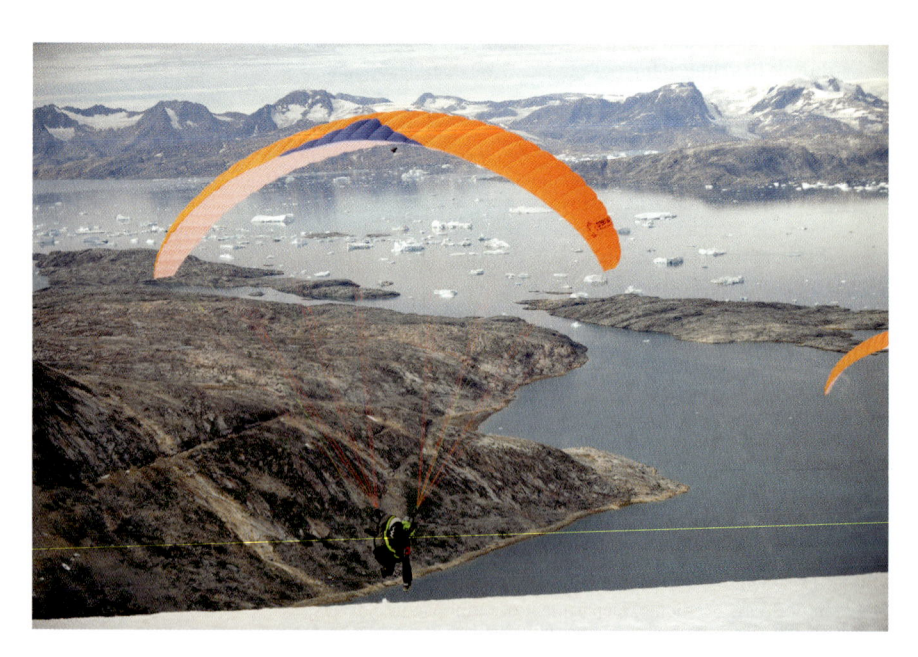

Fig. 12.1 A typical modern ram-air design paraglider (Photo courtesy of Profly.org)

ram-air design (Fig. 12.1). French engineer Pierre Lemoigne produced, in 1961, an improved parachute design that enabled it to be towed by boat or vehicle and by so gain altitude – leading to parasailing/parascending activity.

In 1965, David Barish, while developing the Sail Wing for NASA space capsules recovery, conducted tests on Hunter mountain, New York, after which he went on to promote a summer activity for ski resorts called "slope soaring." The term "paraglider" was first originated by NASA in the early 1960s, and "paragliding" was first used in the early 1970s to describe foot launching of gliding parachutes.

The first flight manual – *The Paragliding Manual* – was written and issued in 1985 by Patrick Gilligan from Canada and Bertrand Dubuis from Switzerland, officially coining the term "paragliding."

Since 1978, when "parapente" ("pente" being French for slope) was born in Mieussy/France, there has been consistent evolution in terms of equipment and different terrains and altitudes paraglided from, leading to continuous increase in the number of paragliding pilots and along side, a growing popularity of the sport.

The evolution of the sport has created a separation between recreational and competitive flying and brought about the need for a platform for competitive pilots.

The first World Championship was held in Kössen, Austria, in 1989, emphasizing the popularity this sport has gained.

Equipment

The paraglider, an advanced form of the parachute, consists of an upper and lower sail, with "ribs" dividing it into numerous separate compartments ("cells") that are stabilized by air pressure. Accurate maneuvers are possible with the aid of two steering lines (also known as "breaks") attached to the rear corners of the parachute. Incoming air (through ram-air pressure) keeps the wing inflated and maintains its shape by leaving most of the cells open only at the leading edge. Once inflated, the wing's cross section is formed into the typical teardrop aerofoil shape.

There are more modern paragliders, known as inflatable parafoils. These are usually ones composed of higher performance wings, in which the cells of the leading edge are closed, forming a cleaner aerodynamic airfoil. These cells are kept inflated by the internal pressure of the wing, similar to the wingtips.

The pilot is supported underneath the wing by a network of strings ("lines"), gathered into two sets (left and right risers) and are connected to the pilot's harness by two carabiners (Fig. 12.2a, b). The harness offers support in both the standing and sitting positions. Modern harnesses are designed to be as comfortable as a lounge chair in the sitting position and can even arrive with an adjustable "lumbar support." A reserve parachute is also typically connected to the paragliding harness.

Paraglider wing typically consists of a surface area of 20–35 sq. m (220–380 sq. ft.) with a span of 8–12 m and weigh 3–7 kg. The total weight of the wing, harness, reserve, helmet, and other related instruments varies from 12 to 22 kg.

Fig. 12.2 (**a**) The pilot is supported underneath the wing by a network of strings ("lines"), divided to left and right risers, and connected to the pilot's harness by two carabiners. (**b**) Using the lines to steer (Photos courtesy of Profly.org)

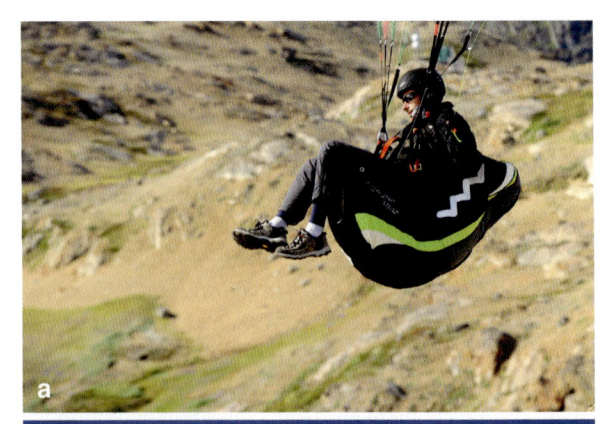

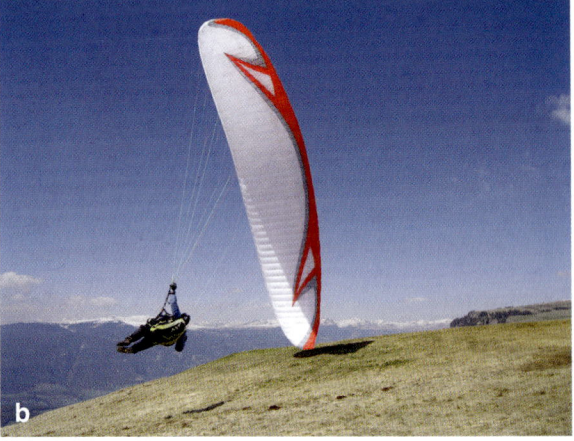

The speed range of paragliders is from 20 to 75 km/h. Beginner and recreational wings sitting in the lower end of the range while high-performance wings are in the upper part of it. The glide ratio of paragliders (the ratio between the horizontal and vertical distance the glider travels at a given speed) ranges from 6:1 for recreational wings (10 m of vertical/altitude lost for every 60 m of forward flying) to about 10:1 for modern competition models. For comparison, a typical skydiving parachute will achieve about 3:1 glide ratio. A hang glider will achieve about 15:1 glide ratio. An idling (gliding) Cessna 152 (a small airplane) will achieve 9:1. Some sailplanes can achieve a glide ratio of up to 72:1.

Modern paraglider wings are made of high-performance nonporous fabrics with ultrahigh-molecular-weight polyethylene fibers or Kevlar/aramid lines – a class of heat-resistant and strong synthetic fibers.

Tandem paragliders, designed to carry the pilot and one passenger, are larger but otherwise similar. They usually fly faster with higher trim speeds, are more resistant to collapse, and have a slightly higher sink rate compared to solo paragliders.

Paragliders, in contrast with skydiving parachutes, are used primarily for ascending. Paragliders are categorized by canopy manufacturers worldwide as "ascending parachutes" and are designed for "free flying" – meaning flight without a tether (as opposed to flying with a tether – in parasailing). However, in areas without high launch points, paragliders may be released after being towed by a ground vehicle or a stationary winch, in order to create a similar effect of "face wind" to a mountain launch. Such tethered launches can enable a paraglider pilot to gain major altitude and use higher starting points (even higher than many mountains offer), creating similar opportunities to catch thermals and remain airborne by "thermaling" and other forms of lift.

As with other forms of free flight, paragliding requires the significant skill and training required for aircraft control, including aeronautical theory, meteorological knowledge and forecasting, personal/emotional safety considerations, adherence to applicable US Federal Aviation Regulations, and knowledge of equipment care and maintenance.

Variometer – When gliding, humans can sense the acceleration when they first hit a thermal but cannot detect the difference between constant rising air and constant sinking air (as opposed to birds). A variometer is a device used to inform the pilot of the near instantaneous (rather than averaged) rate of descent or climb. Variometers measure the rate of change of altitude by detecting the change in air pressure (static pressure) as altitude changes. Modern variometers are capable of detecting rates of climb or sink of 1 cm/s. A variometer indicates climb rate (or sink rate) with short audio signals and/or a visual display and helps the pilot to find and remain in the "core" of a thermal in order to maximize height gain. The more advanced variometers have an integrated GPS, which also enables to record the flight in three dimensions, download, and store it after landing. GPS digitally signed tracks are now used as proof for record claims, and that way, points have been correctly passed (sets of coordinates that identify a point in physical space), replacing the former methods of "above the spot" photo documentation.

GPS – In addition to the above, GPS (Global Positioning System) enables to analyze flying technique by viewing flight tracks when back on the ground, determining drift due to the prevailing wind when flying at altitude, avoiding restricted airspace by providing position information, and location identification for retrieval teams in cases of landing in unfamiliar territory. GPS data, in a more recent use, has enabled pilots to share 3D tracks of their flights on Google Earth, allowing detailed "postflight" analysis and comparisons between competing pilots.

Radio – Radio equipment is used by pilots to support their training, communicate with other pilots, and to report and alert landing intentions and locations. Paraglider pilots often install microphones controlled by a Push-To-Talk (PTT) switch in their helmets either fixed to the outside of the helmet or strapped to a finger. Not frequently, pilots use radios to communicate with airport control towers or air traffic controllers. A cell phone is also very useful, in case of a land away from original point of destination and the need for pickup.

Control, Maneuvers, and Basic Terms

Steering

The steering lines provide the primary and most general means of control in a paraglider and are used to adjust speed, to steer (in addition to weight shift), and to flare (during landing).

The risers connecting to the rear of the wing, via multiple lines, can also be manipulated for steering if the brakes have been severed or are otherwise unavailable.

The "speed bar," also termed "accelerator," is a kind of foot control which attaches to the paragliding harness and connects to the leading edge of the paraglider wing, used to increase speed, by decreasing the wing's angle of attack.

Pilots may encounter descending problems as in cases of thermals with exceptional lift potential or in cases of unexpected weather changes. In this case, the pilot will need to rapidly reduce his altitude in one of various possible techniques. One of these would be a spiral dive, which although being very efficient, places greater loads on the wing than other techniques do. It is initiated by constant pulling and holding down of the brake on one side. This action narrows the turn radius and forms a spiral rotation in which high sink rates can be reached. It offers the most rapid rate of descent at 10–15 m/s and requires the highest level of skill from the pilot to be executed safely. This technique puts/subjects strong G-forces on the wing and glider and might induce blackouts, as well as disorientation caused by rotation.

Launching

There are three methods of launching: forward, reverse, and towed launch. Each method is suitable for different wind conditions and landscapes. In a forward launch, in low winds, the pilot runs forward so that air pressure generated by the forward movement inflates the wing (Fig. 12.3). In a reverse launch, used in higher winds, particularly ridge soaring, the pilot faces the wing to bring it up into a flying position and then completes the launch by turning under the wing. Reverse launches have a number of advantages over a forward launch. In the presence of wind, there is danger of being tugged toward the wing, and facing the wing makes it easier to resist this force and safer in case the pilot slips. Reverse launches are normally attempted with a reasonable wind speed making the ground speed required to pressurize the wing much lower – the pilot is initially launching while walking forward (as opposed to running backward). In flatter landscapes, pilots can also be launched using a tow (towed launch). A release cord is pulled at full height, and the towline falls away. This requires separate training. There are two major towing methods: pay-in (stationary winch that pulls the pilot in the air) and pay-out towing (the line is payed out by a moving car or a boat). "Static" towing is another form of towing involving a moving object, like a car or a boat, attached to a paraglider with a fixed length line. This is a very dangerous method because now the forces on the line have

Fig. 12.3 Forward launching: The wing is inflated by air pressure (**a**) generated by the pilot's forward running movement (**b**) (Photos courtesy of Profly.org)

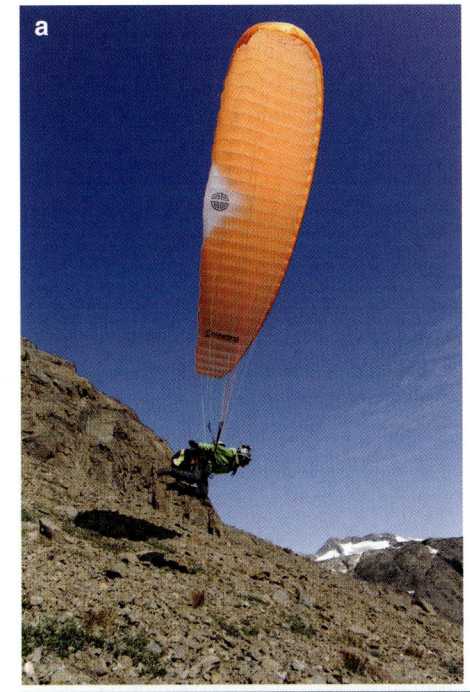

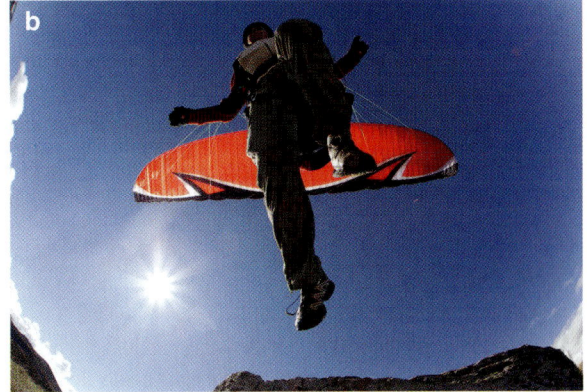

to be controlled by the moving object itself, which is almost impossible. Static line towing is forbidden in most countries and should be avoided at all cost, as it comprises great risk of injury.

Landing

The pilot sets up for approach into wind, and just before touching the ground, "flares" the wing to minimize vertical speed. The aim is to gently go from 0 % brake at around 2 m to 100 % brake when touching the ground. Some pilots apply momentary braking (50 % for around 2 s) at around 4 m before touching ground, then released for forward pendular momentum to gain speed for flaring more effectively and reducing vertical speed before final approach to the ground. Adjustments are to be made according to wind intensity.

Slope Soaring

Whether its a dune or ridge, air is forced up as it passes over the slope, providing lift. Pilots fly along the length of a slope using the lift created. Very little wind and slight lift are enough just to stay airborne as with too much wind, there is a risk of being "blown back" over the slope.

Thermal Flying

The sun tends to warm some features more than others (such as rock faces or large buildings), and these create thermals which rise through the air. These can be simple rising columns of air, or, more often, they are blown sideways due to the wind, breaking off from the source, with a new thermal forming later. Pilots try to find the core of the thermal, which is its strongest part, where the air is rising the fastest. Thermals are not innocent from danger, as there is often a strong sink surrounding thermals and also strong turbulence which might result in wing collapses while trying to enter a strong thermal. Once inside a thermal, shear forces decrease and the lift tends to become smoother.

Cross-Country Flying

Cross-country flying ("XC") is basically gliding from one thermal to the next. After gaining altitude in a thermal, a pilot can glide down to the next available thermal. Potential thermals can be identified by land features, which typically generate thermals, or by cumulus clouds (clouds with noticeable vertical development and clearly defined edges) which mark the top of a rising column of warm, humid air. Pilots are also required proper familiarity with air law, flying regulations, aviation maps indicating restricted airspace, etc., in many flying areas.

Collapse (In-Flight Deflation)

The shape of the wing (airfoil) is formed by the moving air entering and inflating the wing and in turbulent air, part or all of the wing (airfoil) can deflate (collapse). In severe collapses, experience is of essence and pilot training and practice regarding correct response to deflations is necessary. For the rare situations when recovery from a collapse is not possible (or in other threatening situations such as a spin), most pilots carry a reserve parachute. If a wing deflation occurs at a low altitude, i.e., shortly after takeoff or just before landing, the pilot might not have enough altitude remaining to successfully deploy and stabilize by a reserve parachute (the minimum altitude for this being approximately 60–120 m).

Low altitude wing failure can result in serious injury or even death due to ground impact velocity. These complications and other dangers are minimized by flying a suitable glider and choosing appropriate weather conditions and locations for the pilot's skill and experience level.

Competitive Flying Disciplines

- *Cross-country leagues* – annual leagues for the greatest distance "XC" flying.
- *"Comps"* – competitive flying based on completing a number of tasks such as flying around set way points.
- *Accuracy* – spot landing competitions where pilots land on targets with a 3-cm center spot out to a full 10-m circle.
- *"Acro"* – aero-acrobatic maneuvers and stunt flying; heart-stopping tricks (i.e., "helicopters," "wingovers," "synchro spirals," and "infinity tumbles") (Fig. 12.4).
- *National/international records* – despite continually improving gliders, new records have become ever more difficult to achieve. Aside from longest distance and highest altitude, examples include distance to declared goal, distance over triangular course, speed over 100-km triangular course, etc.

Competitive flying is done using high-performance wings which demand far more skill to fly than their recreational counterparts, but which are far more responsive and offer greater feedback to the pilot, as well as flying faster with better glide ratios.

Injuries

The growing popularity of the sport has brought a consequent risk of injuries. Paragliding accidents present a completely new injury pattern, which is not comparable to injuries associated with other air sports or even traffic accidents [2–4]. Most accidents are caused by pilot errors (Table 12.2), unpredictable meteorological changes, or wrong appreciation of environmental conditions; material defects are a rare cause. These accidents may occur in difficult terrain making rescue operations often beyond the capacities of ground rescue services, thus requiring helicopter rescue operations.

Only few publications had been carried out to cover paragliding injuries.

The majority of injuries in paragliding accidents are spinal injuries, located most frequently in the thoracolumbar region, followed closely, and in some reports even

Fig. 12.4 A tumble – an aero-acrobatic maneuver and stunt flying (Photos courtesy of Profly.org)

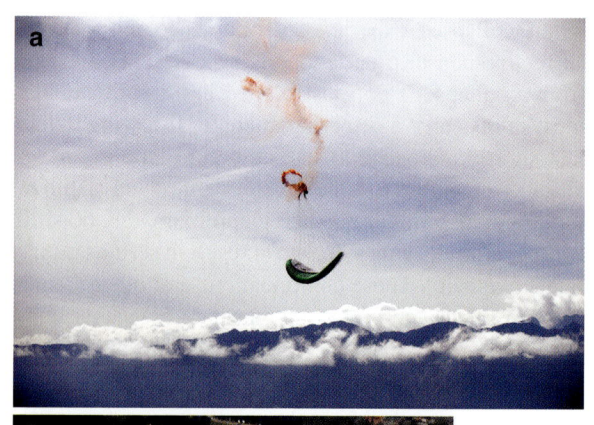

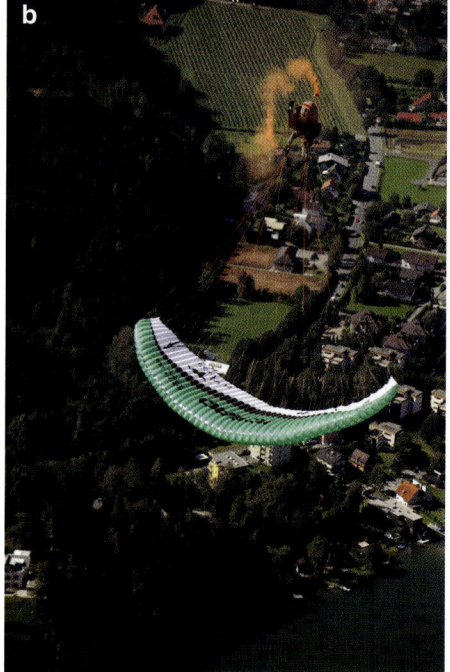

exceeded, by lower extremities injuries (Table 12.1). This is attributed to the fact that most accidents occur during the landing phase, in which large axial compression forces bear on the pilot upon ground contact, predisposing to compression fractures of the thoracolumbar spine and hindfoot (Fig. 12.7). The cervical spine is uncommonly involved as whiplash injuries do not occur in a typical paragliding crash.

Ankle injuries, which are also common, are usually a result of a combination of compression and rotation forces such as pronation/supination of the joint.

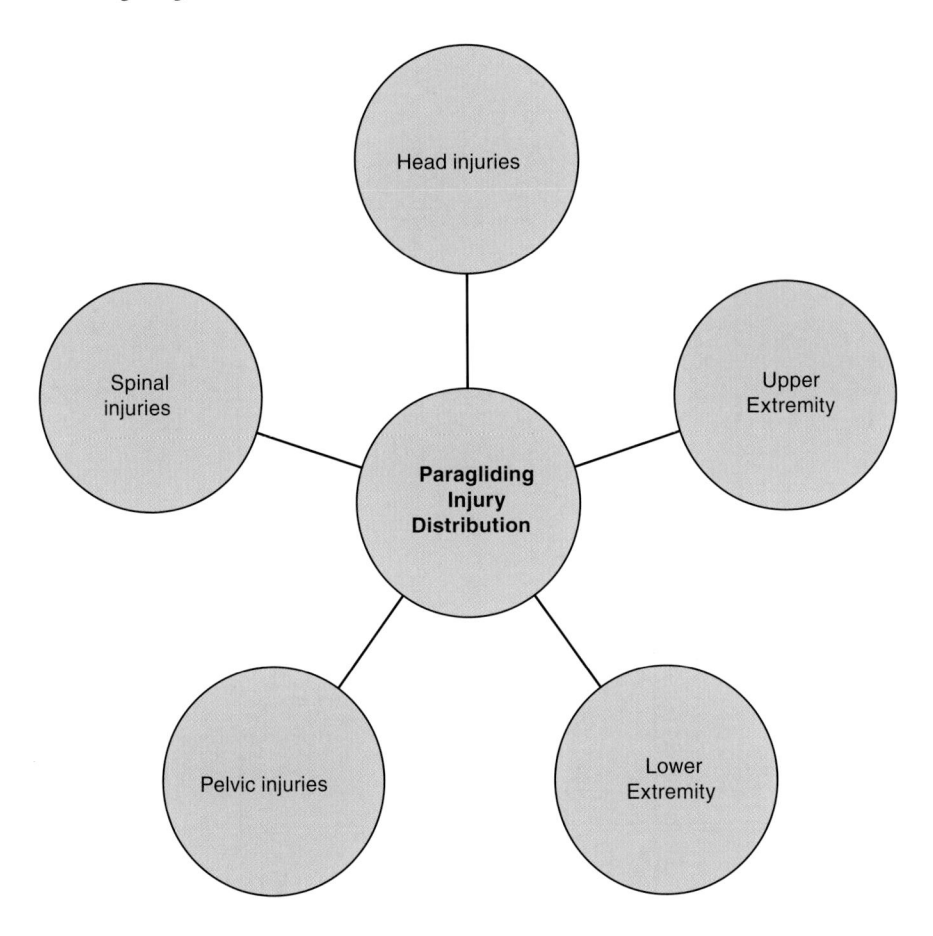

Paragliding Injury Distribution diagram with: Head injuries, Upper Extremity, Lower Extremity, Pelvic injuries, Spinal injuries.

It is not uncommon for paragliding accidents to present as a combined multiple trauma injuries, following the high energy underlying mechanism [5].

Spinal Injuries and Related Mechanism

An analysis of 218 paragliding accidents (283 injuries) in Germany, Austria, and Switzerland between 1987 and 1989 revealed a rate of 34.9 % (99) spinal injuries [6]. The majority of these injuries were located in the lumbar spine (61 fractures, 10 neurological complications). The thoracic spine followed with 25 fractures and 3 neurological complications. The cervical spine was involved in 5 cases (4 fractures, 1 fracture-dislocation which was fatal) and the sacrum in 3 (all fractures). Fasching et al. reported a distribution of 48.5 % spinal injuries (with an 85 % vertebral fracture rate and the lumbar spine being, again, the most injured region) in 70

Table 12.1 Paragliding injuries distribution

	Publication year	Years (injuries)	Country	Accidents	Injuries (n)	Spinal injuries	Pelvic injuries	Lower-limb injuries	Upper extremity injuries	Head injuries
Kruger-Franke et al.	1991	1987–1989		218	283	34.9 % (99)		41.3 % (117)	13.4 % (38)	5.3 % (15)
Zeller et al.	1992		Germany	376	489	25.6 % (125)	3.7 % (18)	46.1 % (221)	17.3 % (84)	5.4 % (26)
Fasching et al.	1997	1987–1991		70	70	48.5 % (34)		54 % (38)	21 % (15)	24.2 % (17)
Schulze et al.	2000	1994–1998	Germany, Switzerland	64		62.5 % (40)	18.8 % (12)	28.4 % (18)		
Lautenschlager et al.	1993	1990	Switzerland		86	36 % (31)	No data	35 % (30)	No data	
Gauler Schulze et al.	2002	1997–1999	Germany	409		34.7 % (142)				
Hasler et al.	2012	2000–2009	Switzerland	144	219	51.3 % (74)	9.7 % (14)			14.5 % (21)

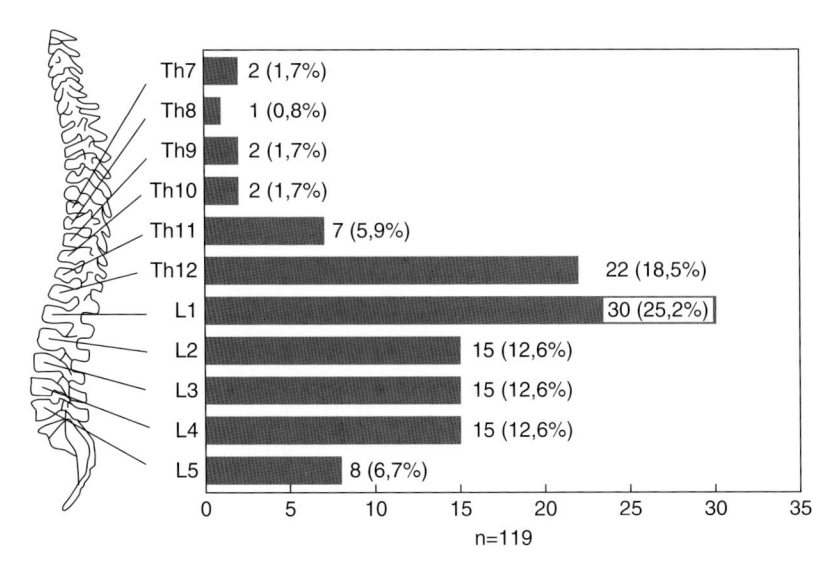

Fig. 12.5 An example of vertebral fracture distribution in 376 accidents in Germany in 1992 (Image was printed with permission from: Zeller et al. [9])

paragliding accidents in Austria between 1987 and 1991 [5]. Forty-six percent of the involved pilots suffered from combined/multiple injuries. A similar distribution of spinal injury rate (46 %) was reported also by Krauss and Mischkowsky [7]. Lautenschlager and fellows gathered a series of 86 injuries associated with paragliding during 1990 in Switzerland, out of which 36 % (31) were spinal injuries [8].

A retrospective study of 376 paragliding accidents in Germany with 489 injuries showed 25.6 % ($n=125$) were located in the spine, with thoracolumbar fractures in 119 pilots (24 % of all injuries) [9]. The most common type of injury was a compression fracture (41.5 %), and the most common vertebrae involved being L1 ($n=30$) followed by T12 ($n=22$) (Fig. 12.5).

Since the early days of paragliding and associated injury data collection, it became evident that the spine is the "Achilles heel" of the sport, sustaining the majority of impact during accidents and consequent injuries (Table 12.1).

When evaluating data about spinal injuries for assessment of spinal cord injury and its prognosis, Gauler et al. showed that there is a high recovery potential if the initial bony spinal canal occlusion is <70 % [10]. As other studies, in their series of 41 patients between 1991 and 2001, they also noted that vertebral fractures peaked in the thoracolumbar region (74 % of fractures were localized between T11 and L3 vertebrae), with L1 vertebrae most frequently affected (30 %). Combination with lower-limb fractures was characteristic for paragliding spinal cord injury. Schulze et al. found 142 spinal injuries out of 409 paragliding accidents analyzed in Germany between 1997 and 1999, predominantly compression fractures of the thoracolumbar spine. Shulze et al. reported a rate of 62.5 % spinal fracture in 64 paragliding accidents between 1994 and 1998 [11]. A series of 144 accidents (219 injuries) gathered in Switzerland between 2000 and 2009 showed spinal involvement in 51.3 % of

Fig. 12.6 Roy-Camille classification of sacral fractures. *Type 1*, flexion fracture; *Type 2*, flexion with posterior displacement and *Type 3*, extension with displacement of S1 and S2 (Image was printed with permission from: Hasler et al. [12])

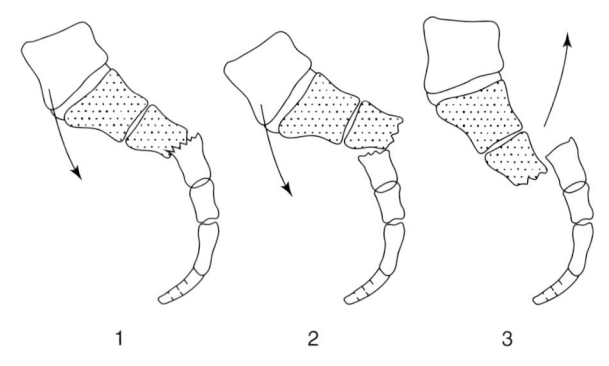

accidents ($n=74$) and 33.7 % of all injuries [12]. The thoracolumbar region was the most affected. Two paragliders suffered injuries resulting in paraplegia, and one suffered from quadriplegia. The most striking finding in this series was the high frequency of spino-pelvic dissociations, with 5.5 % ($n=8$, a 21-fold higher odds ratio than in the general trauma population), and the associated high rate of neurological damage. All patients in this subgroup received surgical management and neurological findings varied from strained but intact nerve roots, to nerve root compression by fracture fragments, and even disruption of all roots below L5 in one patient. When trying to understand the mechanism of sacral fractures in spino-pelvic dissociation injuries using the Roy-Camille classification system [13], it is hypothesized that the fracture pattern is predetermined by the position of the lumbar spine at the time of the axial impact (Fig. 12.6). Types 1 and 2 are considered flexion fractures causing posterior displacement and occur when the lumbar spine is in a kyphotic position (a spontaneous position for protection during landing). Type 3 is considered an extension fracture causing anterior displacement, occurring as a result of impact in a lordotic position. In this series, 2 cases were type 1 fractures, 2 type 2, and 4 cases were type 3 fractures.

Lower Extremities Injuries

Kruger-Franke et al. reported a distribution of 117 lower extremity injuries out of 283 (41.3 %) in their series [6]. The most frequently involved region was the ankle joint, making up for 60 reported injuries (21.2 % of all injuries), out of which 18 were fractures, 12 fractures-dislocations, and 30 ligamentous injuries. Forty-five of the 60 resulted in operative treatment. Zeller et al. found a 46.1 % rate ($n=221$) of lower extremity injuries in their retrospective study of 376 paragliding accidents (489 injuries) [9]. One hundred and twenty cases involved ankle fractures or ligamentous injuries. Twelve pilots suffered ankle fracture-dislocation. Fractures of the tibia and fibula occurred in 39 pilots. Meniscal and ligament injuries of the knee occurred in 34 pilots. Fasching et al. reported a distribution of 54 % (38) lower extremities injuries (with an 84 % fracture rate) [5]. An analysis of 64 accidents between 1994 and 1998 reported by Schulze et al. revealed a 28.4 % (18) of lower extremity injuries [8], mainly affecting the ankle joint or tarsal bones. A 35 % (30) rate was reported by Lautenschlager et al. out of 86 injuries. Fifteen of the cases were severe malleolar fractures that required operative management. Gauler et al., in a retrospective analysis of 41 spinal cord injuries after paragliding accidents between 1991 and 2001, reported 29 non-vertebral fractures in 23 patients, out of which 13 fractures were located in the lower extremities (18.5 % of all injuries) – 6 talocalcaneal, 5 tibial, and 2 femoral [10].

Upper Extremity Injuries

In their analysis of 283 paragliding injuries, Kruger-Franke et al. also reported a 13.4 % rate (38) of upper extremity injuries [6]. Thirteen of those were distal radius fracture, while the rest consisted of acromioclavicular joint separation, shoulder dislocations, elbow fracture-dislocation, combined radius and ulna fractures, carpal and metacarpal fractures, rotator cuff injuries, and other soft tissue injuries. Zeller et al. described upper extremity paragliding injuries as mostly rebound injuries, caused after initially striking the ground. They reported a 17.3 % ($n=85$) distribution in their series of 489 injuries [9]. The hand and forearm were the most commonly involved regions (47 injuries), but shoulder dislocation was also common and was attributed to the special movement carried out when pulling up the canopy. A distribution of 21 % upper extremity injuries was reported by Fasching et al. in a 70 paragliding accidents analysis. Gauler et al. reported 5 upper extremity fractures (1 clavicle, 4 forearm) associated with 41 spinal cord injuries, representing 7.1 % of all injuries (70 injuries in total) [10].

Other Associated Injuries

Head Injuries

Kruger-Franke et al. reported 15 head injuries out of 283 injuries in 218 paragliding accidents [6]. These consisted of 7 concussions (1 fatal), 4 fractures, and 4 lacerations. Zeller et al. reported 26 head injuries in a series of 489 injuries in 376 paragliding accidents in Germany [9]. Due to German helmet regulations, all pilots wore a helmet, with one exception that crashed from about 150 m and was luckily slowed down by trees and was only concussed. Most head injuries were considered minor with the majority being cuts, nose fractures, and loss of teeth. Concussion was reported in 11 cases. Four had signs of brain contusion and one had irreversible brain damage. Fasching et al., in their series of 70 paragliding accidents, reported 24.2 % suffered from head injuries [5]. Other than this series, head injuries were less reported over the years, making it difficult to gather any proper epidemiological data about this type of injury.

Thoracic and Abdominal Injuries

These injuries are uncommon in paragliding, although there have been reports of several cases of hemothorax and pneumothorax, myocardial contusion, and intra-abdominal lesions (rupture of urinary bladder and gut, liver contusion with bleeding). An interesting series of three cases of traumatic rupture of the aorta (descending aorta) secondary to paragliding blunt trauma was reported between 1998 and 2000 [14]. The pathophysiologic mechanism is related to sudden brusque deceleration and chest crushing. In all three cases, the aortic rupture was accompanied by multiple associated injuries, but this injury draws a great deal of attention because of the very high mortality rate it carries, although in this series all patients survived after a prompt surgical procedures and no postoperative complications. The authors concluded that in order to control such injuries, in victims of severe paragliding accidents, the inclusion of spiral CT in the routine ER radiologic evaluation should be mandatory to rule out traumatic aortic rupture.

Pelvic Injuries

There are few reports of pelvic injury distribution in the literature. Nevertheless, this does not represent the true prevalence of these injuries and their importance (regarding severity and residual damage) when evaluating an injured paragliding pilot. One series, by Zeller et al., reported a 3.7 % rate of pelvic injuries ($n=18$) in a retrospective study of 489 injuries in 376 paragliding accidents [9]. Schulze et al. reported 18.8 % ($n=12$) pelvic fractures in a series of 64 paragliding accidents. In another series of 144 accidents analyzed by Hasler et al., 14 pelvic ring fractures (9.7 %) were recorded, all of which required surgery. Additional eight pilots suffered from spino-pelvic dissociation as discussed in a previous section [12].

Soft Tissue Injuries

Muscle, tendon, and ligament injuries varying from strains to ruptures of different degrees are less commonly reported. This might be attributed to the larger "shade" casted by more life-threatening injuries or potentially debilitating osseous injuries which draw more attention in theses multiple trauma series. Some soft tissue injuries are reported under lower and upper extremity injuries categories (i.e., ankle sprains, rotator cuff injuries), but the true rate of these injuries is probably higher than reported, apart from sporadic reports, as in a case of a pilot with a bilateral rupture of the rectus femoris muscle that occurred due to a landing maneuver [15].

Fatality

Between 1986 and 1989, 39 pilots' fatalities were reported in Germany and Switzerland as a result of paragliding accidents, mostly from multiple injuries [16, 17]. In their series of 218 paragliding accidents between 1987 and 1989, Kruger-Franke et al. reported on two accidents which resulted in death (one from head trauma and one suffered a fracture-dislocation of the cervical spine) [6]. Lautenschlager et al. reported one fatal accident (due to a ruptured lung) in 86 accidents during 1990 [8]. Schulze et al. gathered information of 409 accidents in Germany between 1997 and 1999, which revealed 25 fatal accidents during that period (10 in 1997, 8 in 1998, and 7 in 1999, representing 0.06, 0.04, and 0.03 % of licensed paragliding pilots in Germany in those years, respectively) [18]. Of 144 paragliding accidents in Switzerland between 2000 and 2009, only one accident was reported fatal [12].

Injury Patterns and Causes

As mentioned previously, most paragliding accidents are the result of pilot error (Table 12.2). Other important factors are awareness of potential risk factors, unexpected weather conditions, and level of training and experience. Equipment failure is a rare cause.

Paragliding accidents can occur in different phases of flying, from takeoff/launch to landing (Fig. 12.7), whereas each phase may differ in the cause of accidents, the incidence of accidents (Fig. 12.8), injury patterns and mechanisms, and injuries severity.

Takeoff/Launching Accidents

Accidents during takeoff occur often in uneven terrain. Launching with a paraglider often requires a fast run downhill until the sail expands and provides sufficient lift. A terrain with rocks, stones, mud, holes, and bushes is very difficult for the pilot who is forced to pay attention where the feet are placed while making sure the paraglider has opened properly, making it a more stressful and demanding procedure. Failure to control these parameters simultaneously may lead to an inadequately inflated glider's takeoff, resulting in a crash.

The rates of accidents which had occurred during the takeoff phase vary between different reports. Geyer et al. reported a rate of 38 % in 48 paragliding accidents in 1989 [16]. Schulze et al. reported an 11.1 % takeoff incidents rate out of 64 paragliding accidents [11], whereas Fasching et al. reported a 42 % rate in a retrospective analysis of 70 paragliding accidents [5]. Lautenschlager et al. reported 26 % of accidents happened during launching in their series of 86 paragliding-associated injuries [8], whereas Kruger-Franke et al. showed a lower rate of 12.8 % in a larger series of 218 paragliding accidents [6]. In their series of 376 accidents, Zeller et al. reported 35.1 % ($n=132$) of all accidents to occur during takeoff, with the most common injuries located to the ankle, with some affecting the upper extremity [9]. Major spinal injuries occurred in this phase when the pilot sat back too early due to overestimation of the lifting airstream, crashing on his buttocks. They also reported that unexpected crosswinds resulted in the most severe trauma.

Table 12.2 Accident mechanisms and main cause

	Publication year	Years	Country	Accidents	Landing	Flight	Takeoff	Main cause
Reymond et al.	1988	1985–1987	Switzerland	100	Majority		Most severe	Pilot error
Geyer and Beyer	1989			48	32 % (15)		38 % (18)	
Kruger-Franke et al.	1991	1987–1989	Germany, Austria, Switzerland	218	83 % (181)	4.1 % (9)	12.8 % (28)	
Zeller et al.	1992		Germany	376	48.7 % (183)	16.2 % (61)	35.1 % (132)	Pilot error
Lautenschlager et al.	1993	1990	Switzerland	86	60 % (52)	14 % (12)	26 % (22)	Pilot error
Fasching et al.	1997	1987–1991	Austria	70	13 % (6)	44 % (20)	42 % (19)	Pilot error 95.7 % (67)
Schulze et al.	2000	1994–1998	Germany, Switzerland	64	46 % (30)	42.9 % (27)	11.1 % (7)	Paraglider handling
Schulze et al.	2002	1997–1999	Germany	409				Airfoil collapse or deflation
Rekand et al.	2008	1997–2006	Norway	9	100 %			

12 Paragliding

Fig. 12.7 Injury mechanisms: (**a**) contact with the ground, (**b**) crash after stalling, and (**c**) landing with straight legs (Image was printed with permission from: Zeller et al. [9])

Ground Contact

Crash after Stall

Landing with Straight Legs

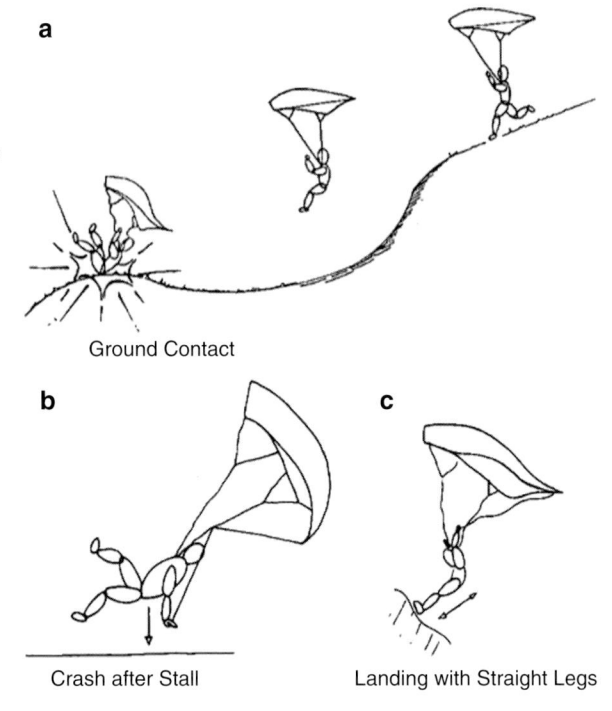

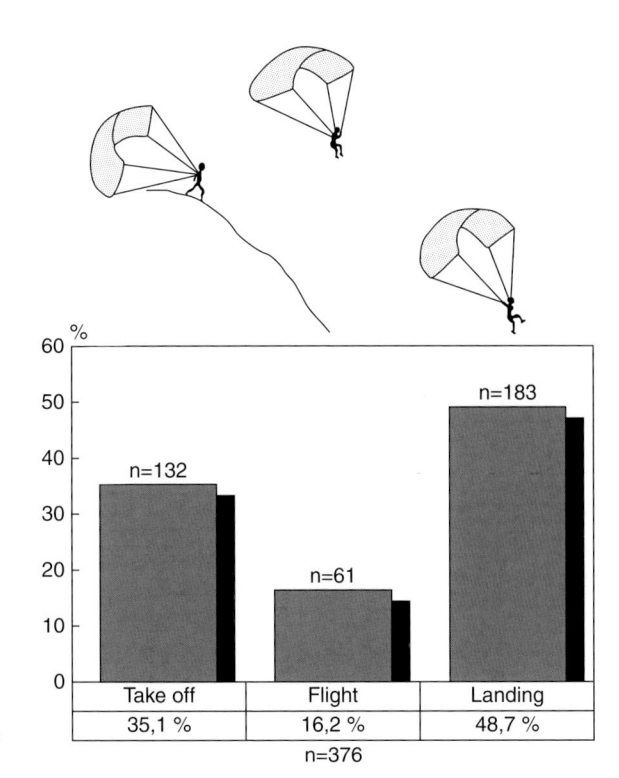

Fig. 12.8 Accidents distribution during different flight phases (Image was printed with permission from: Zeller et al. [9])

	Take off	Flight	Landing
	35,1 %	16,2 %	48,7 %

n=132 (Take off)
n=61 (Flight)
n=183 (Landing)
n=376

Another analysis by Schulze et al. of 409 accidents revealed 16–28 % occurred during starting procedures [18], with causes varying from collisions with obstacles during takeoff, mistakes during takeoff (the most common being getting into the harness before taking-off, resulting in further contact with the ground), incomplete preflight check resulting in unfastened leg loops, and taking off with tangled or knotted lines. There were some cases of backlash from towing cord breaking or after being cut.

In-Flight Accidents

Flight accidents, as launching and landing accidents, can be influenced by factors such as weather changes, pilot's level of experience and training (especially the ability to adjust and maneuver through unexpected extreme conditions), and rarely equipment failure. Canopy collapse or turbulence can lead to a stall, which if not handled fast, results in crashes from a great height, potentially leading to multiple injuries. In their analysis of 218 accidents in Germany, Austria, and Switzerland between 1987 and 1989, Kruger-Franke et al. found only 4.1 % (9) occurred during the flight phase [6]. A similar distribution pattern was recorded by Zeller et al. with 16 % ($n=61$) of all accidents occurring during the flight phase in their series of 376 accidents [9]. A series of 86 paragliding accidents gathered in Switzerland in 1990 by Lautenschlager et al. revealed a 14 % ($n=12$) rate of in-flight accidents [8]. Other reports showed a different incidence in flight accident, as Fasching et al. showed in their series of 70 accidents in Austria between 1987 and 1991, with 44 % (20) occurring during the flight phase [5]. A similar incidence was reported by Schulze et al. in a series of 64 accidents, with 42.9 % (27) occurring in the flight phase [11].

Landing Accidents

Lang [19] and Reymond [17] pointed out that a majority of all injuries occurred during the landing phase, primarily as a result of forceful landings. Main causes were conditions' misjudgment, pilot's inability to adjust to abrupt changes in the thermals and wind conditions, and other technical errors. These can all lead to incorrect or uncontrolled landing. In a series of 64 paragliding accidents between 1994 and 1998, main reported causes were paraglider handling or general lack of awareness about potential risk factors [11]. In this series, 46 % occurred during landing, in comparison to 42.9 % which occurred during flight and 11.1 % during takeoff. A more distinct pattern was revealed in a European study examining 218 paragliding accidents, where 83 % (181) occurred during landing [6]. In another large series analyzing 376 accidents, Zeller et al. found 48.7 % ($n=183$) to occur during landing.

Lautenschlager analyzed 86 injuries associated with paragliding in Switzerland in 1990 [8], revealing 60 % of accidents happened during the landing phase, compared to 26 % at launching, and 14 % during flight. Most accidents occurred due to in-flight error of judgment such as incorrect estimation of wind conditions and a choice of unfavorable landing sites. Only one accident was a result of equipment failure (a ruptured steering line). Improper correlation between paraglider type and pilot's weight and experience was found in more than a third of all accidents in this analysis.

A review of 200 cases of paragliding accidents in high-mountain areas implicated that more frequent accidents happen during landing. This was also confirmed by another review of 39 paragliding accidents in Switzerland where the most severe injuries occurred immediately after taking off [17]. This review also showed a correlation between the altitude, the wind velocity, and the injury severity.

In contrary to the above, Geyer et al. found 32 % of the 48 paragliding-related injuries studied to occur during landing, while 38 % occurred during takeoff [16]. An even more reversed trend was evident in a retrospective analysis of 70 paragliding accidents, where only 13 % (6) occurred during landing [5].

Main Cause of Accidents

A more thorough analysis of paragliding accident's causes was performed in 409 accidents between 1997 and 1999 in Germany [18]:

- Collapse of the glider was the most common cause of accident, with an asymmetric collapse (85.1 %) being more common than a frontal collapse (15.9 %).
- Collapse or deflation of the airfoil was the cause in 133 cases (32.5 %). In 59.9 % of accidents, failure to restore the canopy shape after deflation led to the pilot hitting either an obstacle or the ground.
- About one-third (30.1 %) of accidents were caused by incorrect use of the break lines resulting in a stall.
- Over-steering or pilot error was the cause in 57 cases (13.9 %).

Incorrect break line handling caused airflow interruption (invariably a pilot error) — that is, in rapid descent maneuvers or parachutal flight. A paraglider is normally landed by stalling it just above the ground. Poorly trained pilots may perform this maneuver incorrectly, especially at too great of a height, resulting in a "straight down falling" and hard landing. Newer generation of gliders presented a recent problem which was that they could become locked into a spiral after intentional performance of this maneuver by a pilot not trained properly to counteract it on the model being used, emphasizing again the need of correlation between the paraglider used and the pilot's experience and training.

- Collision with an obstacle was the cause in 49 cases (12 %) occurring during takeoff, while soaring close to cliffs, and, most often, during landing. In 78 % of cases, a tree was the obstacle involved. More uncommon, and dangerous, were collisions with cable cars or power lines (6 % of accidents). The final 16 % involved buildings, vehicles, or other obstacles.

- Mistakes during takeoff accounted for 42 of the cases (10.3 %), where most common mistakes were made while getting into the harness before taking off, resulting in further contact with the ground.
- *Mistakes during landing* accounted for 56 of the cases (13.7 %), with causes varying between:
  - *Incorrect landing approaches* (too high or too low)
  - *Erroneous correction of the direction*
  - *Fast curves close to the ground*
  - *Landing with a tailwind*

Difficult landing conditions, such as particularly strong winds, thermal activity, small landing areas, and obstacles on the edge of the landing area, resulted in miscalculations. During actual landing itself, the errors were:

- Not getting out of the harness quickly enough (delaying the ability to place feet properly on the ground)
- Braking too hard
- Miscalculation of obstacles leading to a crash landing
  - *Misjudgment of the weather* has led to 20 of the cases (4.9 %) with the most common problems being underestimating wind velocity and meteorological miscalculations.
  - *Incomplete preflight check* was the cause in 20 cases (4.9 %), with mistakes such as pilots not fastening the leg loops resulting in falling out on takeoff, and taking off with tangled or knotted lines.
  - A more rare cause of accident was loss of the emergency parachute during the flight because it was not secured properly although needed later.
  - Mid-air collisions occurred in nine cases (2.2 %).
  - Problems with the winch (the device used to let out the paraglider in a towed launch) were the cause in nine of the cases (2.2 %).
  - Equipment problems were responsible for two of the cases (0.5 %), a result of age related performance changes of the gliders.

After analyzing 376 paragliding accidents in Germany, Zeller et al. described two main injury mechanisms:

1. Falls during running on the ground in the takeoff phase or after landing, which resulted in low-energy trauma and usually minor damage
2. Falls from various heights, resulting in landing on straight legs or buttocks

The majority of accidents in this series were due to pilot error, and most injuries were a result of mishandling of the sail, which could have been avoided with appropriate training, more experience, and awareness. Sail collapse or complete stall due to turbulence and wind changes was found to be the primary cause of crash in 19 % ($n=71$) of all accidents in this series [9].

Another retrospective study of nine paragliding accidents between 1997 and 2006 pointed causes were landing problems combined with unexpected whirls, technical problems, and limited experience with unexpected events [20].

In terms of terrain in which accidents occur, most accidents occur in high-mountain areas, whereas flights in lowland areas are considered significantly less dangerous.

Safety Requirements and Prevention

Pilot error has been emphasized in previous sections as the main cause of accidents, being derived from pilot's skill level and judgment. However, there are additional factors influencing flight safety and injury risk. Equipment failure is a rare cause of accidents and injuries. The average paraglider has around 30 lines connected to the risers, each one strong enough to support the full weight of a pilot individually. When assessing weather conditions, turbulence, or conditions conducive to turbulence generation is a primary factor in determining the safety degree.

There are several safety precautions regarding weather conditions which should be emphasized:

1. Excessive wind speed of over 24 km/h (15 mph) should be avoided, and most pilots will refrain from taking off in conditions more windy than that. The limit of 15 mph is quite arbitrary, as it also depends on local parameters. There are sites where people can fly safely at 20-mph winds, whereas at other sites 10 mph may be at risk. High winds may also increase the effect of mechanical turbulence, thus elevating the risk of collapses while in flight and the risk of accidents.
2. Wind direction that will not allow a takeoff (or landing) into the wind should be avoided, and pilots should avoid tailwind takeoffs at all cost.

Flying into heavy rain or snow should also be avoided since the paraglider wing is made from fabric and can absorb moisture, thus affecting the weight of the wing which is critical to its performance, making it less controllable, less stable, and reducing its ability to recover into normal flight. Additional important safety precautions are as follows:

- Preflight check should be a mandatory routine and should include a thorough inspection of all the equipment, including the reserve parachute and protective gear.
- Protective helmets and sturdy footwear reaching above the ankle joint are indispensable equipment. Use of protective gloves is highly recommended.
- New generation back protection devices provide the best prophylaxis for pilots against pelvic and spinal cord injuries [11]. Foam multichamber and airbag harnesses are considered the best protection against spinal and pelvic fractures. The

number of vertebral fractures decreased significantly between 2000 and 2003 in Germany and Austria through the introduction (and enforcement) of a spine protector system [21]. Together with adaptation of beginners and intermediate wings for respective levels, this area holds the most promise for reducing injury risk in the future.
- Careful prelaunch observation of other pilots in the air to evaluate conditions.

Pilots who want to stretch themselves into more challenging conditions can take part in advanced courses which simulate different flying incidents, teaching pilots how to cope with hazardous situations which may arise during flight. In these courses, pilots deliberately induce (under guidance) major collapses, stalls, spins, etc., in order to learn recovery techniques and maneuvers.

Level of Training

There are only a few series which evaluated the training level of pilots in accidents. However, it is widely accepted that further performance and safety training (to the initial basic training) and flight experience are important to handle unexpected conditions and events. In a subjective analysis in different series, the majority of pilots stated that the accidents they were involve in could have been avoided with better training, more experience and awareness, and sufficient preparation. The exact impact of these factors on safety and lowering injury occurrence and severity is unknown, but it has been shown that beginners and recreational pilots with less than 100 flights (40 %) were the most accident-prone group out of 409 accidents [18]. In this group, the number of accidents that occurred during takeoff and landing as well as due to over-steering was above average; as opposed to the reasonably experienced pilots group with up to 200 flights (27 %), there was no predominant cause of accident. Irrespective of the number of completed flights, the 2 years immediately after gaining the pilot's license were the most dangerous period, as well as the training period, during which the number of accidents was above average.

An important aspect that requires attention is adjusting the appropriate paraglider to the pilot's level of training. For instance, high-performance paragliders are very sensitive and require an experienced pilot, as small mistakes may result in drastic unwanted effects. The desire for longer flights often motivates pilots to use too large surface area gliders, leading elevating the risk for a more unstable flight. Accurate equipment choice and increased attention to environmental factors are recommended in order to reduce the frequency and severity of paragliding injuries.

Summary

As the sport of paragliding is increasing in popularity, the number of injuries encountered by physicians is likely to grow as a consequence. Therefore, recognition and understanding of common paragliding injuries and mechanisms may enable to provide a fast and accurate diagnosis and a better treatment.

The spine has been described as the "Achilles" heel of the sport, with higher injury rates than any other sport, and together with lower-limb injuries, they comprise the most common injuries in paragliding. The use of a spine protector system significantly lowers the incidence of vertebral fractures and should be an inseparable part of the paraglider's pilot essential gear set, alongside with a helmet, an ankle protecting system, and shock absorbing shoes.

Most injuries occur during the landing phase and pilot error is the main reason for most injuries, underlining the need for constant and better performance and safety training. Extreme flight conditions should be simulated and discussed more thoroughly and better awareness and recognition of danger should be emphasized. Injuries in paragliding can be reduced by correlating the appropriate gliders to pilots, according to their level of training, experience, and physical features.

The role of the physician, especially in areas where paragliding is more popular, should encourage application of safe flight precautions and the use of protective equipment.

References

1. Jalbert DC. Inventor multicell parachute canopy. US patent 2734706. 1952.
2. Katoh S, Shingu H, Ikata T, Iwatsubo E. Sports-related spinal cord injury in Japan (from the nationwide spinal cord injury registry between 1990 and 1992). Spinal Cord. 1996;34(7):416–21.
3. Dawson M, Asghar M, Pryke S, Slater N. Civilian parachute injuries; 10 years on and no lessons learned. Injury. 1998;29(8):573–5.
4. Schmitt H, Gerner HJ. Paralysis from sport and diving accidents. Clin J Sport Med. 2001;11(1):17–22.
5. Fasching G, Schippinger G, Pretscher R. Paragliding accidents in remote areas. Wilderness Environ Med. 1997;8(3):129–33.
6. Kruger-Franke M, Siebert CH, Pforringer W. Paragliding injuries. Br J Sports Med. 1991;25(2):98–101.
7. Krauss U, Mischkowsky T. The severely injured paraglider: analysis of 122 cases. Unfallchirurg. 1993;96:299–304.
8. Lautenschlager S, Karli U, Matter P. Paragliding accidents – a prospective analysis in Swiss mountain regions. Z Unfallchir Versicherungsmed. 1993;Suppl 1:55–65.
9. Zeller T, Billing A, Lob G. Injuries in paragliding. Int Orthop. Springer-Verlag. 1992;16(3):255–9.
10. Gauler R, Moulin P, Koch HG, et al. Paragliding accidents with spinal cord injury: 10 years' experience at a single institution. Spine (Phila Pa 1976). 2006;31(10):1125–30.
11. Schulze W, Hesse B, Blatter G, Schmidtler B, Muhr G. Pattern of injuries and prophylaxis in paragliding. Sportverletz Sportschaden. 2000;14(2):41–9.
12. Hasler RM, Huttner HE, Keel MJ, et al. Spinal and pelvic injuries in airborne sports: a retrospective analysis from a major Swiss trauma centre. Injury. Elsevier. 2012;43(4):440–5.
13. Roy-Camille R, Saillant G, Gagna G, Mazel C. Transverse fracture of the upper sacrum. Suicidal jumper's fracture. Spine (Phila Pa 1976). 1985;10(9):838–45.
14. Navarrete-Navarro P, Macias I, Lopez-Mutuberria MT, et al. Traumatic rupture of aorta should be ruled out in severe injuries from paragliding: report of three cases. J Trauma. 2002;52(3):567–70.

15. Schulze Bertelsbeck D, Veelken D. Paragliding-associated bilateral partial rupture of the rectus femoris muscle. Unfallchirurg. 2004;107(12):1196–8.
16. Geyer M, Beyer M. Verletzungen beim gleitschirmfliegen. Unfallchirurg. 1989;92:346–51.
17. Reymond MA, de Gottrau P, Fournier PE, Arnold T, Jacomet H, Rigo M. Traumatology in hang-gliding accidents. Studies based on 100 cases. Chirurg. 1988;59(11):777–81.
18. Schulze W, Richter J, Schulze B, Esenwein SA, Buttner-Janz K. Injury prophylaxis in paragliding. Br J Sports Med. 2002;36(5):365–9.
19. Lang T, Dengg C, Gabl M. Der Unfall mit dem 'gleitschirm'. Sportverletz Sportschaden. 1988; 2:115–9.
20. Rekand T, Schaanning EE, Varga V, Schattel U, Gronning M. Spinal cord injuries among paragliders in Norway. Spinal Cord. 2008;46(6):412–6.
21. Bohnsack M, Schroter E. Injury patterns and typical stress situations in paragliding. Orthopade. 2005;34(5):411–8.

Chapter 13
Mountain, Sky, and Endurance Running

Denise Park and Michael R. Carmont

Contents

Origins of Mountain Running and Its Development	274
Background	274
Mountain Running	274
Skyrunning	275
Endurance Running	277
The Equipment Used: Essential and Safety Requirements/Considerations	278
Clothing	278
Footwear	279
Climate	280
Food and Drink	280
Altitude	280
Safety Requirements	281
Injury Demographics, Mechanisms, and Rates	281
Injury Rates	281
Fatalities	283
Specific Types of Injury	285
Runner's Knee	285
Common Treatments (Conservative/Surgical) and Rehabilitation	289
Causes of Injury	289
Treatment	291
Acute Injury	292
Chronic Injury	293
Conservative Physiotherapy Treatment	293
Proposed Preventative Measures (Training and Equipment Wise):	
Injury and Illness	294
Acute Mountain Sickness (AMS)	299
References	299

D. Park, M.Sc., MCSP, SRP, Grad Dip Phys (✉)
Musculoskeletal Chartered Physiotherapist, Denise Park Practice, Clitheroe, UK
e-mail: denisephysio@hotmail.com

M.R. Carmont, FRCS (Tr&Orth)
The Department of Orthopaedic Surgery, Princess Royal Hospital,
Shrewsbury and Telford NHS Trust, Telford, UK

The Department of Orthopaedic Surgery, The Northern General Hospital,
Sheffield Teaching Hospitals NHS Foundation Trust, Sheffield, UK
e-mail: mcarmont@hotmail.com

Origins of Mountain Running and Its Development

Background

- Running is one of man's greatest natural abilities and has been essential to the survival of the human race. An individual's ability to run longer, faster, uphill, or downhill has been advantageous in war and conflict, escaping danger, hunting for food, and as in the first marathon – carrying messages. Running first took place over a multitude of terrains – mountains, rivers, forests, and deserts, and did not involve any specialist equipment – there were no tarmac roads or asphalt tracks, and many individuals ran barefoot.
- While it is no longer essential to run well to survive, many individuals still have the passion to run in challenging natural environments. Personal achievement, world ranking, prize money, and medals have replaced the goal of survival, but it is man's battle against the extremes of nature which still continues to drive the athletes competing in mountain, skyrunning, and endurance races.
- While these three areas overlap at times, each has a slightly different philosophy with different governing bodies regulating national and international events.

Mountain Running

Mountain running is a worldwide sport, and its origins can be traced for hundreds of years. While the term "mountain running" is used globally, it is often referred to as fell running in England (after the Norwegian word for mountain – fjell), hill running in Scotland, and trail running in America.

There is a pre-Christian folk tale that Irish hero Fionn MacCumhaill staged a female-only race up and down the Slievenamon Mountain in County Tipperary, Ireland, to select his wife. The first actual recorded "hill" race occurred in Scotland around 1,068 when the race was used as an interview process by King Malcolm II to appoint servants or guides [1].

There are many stories that mountain racing developed in England as shepherds and professional mountain guides challenged each other to race on the fells. Races were often referred to as guide races, and records are available from the Grasmere Guides Race from the early 1850s. These professional "guide races" had restricted entries until 1995 when they finally became open to other competitors. The Burnsall Fell Race is regarded as the oldest non-guide race in England, allegedly being first staged in 1850, but the press reports are only available from 1882. Other documented mountain races date back to the Sugarloaf (Ireland) in 1873, the Ben Nevis Race (Scotland) in 1895, and the Mount Washington Race (USA) in 1921.

The first Mountain Running Committee was created in Italy in 1968, and in 1971 the Fell Runners Association (FRA) was formed in Great Britain. The International Committee for Mountain Running (ICMR), formed in 1984, organized the first World Cup being held the same year. The year 1999 saw this organization being renamed the World Mountain Running Association (WMRA), and 3 years later, in 2002, it gained the approval from the IAAF (International Association of Athletic Federations) to organize international competitions.

The European and World Mountain Running Championship courses alternate annually between an uphill course and an up- and downhill course, allowing the competitors to be tested over different disciplines. The championship courses vary between 11–13 km for senior men and 7–10 km for senior women, with height differences of between 500 and 900 m and peaks of above 1,500 m. Junior athletes also entered the international field in 2007.

Other non-championship races take place over a variety of distances, terrains, and ascents/descents. Many take place over summer in winter ski areas, where high-level facilities allow races to finish with an ascent with ski lifts being available for easy transportation back down the mountain, or a descent into a mountain village. Some are over rough terrain, whereas others take place on established mountain paths. The courses are usually well marked and do not require navigational skills, although in England, it is often the responsibility of the runner to calculate the fastest route from the start to the finish line, checking in at various points en route.

The Sierre-Zinal race in Switzerland, also called the race of five 4,000-m peaks, is considered to be one of the finest mountain races in the world and is the oldest mountain race in its category in Europe. It is 31 km with 2,200 m of ascent and 800 m descent. Jonathon Wyatt, race record holder and six times world champion, wrote "Every (mountain) runner must participate in this legendary race at least once in their lifetime" (Fig. 13.1 and 13.2).

Skyrunning

Skyrunning is the discipline of running in mountains above 2,000 m, where the incline exceeds 30 % but the climbing difficulty does not exceed II° grade (hiking up a steep trail). It differs from mountain running in that it takes place at altitude, the courses can be more technical, they avoid asphalt paths (some mountain races are almost entirely on asphalt roads, e.g., the Mount Washington Race), and they tend to include more downhill sections.

The sport is divided into the following categories:

- *Skymarathon* – races with a minimum of 2,000 m total elevation gain reaching or exceeding 4,000-m altitude. Between 30 and 42 km, with terrain incorporating paths, trails, moraine, rock, or snow.

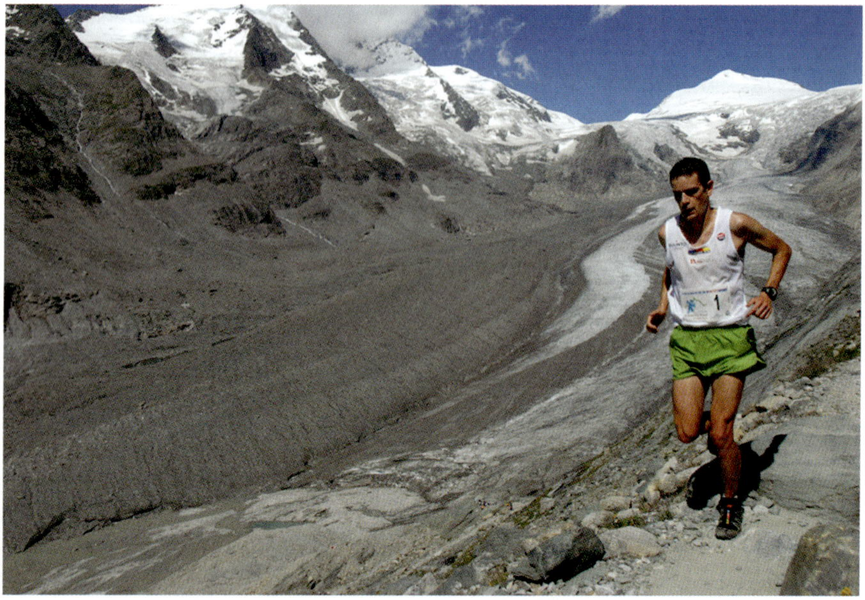

Fig. 13.1 Jonathan Wyatt, Grossglockner Race, 2007 (Photo courtesy of Peter Hartley)

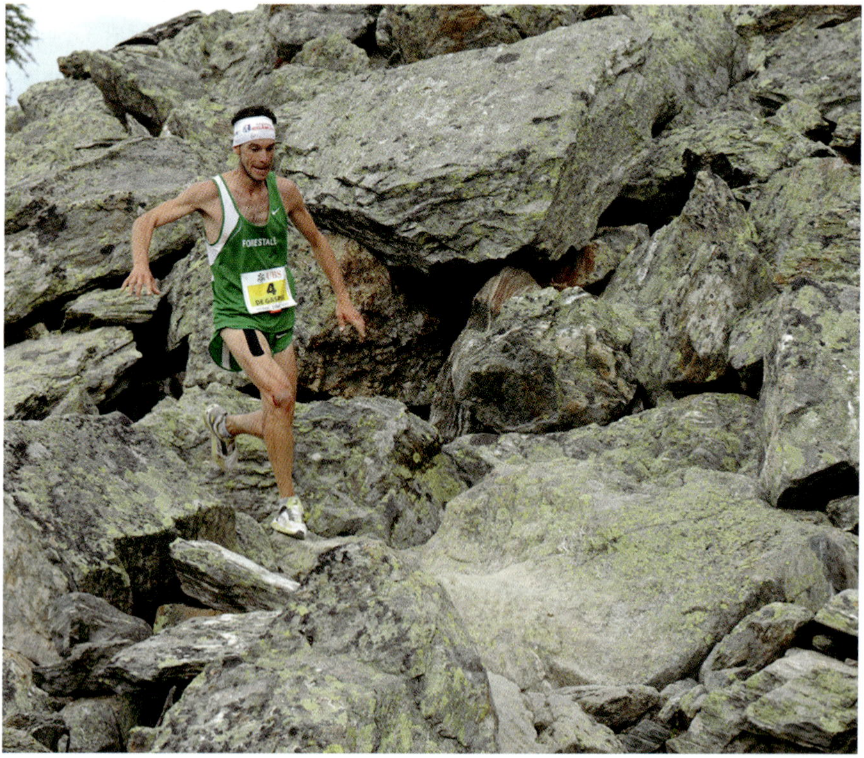

Fig. 13.2 Marco Di Gasperi (six-time world champion and record holder of Mount Kinabalu Climbathon), on target to win Sierre-Zinal Race 2011 (Photo courtesy of Peter Hartley)

- *Ultra skymarathon* – races that exceed the parameters for a skymarathon by more than 5 %.
- *Skyraces* – races between 2,000 and 4,000 m, and between 20 and 30 km.
- *Vertical kilometer* – races with 1,000-m vertical climb over variable terrain with a substantial incline, not exceeding 5 km in length. These races are categorized into three altitude levels.
- *Skyspeed* – races with 100 m or more vertical climb and more than 33 % incline.
- *Skyraid* – team skyrunning races over long distances which incorporate other sports such as cycling, skiing, and climbing.

The Federation for Sport at Altitude (FSA) was founded in 1995 and was transformed into the International Federation for Skyrunning (IFS) in 2008. A circuit of international standard races in varying countries is selected by the IFS which are open to individuals affiliated to a national sports or mountain federation/association. Approximately 30,000 athletes participate in the official skyrunning races annually with up to 54 countries being represented. The FSA is also responsible for carrying out scientific research on athletes both at altitude and in the laboratory.

The Mount Kinabalu International Climbathon has the reputation as the world's toughest race and is the steepest race on the sky circuit ascending from 1,866 m to the summit of Mount Kinabalu at 4,095 m. It rises along paths and slippery steps until the summit where runners use fixed ropes for assistance. The first climbathon was inaugurated in 1987 when Sabah Parks tried to find new recruits for the rapid rescue team – where an individual's fitness was essential to help bring injured climbers off the mountain as quickly as possible. Entry was initially restricted to Malaysians, but the following year was opened for international participation. The race record is held by six-time world champion mountain runner, Marco di Gasperi, in 2 h 33 min and 56 s (2010).

Endurance Running

Endurance races often take competitors to the extremes of nature – temperature (−30 to 56 °C), altitude (up to 5,184 m), terrain (on- or off-road, desert, glacier, or jungle), isolation – or a combination of any. The competitors have the desire to overcome what appears to be seemingly impossible physically and mentally, with the event sometimes being more of a personal challenge.

The races take place in some of the remotest parts of the world (the Sahara Desert (Fig. 13.3), the Himalayas, and both Arctic and Antarctic Circles) and vary in distance from that of a marathon (26.2 miles) to hundreds of kilometers. The world's longest certified race is the Sri Chinmoy's 3,100-mile race.

Endurance races can be categorized into:

- *Ultramarathons* (e.g., Comrades Marathon)
- *Ultra-trails* (e.g., Ultra-Trail du Tour du Mont-Blanc)
- *Trail/mountain marathons* (e.g., Everest Marathon)
- *Multistage footraces* (e.g., Transalpine Run)

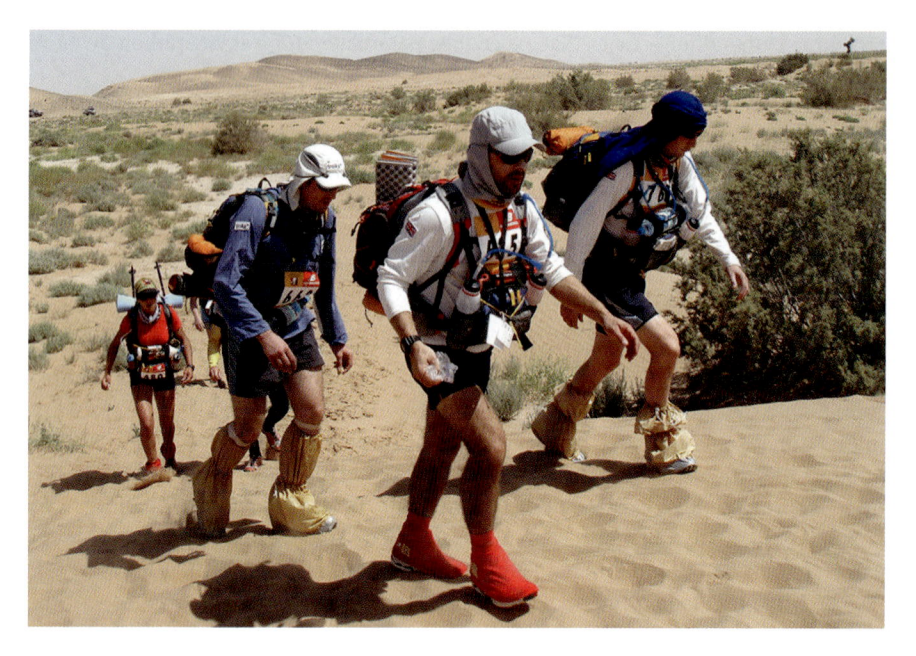

Fig. 13.3 Marathon de Sables 2007 (Photo courtesy of Steven Worralio)

The International Association of Ultrarunners (IAU) came into existence in 1984, and there are now more than 1,000 ultra races around the world, with over 100,000 runners. The IAAF granted its patronage to the IAU in 1988, and the 100-km race became a standard distance recognized by the federation.

The Equipment Used: Essential and Safety Requirements/Considerations

Mountain running attracts competitors with a wide range of abilities and experiences. Individuals with limited experience are more at risk in the challenging conditions, and it is essential that runners take responsibility for their own safety. If injury causes a runner to stop running or slow down, body heat can be lost very quickly, creating a high risk of hypothermia.

The two items of equipment essential to mountain running are appropriate clothing and footwear. Equipment must be lightweight and comfortable to the individual so as not to impede running, but it must be durable and functional to be effective (Fig. 13.4).

Clothing

With the advent of modern fabrics, there are now vast selections of garments available. It is important to consider body temperature and dryness from both the

Mountain Marathon kit list

- Warm trousers or leggings
- Shirt or thermal top
- Sweater or fleece top
- Waterproof over trousers (taped seams)
- Waterproof jacket (taped seams)
- Socks, gloves and hat
- Head torch
- Whistle
- Food For 36 h
- Additional emergency rations
- Compass (GPS not allowed)
- Sleeping bag
- Sleeping bag
- Footwear with adequate grip for fell conditions
- Space blanket or large heavy gauge polythene bag
- Rucksack
- First-aid, a minimum of a crepe bandage and small wound dressings.
- Pen or pencil
- Tent with sewn-in groundsheet
- Cooking stove with enough fuel at the end of day 2 to make a hot drink.

Fig. 13.4 Mountain marathon kit list

inside (perspiration) and the outside (precipitation). Layering of *clothing* allows the runner to adapt clothing in response to changes in temperature and weather conditions, which occur rapidly at altitude or in mountainous conditions. Technological breakthroughs have enabled garments to be produced that are breathable, windproof, waterproof, lightweight, antibacterial, lightweight, and that wick away any personal moisture. Runners must carefully assess conditions before selecting appropriate apparel for both training and racing as this could be crucial for safety. In good weather, a lightweight running vest and shorts might be sufficient, whereas waterproof, full body protection may be necessary in adverse conditions.

Footwear

When selecting *footwear,* the runner needs to take into account:

- Terrain
- Distance
- Biomechanics (especially if they have a tendency to pronate or supinate)
- Personal weight
- Foot width
- Gender (some shoes are now manufactured on a narrower last more suitable for females)
- Any preexisting medical conditions which would suggest a particular shoe might be more beneficial – e.g., a runner with osteoarthritis or rheumatoid arthritis would benefit from more cushioning
- The weight and unique design features of a particular shoe at higher levels of competition

The shoe needs to provide flexibility and speed, but comfort, traction, support, stability, motion control, cushioning, breathability, and, at times, protection from rocks must be considered. Sometimes advanced lacing or webbing systems are used to help hold the foot stable within the shoe, and various soles have been developed ranging from pyramid "studs" for mud to a "sticky rubber" for grip on wet rock. The shoe uppers need to be quick drying and allow any water collecting in the shoe to easily seep back out. The most suitable shoe for a short race through mud is completely different to that for tricky rocky terrain or a 2-day event carrying overnight equipment. Runners often have several pairs of running shoes to suit the varying conditions. Some of the market leaders are Salomon, Inov-8, Montrail, Walsh, and La Sportiva.

Climate

The *climate* is a serious factor, and representatives from the various committees and race organizers must decide whether weather conditions are suitable for races to proceed as planned. Where adverse weather conditions could endanger competitors, marshals, or volunteers assisting at the race, the race may be abandoned or a safer alternative course is used. It is the responsibility of the race organizers to make sure that the course is as safe as possible and not unnecessarily dangerous.

Food and Drink

A runner may need to carry food and drink while racing or on long-training runs to avoid hypoglycemia or dehydration. It is a race requirement in some events, but athletes are generally advised to carry sufficient supplies whenever they are racing for longer than 1 h [1].

Altitude

The skyrunning races and some of the mountain and endurance events involve racing at *altitude*. When the athlete resides at a much lower level and has little time to acclimatize, they must be very careful in appropriate race preparation. Athletes often train at altitude to benefit from the physiological adaptations when racing at sea level, but racing at altitude is the opposite extreme and places serious demands on the body. The effects of altitude on the heart generally begin around approximately 1,000 m (3,048 ft) above sea level. Runners are advised to train at altitude of approximately 8,000 ft for at least 4–5 days before running above 13,000 ft, although if they live above 6,500 ft is not always necessary. The guidelines suggest that once above an altitude of 2,500 m, the altitude at which one sleeps should not be increased by more than 600 m in 24 h, and that an extra day should be added for acclimatization for every increase of 600–1,200 m in this altitude [2].

Altitude and acclimatization are taken very seriously by organizers of races such as the Everest Mountain Marathon. This race is preceded by a 15-day trek in the Everest region to allow for acclimatization, all while under careful medical supervision [3]. Physical fitness is not protective against high-altitude illness [2], but instead it seems to be influenced by the rate of ascent, the altitude achieved, the height at which the person sleeps (sleeping altitude), and the individual's physiology. Skyrunners may adapt their running style when racing at altitude by generally slowing down, shortening their stride, and walking where the gradient exceeds 25 %.

Safety Requirements

The WMRA does not impose any specific *safety requirements*, but the Fell Runners Association in England, the International Ski Federation, and races such as the Original Mountain Marathon (OMM), which is a 2-day mountain marathon, all carry their own regulations. These recommendations are made with the safety of the runner being the main priority (Fig. 13.4).

The FRA requires competitors to arrive at races prepared to carry body cover appropriate for the weather conditions, a map, compass, and whistle, and emergency food in long races. Race organizers can also impose additional safety requirements or waive some of the requirements in settled, fine weather.

In skyrunning races, the use of ski poles is permitted, although this is regulated by each race organizer. It is compulsory to have windproof jackets, trail-running shoes, and socks, plus it may be a requirement to carry tights, gloves, water, helmets, and sunglasses. The recommended equipment for each skyrunning race is stated in the race briefing.

The 2008 Original Mountain Marathon in England suffered from sudden adverse weather conditions. The race had over 2,000 competitors scattered over the fells and had to be abandoned due to torrential rain and high winds. Previous experience of the competitors – a requisite to participating in the event – along with the safety equipment carried by the athletes ensued there were no fatalities and only one reported injury.

Injury Demographics, Mechanisms, and Rates

Injury Rates

As yet there are few published studies regarding the frequency and type of injuries specifically experienced by mountain runners, although a systematic review published in 2007 reported on the incidence and determinants of lower extremity running injuries in long-distance runners [4]. The literature published on ultra races, the Marathon Des Sables and the World Deca Iron Triathlon, has focused on weight and body water composition changes related to performance and is probably beyond the scope of this text [5, 6]. Analysis of the presenting complications reported by the 69 competitors in the 219-km Al Andalus 5-day ultramarathon stage race showed that in this competition over half (56.5 %) reported injuries. The majority of these were minor with foot blisters comprising 33.3 % and chafing 9 %. Lower limb musculoskeletal injuries accounted for 22.2 % and predominantly affected the knee [7]. Van Gent's review included studies where subjects ran >5 km per training or race, which, while useful, is not totally representative of mountain, sky, and ultradistance running.

Park has conducted a questionnaire survey of the injuries experienced by mountain, sky, and endurance runners over a 6 months period identified sites of injury, possible causes, and subsequent treatments received. As the runners were unable to be medically assessed and diagnosed accurately, they were asked to stipulate the area of injury rather than the specific medical diagnosis. The survey population comprised of 200 runners from 11 countries −100 competing at international level including 6 previous world champions and 100 "club" runners.

Of the 200 responses, 142 runners (71 %) reported at least one injury during the previous 6 months, although this was not necessarily representative of the frequency of injuries in the sport. Twenty-seven percent of the runners reported more than one injury suggesting some may have been compensatory.

For the male athletes, the number of injuries increased as the standard of the athlete decreased (33 % of non-GB international athletes reported injuries, compared to 89 % of club athletes). Van Gent similarly found that an increase in training distance per week appeared to protect the individual against knee injuries, rather than being causative [4].

The most commonly reported injury in Park's survey was to the knee (22 %), followed by the shin or calf muscles (15 %), foot (14 %), ankle (12 %), thigh muscles – hamstrings or quadriceps (10 %), pelvis/buttocks (9 %), Achilles tendon (9 %), spine (8 %), and upper body (1 %) (Fig. 13.5). The majority of these injuries were overuse in nature particularly tendinopathy and tenosynovitis.

The males had a much higher incidence of knee injuries compared to the females (Table 13.1) despite studies suggesting females experience a higher incidence of sports-related knee pain [8]. Females reported more foot injuries, although the reasons why require further investigation.

The higher incidence of male knee injuries could be because:

- Mountain runners do not have a repetitive running style, so factors such as the Q-angle may not be as relevant.
- Males may land with more impact, particularly when running downhill (taller or heavier subjects are at a greater relative risk of injury because of the greater forces acting on the bones, muscles, and connective tissue) [9].
- Males may be more reckless when descending, although clearly this is objective.
- Females tend to be more diligent and incorporate core stability and Pilates type exercises into their training schedule, which could be particularly beneficial to lower limb biomechanics when running downhill [10].

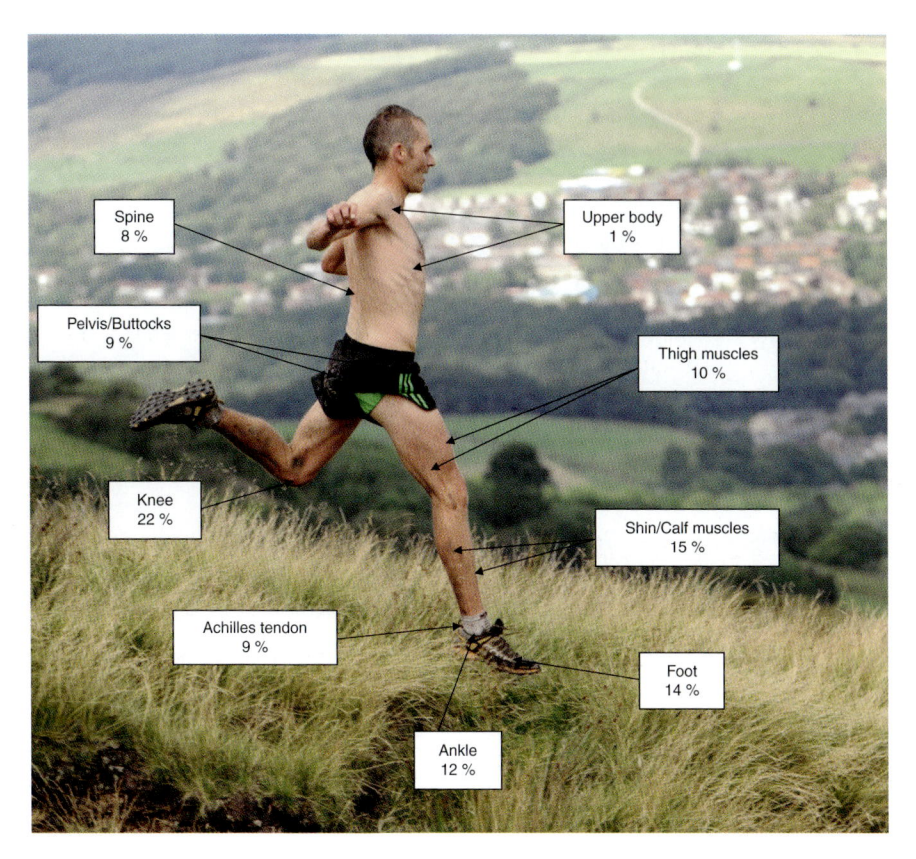

Fig. 13.5 Percentage of injured areas experienced by mountain runners (Photo courtesy of Peter Hartley)

Fatalities

Fatalities due to mountain running are rare, but adverse weather conditions while training or racing can result in exposure, fatigue, hypothermia, and occasional tragedy.

In 2008, 2 runners were killed and 6 seriously affected in the Zugspitze Mountain Race in Germany. A sudden change in weather brought temperatures below freezing point, with strong gusts of wind and snow. Five hundred runners were competing in the race, most of them only clad in t-shirts and shorts, but the fitness of the individuals involved helped most of them cope with the extreme conditions [11].

There have been very few deaths reported when weather has not played a major factor, but the consensus of opinion is that these deaths have been due to other pre-existing conditions such as heart disease or congenital abnormalities. While this has been proven in road marathon running, no specific studies are available relating to mountain running [12].

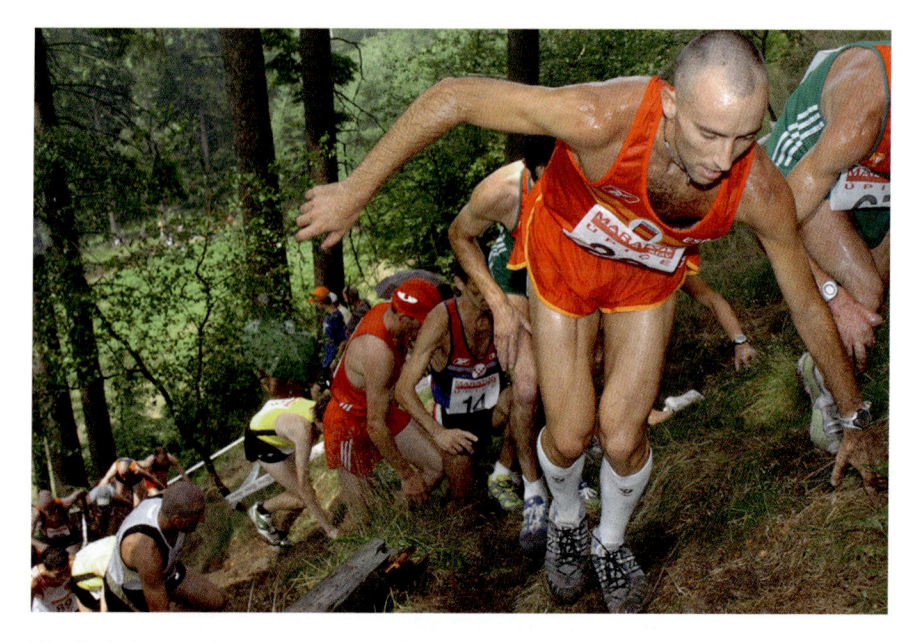

Fig. 13.6 European Mountain Running Championships 2006 (Photo courtesy of Peter Hartley)

Table 13.1 Frequency of injuries

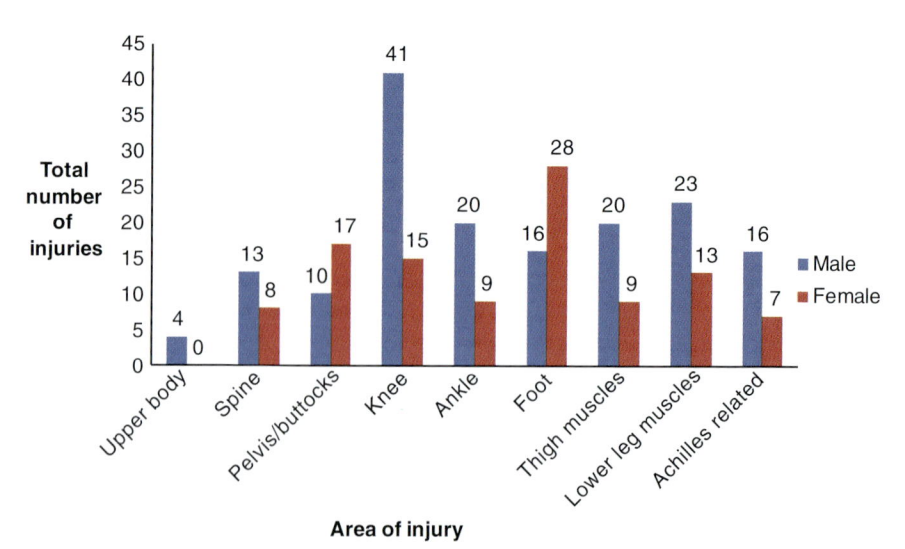

Frequency of injuries – male/female

Area of injury	Male	Female
Upper body	4	0
Spine	13	8
Pelvis/buttocks	10	17
Knee	41	15
Ankle	20	9
Foot	16	28
Thigh muscles	20	9
Lower leg muscles	23	13
Achilles related	16	7

Specific Types of Injury

Some injuries occur more frequently in mountain running because of the unique demands placed on the body when running steep ascents or descents. The common injuries associated with running are documented sufficiently in other sports' injury textbooks, but some of the more obscure injuries deserve specific attention.

Runner's Knee

Runner's knee – possibly more aptly named *mountain runner's knee* – is the most frequent injury encountered by those regularly providing medical treatment for mountain runners, with almost a quarter of survey respondents complaining of this problem.

Noakes and Grainger [13] suggested that this is *the* most common injury associated with distance running but, combined with the biomechanics of the knee while mountain running, explains why it is so prevalent. Other textbooks refer to it as patellofemoral stress syndrome, lateral patellar compression syndrome, peripatellar syndrome, and retinaculitis [14].

The symptoms and signs are:

- Pain located around the patella.
- Full, pain-free movement of the knee joint, although pain may be present on maximum flexion due to the stretch on the affected structures (the elicited pain feels more anterior than intra-articular).
- Increase in pain when increased quadriceps recruitment – e.g., cycling stood on the pedals, walking up, and especially downstairs.
- Increased symptoms running downhill.
- Increase in pain after sitting long periods, especially when >90° knee flexion.
- Painful kneeling/squatting.
- Driving may irritate symptoms, especially if stiff pedals or maintaining a sustained position on the accelerator pedal.
- The symptoms often ease while running but may return later in the run.
- Possibly no memorable history of trauma, although there may have been either of the following:

  (a) A single maximal load such as a sudden change in direction
  (b) Multiple submaximal loads causing repetitive microtrauma

On clinical examination, there is:

- Localized tenderness along the border of the patella, often the inferomedial aspect, where the quadriceps retinacula and patellar ligament attach to the patella.
- No other obvious bone lesions/positive joint signs or intra-joint/retropatellar crepitus. Clarke's test (resisted patellar movement) is not necessarily indica-

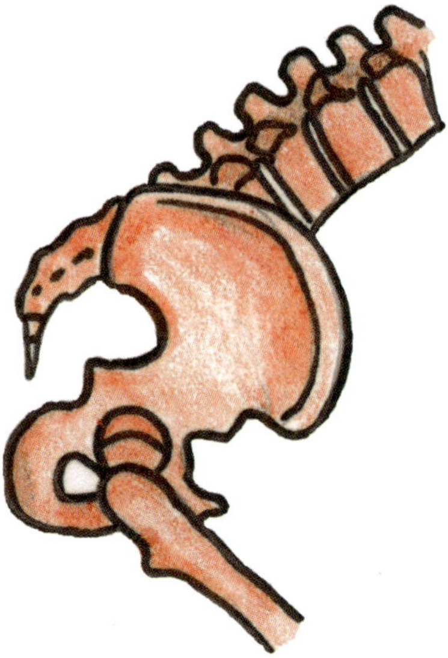

Fig. 13.7 Pelvic tilt in uphill running (Photo courtesy of Peter Hartley)

tive of this condition, as this test is positive in 66 % of subjects with normal knees [15].

Lumbar pain, pelvic pain, buttock pain, and thigh pain are all common in mountain running and often remain misunderstood and misdiagnosed by medical practitioners due to the confusing clinical presentation.

Running up- or downhill alters the pelvic tilt considerably (Fig. 13.6 and 13.7), affecting the body's biomechanics. The structures that are associated with the lumbosacral spine, pelvis, buttocks, and hips (Fig. 13.8 and 13.9) are exposed to unaccustomed stresses which are completely different to those of flat, propulsive road running.

If eccentric loading exceeds eccentric strength (as in downhill running), there is an additional risk of accumulative microtrauma.

While minor lesions are initially asymptomatic, the continuous cycle of repair, reinjury, and re-inflammation ultimately becomes problematic, with compensatory damage occurring in the closely related structures [15].

The possible signs and symptoms are:

- Gradual onset of diffuse pain in the low lumbar region, buttock, groin, or thigh.
- Rest may ease the symptoms, but any return to activity results in a recurrence, often more debilitating.
- Sitting often irritates the symptoms.
- Pain increases while running.
- Training and racing may be possible at a lower level until symptoms become too severe.
- Occasionally the athlete describes a sensation of paresthesia, although it is usually non-segmental and does not relate to any specific dermatome.

13 Mountain, Sky, and Endurance Running

Fig. 13.8 A superior hamstring lesion and the associated structures (Photo courtesy of Peter Hartley)

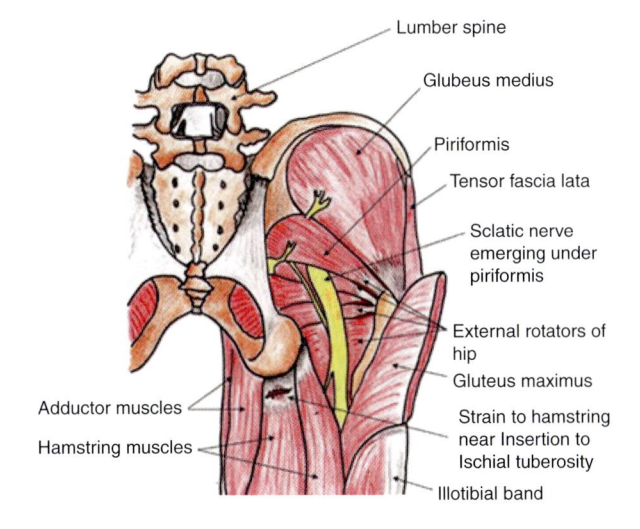

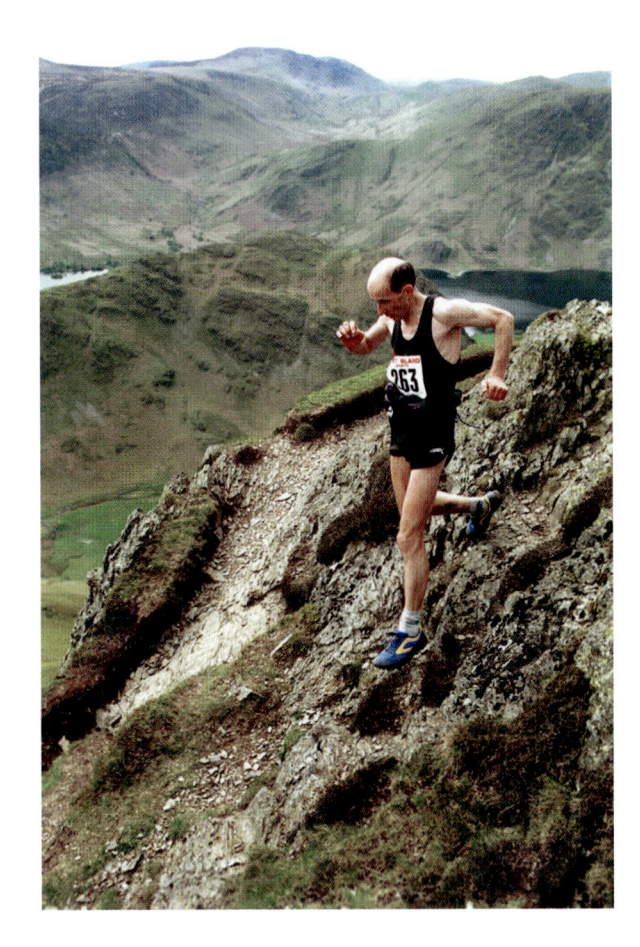

Fig. 13.9 The terrain of an English Fell Race – Ian Holloway descending Sailbeck, 1998 (Photo courtesy of Peter Hartley)

Clinically:

- There may not be any apparent lack of movement in the lumbar region, although hamstring mobility may appear restricted.
- Very tender "knots" may be palpable in the painful regions.
- Muscle weakness may be identifiable, especially when tested eccentrically. A single-leg squat may highlight weakness in the hip abductors or external rotators, which could have a subsequent adverse effect on the lumbar spine, pelvis, and lower limb alignment.

Further investigations do not usually help in the diagnosis of this complex problem, although imaging may occasionally identify a minor disc protrusion or superior hamstring lesions. The MRI report frequently suggests there is nothing untoward, which often causes the runner serious psychological distress. It is important to explain that there may be areas of micro-damage, which have not been identifiable, but the report excludes any serious pathology. The diagnosis of a disc lesion occasionally leads to other associated areas being neglected in the treatment plan, and personal experience has shown that the primary site and the associated areas must be addressed to achieve optimum recovery and avoid any future recurrences.

Tendon injuries are common in running, although mountain running affects different tendons to road running. Flexor hallucis longus (FHL), tibialis posterior, and both peronei tendons are at higher risk around the foot and ankle. FHL tendons have been known to rupture during uphill repetition training sessions. Many of the athletes run on their toes, so the undulating terrain put these structures under considerable stress. Pain is usually localized, and resisted muscle testing of the structure often identifies the problem. If resisted testing is negative (given it is impossible to replicate similar strains within the clinic), palpation is often paramount in locating the site of injury.

In ultramarathon running, the high-mileage training requirement has been associated with ankle extensor tendon tenosynovitis localized at the extensor retinaculum [16, 17]. These comprised 19 % of all injuries sustained during a 1,115-km ultramarathon race from Sydney to Melbourne [16]. Tenosynovitis of the extensor digitorum longus tendon has since been termed ultramarathoner's ankle [16]. A typical ultramarathoner's shuffling gait has been suggested as a causative factor in addition to excessive pronation, tight-fitting shoes, muscle imbalance, eccentric overload, and in one case talar head impingement [17].

Continuous overload means that mountain runners are susceptible to *stress fractures*, with several being reported in the survey. Signs and symptoms are:

- Localized pain which may be bearable at rest, but where running is impossible
- Usually sudden onset, although it can be insidious
- Bony or soft tissue swelling
- Tenderness on palpation
- Pain on impact – hopping, running on the spot, or jumping

Most runners want evidence of the injury due to the enforced period of rest from running, but radiographs may fail to reveal a fracture until at least 3 weeks post-injury when new bone growth is identifiable.

Osteoarthritis and the development of *cardiac damage* are often misconstrued as being prevalent in runners, but this is unproven. Animal and human studies have shown no evidence of increased risk of hip or knee osteoarthritis in subjects carrying out moderate exercise (in the absence of any traumatic injury). Sporting activity has even been shown to have a positive effect as a study of recreational runners who ran 12–14 miles per week for up to 40 years showed no increase in either radiological or symptomatic hip or knee OA [18].

Equally, there has not been any link between extreme strenuous exercise and the development of *cardiac damage*. A study of 23 ultramarathon runners who completed the 100-mile Western States Endurance Run (a race through the Sierra Mountains over rough terrain and extreme temperatures) did not show any signs of race-related cardiac damage [19]. Research has instead suggested that well-trained endurance athletes have only approximately 40 % of their sedentary counterpart's risk of dying from any cardiac problems [20].

Common Treatments (Conservative/Surgical) and Rehabilitation

Clinical effectiveness is achieved by *the right person, doing the right thing, the right way, in the right place, at the right time, with the right result* [21].

The most serious "injury" for the runner is misdiagnosis accompanied by inappropriate advice. Running is unusual because the cause of the problem can often be identified, and treatment is futile if it is not linked to adaptation of genetic, training, or environmental factors contributing to the cause of the injury.

Causes of Injury

Soft tissue injuries are a very common cause of morbidity in both competitive and recreational athletes with most of these conditions being provoked by muscle-tendon overload (or overuse) [22]. The survey (Table 13.2) identified *overuse* as the most frequent cause of injury (34 %) followed by *trauma* (18 %), particularly in the more inexperienced club runner. When overuse is considered the main cause of injury, the athlete should review training intensity and techniques. Van Gent refers to two high-quality studies suggesting training for more than 64 km/week puts male runners at a significant higher risk of injury [4].

Trauma frequently results in injury, but this is to be expected in the challenging conditions. A gradual increase in training to improve stamina, with an improvement in lower limb strength, balance, and coordination can all be beneficial, but the

Table 13.2 Cause of injuries

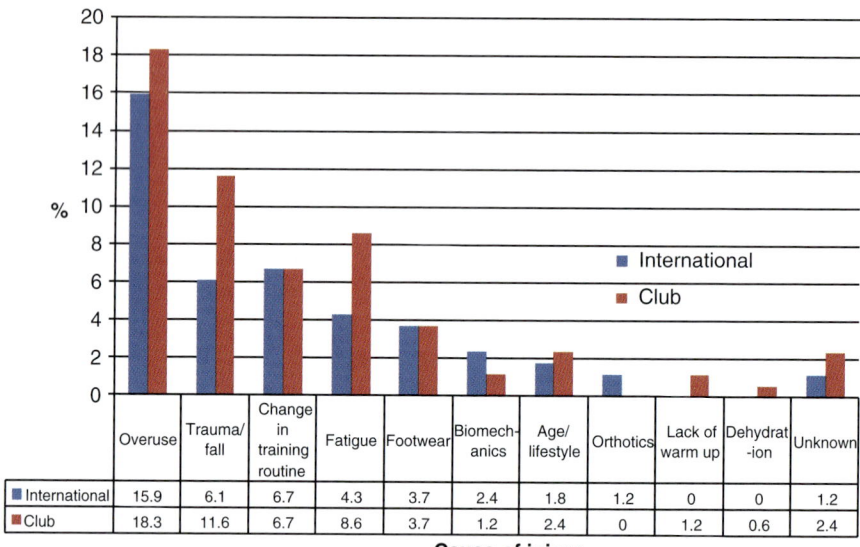

Cause of injuries – international/club

Cause of injury	Overuse	Trauma/fall	Change in training routine	Fatigue	Footwear	Biomechanics	Age/lifestyle	Orthotics	Lack of warm up	Dehydration	Unknown
International	15.9	6.1	6.7	4.3	3.7	2.4	1.8	1.2	0	0	1.2
Club	18.3	11.6	6.7	8.6	3.7	1.2	2.4	0	1.2	0.6	2.4

circumstances in which these injuries occur – often a fall – are usually unpredictable so the athlete can never be totally prepared.

A *change in training program* alters the familiar demands placed on the musculoskeletal system. Duration, intensity, frequency, and recovery times must all be progressed gradually to allow for adaptations to occur and to maintain tissue homeostasis; otherwise, the tissues are susceptible to damage.

Fatigue is more of an issue for the club runner than the international runner. International runners may be full-time athletes or work part time enabling them to focus on appropriate training, racing, and recovery. Club runners are often in full-time employment with family commitments, so frequently neglect the aspects of training which help in the prevention of injuries. It is important to determine whether the individual is running to train, or training to run, and to take this into consideration when planning the treatment regime.

Footwear was found to be attributable for 7 % of the injuries, and inappropriate footwear for the terrain, worn-out or "disfigured" shoes, a recent change in model/style, or simply a change in the type of shoe can all be contributory. Calf- and Achilles-related problems frequently occur when the *change of season* suddenly dictates a change in terrain. Dark, wet nights or the first, sunny spring evenings result in a sudden change of footwear to accommodate more on- or off-road running. The change between flatter mountain-running footwear and more supportive or cushioned road shoes alters the biomechanics of the lower limb structures considerably, exposing the athlete to increased risk of injury.

The use of snowshoes and snow running presents a whole array of biomechanical challenges and should be introduced with extreme caution.

Published research suggests that biomechanical alignment is a major factor in the cause of running injuries, resolved by the use of appropriate *orthotics* [23]. Orthotics are not necessarily the panacea of all running problems and may lead to other problems, e.g., stress fractures.

Mountain runners traverse rough, undulating terrain, with the foot striking the ground in varying positions, unlike road runners. Given orthotics aim to help correct lower-limb biomechanics, the changes in running surface may mean that orthotics are not always appropriate in mountain-running shoes. Runners also prefer to be in close contact with the ground, and an orthotic correction sometimes makes them feel more susceptible to injury, especially anterior talofibular sprains at the ankle.

Mountain-running shoes often provide little support, so basic insoles can help to maintain an improved foot position particularly in those demonstrating excessive pronation or supination. Off-road runners usually incorporate some measurable training sessions on the road or track, and orthotics and/or appropriate footwear should be considered for these circumstances.

Treatment

The conventional treatments for all musculoskeletal injuries should be adopted together with careful examination for predisposing biomechanical aspects. Unless these are addresses, it is likely that the injury or problem will recur [24].

Once the possible cause of injury has been addressed, the appropriate course of treatment is essential (Table 13.3). Seventy-two percent of the injuries reported in mountain runners resolve conservatively with *physiotherapy* treatment. Five (3 %) individuals received *cortisone* injections (although this did not appear to be the appropriate standard care pathway for 2 of the injuries), and 7 (5 %) required *surgery* for obvious orthopedic cases:

- 3 knee meniscal injuries
- 1 ankle fixation
- 1 Haglund's deformity
- 1 acromioclavicular dislocation
- 1 degenerative spinal condition

The results of a survey of mountain runners confirmed popular belief that most mountain-running injuries (91 %) can be resolved with either appropriate *physiotherapy* treatment or with no treatment and *self-management*.

Practitioners dealing with runners need to have an in-depth knowledge of both the musculoskeletal system and the unique demands of the sport. They need to be competent in diagnosing an injury accurately and be aware of the types of running

Table 13.3 Treatment received

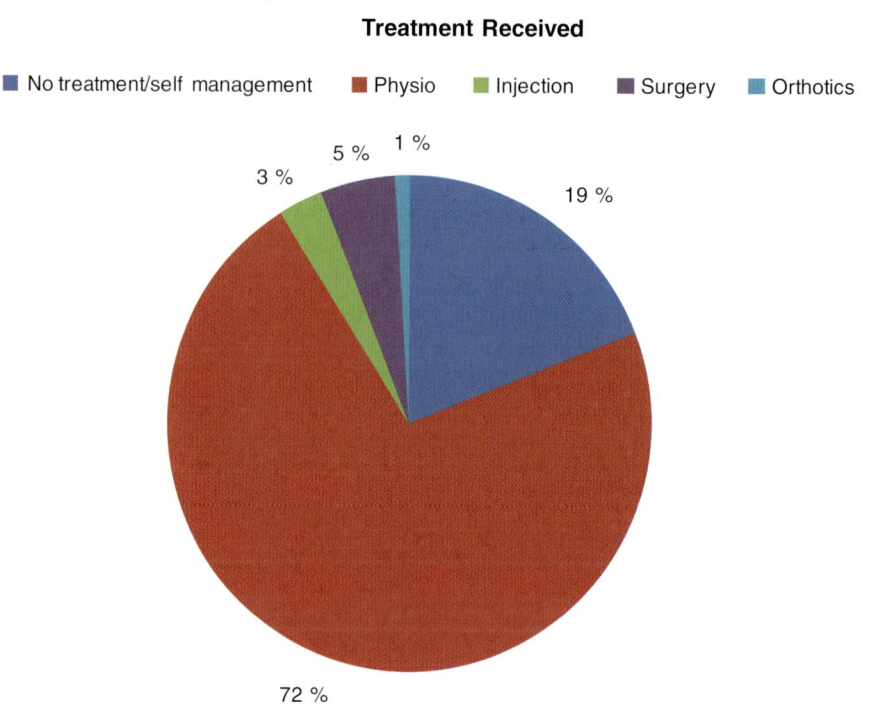

Treatment Received

- No treatment/self management
- Physio
- Injection
- Surgery
- Orthotics

- Physio: 72 %
- No treatment/self management: 19 %
- Injection: 3 %
- Surgery: 5 %
- Orthotics: 1 %

footwear, subtle lower-limb structural abnormalities, and benefits and hazards of in-shoe orthotics [25]. They must also appreciate the differences between the various running styles, especially between road and off-road running.

Acute injuries can often be self-treated, but it is the complex, chronic, often misdiagnosed injuries which are the most troublesome, and often resulting in the runner being advised to refrain from the sport.

Anatomy books have encouraged the concept that the body is constructed of various "single" parts, but in physiological terms, this is inaccurate. New theories suggest that the body is made up of a series of networks, and the position of the bones within these networks is dependent upon the tensional balance between the soft tissue structures [26]. When this tensional balance is disturbed, sometimes as a result of overload and repetitive microtrauma, it can lead to both local and widespread consequences. It is the role of the physiotherapist, using a variety of therapeutic modalities, to address this and rebalance the stresses being transmitted through the connective tissue network.

Acute Injury

Immediately following acute soft tissue injury, the PRICE principle (Protect, Rest, Ice, Compression, and Elevation) should be engaged [27] – cryotherapy (crushed ice) for 10–20 min, two to four times per day for the first 2–3 days. This assists in early mobilization which is essential to promote correct orientation of the regenerating muscle fibers, revascularization, and remodeling of the scar. It also minimizes inactivity-induced atrophy, loss of strength, and extensibility – serious adverse sequelae of prolonged immobilization [28]. A short period of immobilization is needed to accelerate formation of the scar between the stumps of the ruptured myofibers but should not be longer than necessary for the scar to bear the pulling forces without re-rupture (3–5 days was shown to be most effective in a gastrocnemius injury in rats) [29].

Chronic Injury

When areas of micro-damage are not addressed in the early stages, accumulative adhesions become firmer and denser, increasing presenting symptoms. A progressive decrease in flexibility of the affected tissues results in compensatory adaptations, and while some structures become stronger, others weaken. These tissue adaptations lead to increased pain, altered muscle recruitment patterns, and changes in biomechanics so should be avoided wherever possible.

Conservative Physiotherapy Treatment

Clinical diagnosis determines the fine details, but certain principles govern physiotherapeutic management of most musculoskeletal mountain-running injuries.
- *Minimize/Resolve Ongoing Inflammatory Processes and Stimulate/Encourage Healing*
- Use of cryotherapy and electrotherapy including ultrasound, pulsed electromagnetic therapy, laser, and micro-current stimulation.
- *Mobilization of Any Adhesions Within the Connective Tissue Network*
- The following modalities are effective:
  1. Deep transverse cross-frictional massage [30], referred to by Noakes [13] as crucifixional massage. Despite popular belief, this treatment does not need to be particularly vigorous, and gentler frictions are often equally effective.
  2. Myofascial release techniques. Interaction between the myofascial planes of the body dictates that changes in tension within the connective tissue network can produce both local and global adaptations [26]. The role of the fascia within the connective tissue network is currently under close review, and especially the effect of fascial remodeling on both movement patterns and central nervous system plasticity [30].
  3. Acupuncture – recent evidence suggests that acupuncture helps to stimulate realignment of scar tissue, reduce pain, and provide a boost to the healing process, particularly in chronic conditions [31].

- *Stretching to Regain Full Mobility of Both the Injured Tissue and the Connective Tissue Network*
  Extensive research has identified that frequency and repetition of eccentric stretching exercises influences the deposition of collagen [32, 33], and that eccentric training produces superior results when compared to concentric exercises [34]. Langevin's study on rats indicated that frequent sustained stretching of injured tissue induced nuclear remodeling of the fibroblasts within the connective tissue and identified a decrease in mechanosensitivity, a decrease in the production of macrophages and a decrease in collagen deposition [35]. As inflammation and "rest" both impair connective tissue mobility, stretching is essential in the repair of injured tissues.
- *Progressive Resistance Exercises (Isotonic, Isokinetic, and Isometric)*
  These promote restoration of full muscle and joint function and must ultimately include acceleration, deceleration, stopping, hopping, and other controlled movements in both transverse and frontal planes. Kinesio tape has been shown to be beneficial in the rehabilitation of injured muscles, with its effectiveness still undergoing considerable investigation [36]. Key muscles which must be addressed include the deep core abdominal and pelvic muscles, hip rotators, gluteals, quadriceps, hamstrings, and gastrocnemius. Exercises which are particularly beneficial are the "Figure-4" exercise, the "clam," and single-leg squats.

  The Figure-4 exercise is particularly effective in strengthening the external rotators in the buttock. The individual lies prone on the edge of a bed, with one leg unsupported over the edge and the unsupported foot positioned under the knee of the supported leg. The unsupported knee is slowly raised toward the ceiling with the pelvis remaining in contact with the surface. It is a relatively small movement and is particularly effective when done correctly.
- *Continuous Reassessment of Motion Control, Biomechanical Alignment, Strength, Flexibility, Myofascial Mobility, and Sensory and Proprioceptive Awareness*
  This is done throughout the rehabilitation of the injured athlete and is addressed accordingly. Every treatment plan is unique to the athlete, and there is no such thing as a "standard" treatment.

  Rehabilitation is complete when the injured and adjacent associated tissues are restored to full pain-free functional capacity with the individual able to return to pain-free competition [37].

Proposed Preventative Measures (Training and Equipment Wise): Injury and Illness

The following measures should be given careful consideration when helping to minimize the risk of injury:

- Careful planning of training schedules.
- Sensible, progressive training allows for tissue adaptation, and only one parameter should be altered at any given time – volume, intensity, speed, or terrain

(grass, dirt road, track, tarmac, concrete, hills, or camber). Overload is often a precursor to injury, and training diaries can help to identify times of vulnerability.

- *Monitoring of running footwear.*
  Footwear should be:

  (a) Suitable for the conditions.
  (b) Aligned when on a solid base. Both new and worn shoes should be checked.
  (c) Of a reasonable age and condition that the "unique" features of the shoe are still effective, particularly the sole and uppers.
  (d) Continually rotated or changed gradually over a period of time. New footwear affects the biomechanics of the lower limb, and when changed suddenly it has the same effect as a sudden change in training.

- *Improve running style, proprioception (balance), flexibility.*
  These should all be incorporated into the training schedule. Any improvement in running efficiency will both boost performance and reduce risk of injury.

- *Address any obvious biomechanical issues or any muscular imbalances.*
  Training and some races may incorporate road or track running, so gait analysis along with appropriate correction can be beneficial when there is an underlying malalignment problem.

- *Strengthen the core stability and pelvic muscles.*
  The upper and lower body converges at the pelvis where strength and stability is essential to cope with the extremes of mountain running. Weak gluteals result in poor control of hip rotation and adduction, and there is a strong association between gluteal weakness and injury [38].

  A study assessing the effectiveness of hip-strengthening exercises identified that hip adduction, hip internal rotation, and contralateral pelvic drop all decrease significantly following a hip strengthening and movement education program [10]. While this study did not identify any change during a normal running action, it is highly significant in mountain running when a foot strike often resembles a functional single-leg squat.

- *Sufficient warm-up.*
  It is well documented that a warm-up increases respiration and circulation, increases the temperature of the muscles, reduces tissue viscosity, and increases flexibility [14]. It also allows for tissue adaptation with reorganization of the shape and orientation of connective tissue cells. Magnetic resonance images have shown that cells actively reorganize within 5–10 min of a postural change [29], which is an important aspect of the time spent warming up.

- *Wear compression garments during or immediately after running.*
  Distance runners are considered to be at high risk of venous disease [39]. The venous system is put under considerable pressure when the muscle pump is active during prolonged running, but this is suddenly stopped at the end of activity, resulting in venous pooling. A period of time spent warming down helps to minimize these effects, but distance runners are notorious for missing this aspect of training/racing.

As well as compression garments helping to provide support to the vein walls both during and immediately after running, garments which comply with the medically accepted Rall standard have also been shown to:

1. Significantly lower the energy costs during submaximal running – thought to be due to an enhanced circulation and decreased muscle oscillation [40]
2. Significantly decrease delayed onset muscle soreness (DOMS) when compared to those doing similar exercise without compression [41]

- *Do not stretch immediately prior to exercise.*
  Pre-exercise stretching has not been shown to reduce the incidence of injury [42].
- *Be aware of or avoid factors known to increase susceptibility to stress fractures.*
  These are:
  1. Females who are amenorrheic or have menstrual abnormalities.
  2. Repeated loading.
  3. High training volume.
  4. Muscle weakness.
  5. Dietary deficiency – either a low-calcium diet or a vitamin D deficiency. Vitamin D deficiency should be suspected when an athlete experiences multiple stress fractures within a short period. While injured, they are not exposed to their usual amounts of sunlight and tend to train indoors.
  6. Novice runners.
  7. Genetic factors – a high-arched supinated foot, a low-arched pronated foot, or any leg length discrepancy.
  8. Low bone density.
  9. Race – Caucasians are at more risk than runners of African descent [13, 43, 44].
- *Consider effects on the immune system.*
  Many components of the immune system exhibit adverse changes after prolonged, heavy exertion [45]. These immune changes occur in several compartments of the immune system and body (e.g., the skin, upper respiratory tract mucosal tissue, lung, blood, and muscle). Most exercise immunologists believe that it is during this "open window" of impaired immunity (between 3 and 72 h), that viruses and bacteria may gain a foothold, with an increased risk of subclinical and clinical infection. This infection risk may be amplified if other factors related to immune function are present:

  – Exposure to novel pathogens while traveling
  – Lack of sleep
  – Severe mental stress
  – Malnutrition
  – Weight loss

  This is particularly relevant to touring international athletes as a period of illness can be as debilitating as a musculoskeletal injury.

- *Ingest sufficient carbohydrate.*
 The body can manage for approximately 90 min of running before it needs additional supplies, with liver glycogen depletion occurring around 2 h [46]. *Hypoglycemia* reduces the strength of the stimulation from the brain to the muscles, resulting in weaker muscle contractions and decreased performance [47]. Increased carbohydrate consumption in the week leading up to longer races has been shown to help produce faster race times [48] with a prolonged running time prior to exhaustion [49]. However, carbohydrate loading just prior to a long-distance event does not appear to be beneficial [50].

 Hypoglycemia is uncommon in athletes competing in races of up to 56 km [51], provided they ingest sufficient carbohydrates prior to the race and 30–60 g per hour during competition [52]. Various types of carbohydrate can help to maintain blood glucose levels with sports drinks, shakes, bananas, energy bars, and gels all being equally effective [51].
- *Avoid dehydration or overhydration.*
 Fluid should be ingested regularly as dehydration of 3 % of a runner's body weight can affect performance [53]. Prevention is imperative, and it is important to try to avoid more than 1 % dehydration by calculating pre- and postexercise body weight to determine the average weight loss. Runners should be sufficiently hydrated prior to exercise and then should drink regularly during exercise (but not exceeding 400–800 ml/h) [54]. Rather than drinking water, consumption of beverages containing 6 % sucrose appears to significantly improve end-of-exercise performance [54].

 Runners are often encouraged to consume large quantities of water during long-distance events to avoid dehydration, but excessive drinking can be more serious resulting in potentially fatal *hyponatremia*. Inexperienced runners are particularly at risk, with hyponatremia occurring more frequently in women, slower runners (over 4 h marathon time), and in those taking over the counter NSAIDs [55].

 Typically post-race collapse is due to postural hypotension with the skeletal muscle ceasing to assist in venous return, but it can be due to the sudden absorption of excessive fluids into the gastrointestinal tract, resulting in a further dilution of the plasma sodium [56].
- *Maintain a healthy diet.*
 The importance of a healthy diet is often undervalued.

 Runners require a regular *carbohydrate*-rich diet to replenish their muscle and liver glycogen stores. It is recommended to have 5–7 g of carbohydrate/kg of body weight per day on easier training days and 7–12 g on harder training or race days. Without sufficient daily carbohydrates, the runner's performance and recovery can be impaired.

 Protein is necessary to keep the immune, metabolic, digestive, and structural systems healthy. They assist in recovery by preventing muscle breakdown, assist in the contraction and relaxation of muscles, help build ligaments and tendons, support bone, help in the production of insulin which is essential to regulate blood sugars, help maintain the thyroid, and support the immune system. Without sufficient protein, the runner may be plagued by injury or illness. Runners training four to five times per week for 45–60 min need approximately 1.2 g of protein/kg of body weight per day, increasing up to 1.7 g if they are including any strength or cross training.

A certain amount of *fat* is required in the diet in order that the fat-soluble vitamins A, D, E, and K can be absorbed. Omega-3 fatty acids are also thought to act as anti-inflammatories. It is recommended that up to approximately 30 % of the athlete's total daily calorie intake should be from fats – especially unsaturated fats and omega-3 fatty acids.

Vitamins and *minerals* have an impact on the health and performance of the runner. Minerals are essential to cell function controlling the flow of liquids in cell membranes and capillaries, regulating nerve tissue and muscle response, and assisting in the building of blood, nerve muscle, bones, and teeth. While it is thought that supplements should not be necessary for an athlete with a healthy diet, sometimes training, work, low-quality meals and snacks, and low-calorie diets trying to keep body weight low may result in a vitamin or mineral deficiency. Folic acid, the B vitamins, vitamin C, calcium, potassium, magnesium, iron, and zinc are all of importance to the runner, with iron and vitamin B_{12} having particular importance for the vegetarian. If the runner feels their recovery or performance is being seriously affected, a deficiency may be present [1].

- *Be aware of the dangers of training and racing at altitude.*
  The partial pressure of oxygen decreases as altitude increases, and it is this lack of oxygen that reduces the amount of oxygen available to the muscles. The Federation of Sport at Altitude have shown that the lack of oxygen at elevations above 10,000 ft translates to 25–40 % less muscle power, but that competitive running at high altitude does not impose a substantial increase in health risk beyond that encountered at low altitude, provided athletes are well trained, altitude acclimatized, and medically controlled [57].

If an individual is being affected by altitude, they may begin to experience any of the following and should be closely monitored:

- Dehydration
- Shortness of breath
- Light-headedness
- Muscle soreness
- Headache
- Increased heart rate
- Tiredness/fatigue
- Irritability
- Constipation
- Inability to sleep
- Loss of appetite
- Nausea/vomiting
- Flatulence
- Decreased urinary output despite being hydrated

Acute Mountain Sickness (AMS)

The onset of acute mountain sickness (AMS) can begin 6–12 h after being at altitude but becomes more intense after 1–2 days. These symptoms may last a week until the body can acclimatize. High-altitude cerebral edema (HACE) and high-altitude pulmonary edema (HAPE) can occur in extreme cases of AMS, and in these cases the individual should be given supplementary oxygen, appropriate medication, and may need to be brought down from altitude.

A study in 2002 looked at the incidence and prevalence of AMS, HACE, and HAPE during a 10-day race in Colorado [58]. It started at over 9,500 ft, ascended to over 13,500 ft, with 138,800 ft of altitude change during the event. Of the competitors, 4.5 % exhibited signs of altitude illness at the start of the race, with 14 % requiring medical treatment during the race for AMS, HAPE, and HACE. There was no correlation between home altitude, prerace medical assessment scores, and successful completion of the race, but it was concluded that altitude sickness contributed significantly to withdrawal from such events so it should be considered seriously by any individual wanting to compete in events of this nature.

Mountain, altitude, and endurance running are regarded as the ultimate "extreme" of the running world, but they are relatively safe sports when the recommended safety and preventative measures are implemented appropriately.

References

1. Chase AW, Hobbs N. The ultimate guide to trail running. Guilford: Falcon Guides; 2010.
2. Hackett PH, Roach RC. High-altitude illness. N Engl J Med. 2001;345:107–14.
3. Buckler DGW, O'Higgins F. Medical provision and usage for the 1999 Everest marathon. Br J Sports Med. 2000;34:205–9.
4. Van Gent RN, Siem D, Van Miidelkoop M, Van Os AG, Bierma-Zeinstra SMA, Koes BW. Incidence and determinants of lower extremity running injuries in long distance runners: a systematic review. 2007. Br J Sports Med. 2007;41:469–80.
5. Zouhal H, Groussard C, Vincent S, Jacob C, Abderrahman AB, Delamarche P, Gratas-Delamarche A. Athletic performance and weight changes during the "Marathon of Sands" in athletes well trained in endurance. Int J Sports Med. 2009;30:516–21.
6. Knechtle B, Salas Fraire O, Andonie JL, Kohler G. Effect of a multistage ultra-endurance triathlon on body composition: World Challenge Deca Iron Triathlon 2006. Br J Sports Med. 2008;42:121–5.
7. Scheer BV, Murray A. Al Andalus Ultra Trail: an observation of medical interventions during a 219 km, 5 day ultramarathon stage race. Clin J Sport Med. 2011;21:444–6.
8. Dugan SA. Sports-related knee injuries in female athletes: what gives? Am J Phys Med Rehabil. 2005;84:122–30.
9. Van Mechelen W. Running injuries: a review of the epidemiological literature. Sports Med. 1992;14:320–5.
10. Willy RW, Davis IS. The effect of a hip strengthening program on mechanics during running and during a single leg squat. J Orthop Sports Phys Ther. 2011;41:625–32.
11. Spiegel Online International, 7/14/08, tragedy in the Alps – summer snowstorm kills two on Bavarian Mountaintop. www.spiegel.de/international/germany/0,1518,565678,00.html. Accessed on 15 Sep 2012.

12. Marrin BJ, Poliac LC, Roberts WO. Risk for sudden cardiac death associated with marathon running. J Am Coll Cardiol. 1996;28:428–31.
13. Noakes TD, Granger S. Running injuries. Oxford: Oxford University Press; 2003.
14. Noakes TD. The lore of running. Champaign: Human Kinetics; 2003.
15. Livingstone BN. Clinical tests for chondromalacia patellae. Lancet. 1982;ii:210.
16. Fallon KE. Musculoskeletal injuries in the ultramarathon: the 1990 Westfield Sydney to Melbourne run. Br J Sports Med. 1996;30:319–23.
17. Kobayashi M, Sakurai M, Kobayashi T. Extensor digitorum longus tenosynovitis caused by talar head impingement in a ultramarathon runner: a case report. J Orthod Surg. 2007;15:245–7.
18. Molloy MG, Molloy CB. Contact sport and osteoarthritis. Br J Sports Med. 2011;45:275–7.
19. Scott JM, Esch BTA, Shave R, et al. Cardiovascular consequences of completing a 160 km ultramarathon. Med Sci Sports Exerc. 2009;41:26–34.
20. Siscovick DS, Weiss NS, Fletcher RH, Lasky T. The incidence of primary cardiac arrest during vigorous exercise. N Engl J Med. 1984;311:874–7.
21. Graham G. Clinically effective medicine in a rational health service. Health Director. 1996;6:11–2.
22. Hart LE. Exercise and soft tissue injury. Balliere's Clin Rheumatol. 1994;8:137–48.
23. Gross ML, Davlin LB, Evanski PM. Effectiveness of orthotic shoe inserts in the long-distance runner. Am J Sports Med. 1991;19:409–12.
24. Noakes TD. Fenbufen in the treatment of over-use injuries in long-distance runners. S Afr Med J. 1982;61:301.
25. Pinshaw R, Atlas V, Noakes TD. The nature and response to therapy of 196 consecutive injuries seen at a runner's clinic. S Afr Med J. 1984;65:291–7.
26. Myers TW. Anatomy trains. Edinburgh: Elsevier; 2001.
27. Bleakey CM, Glasgow PD, Phillips N, Hanna L, Callaghan MJ, Davison GW, Hopkins TJ, Delahunt E. PRICE guidelines for clinical practice. Sheffield: ACPSM; 2010.
28. Jarvinen T, Kaariainen M, Jarvinen M, Kalimo H. Muscle strain injuries. Curr Opin Rheumatol. 2000;12:155–61.
29. Cyriax JH. Textbook of orthopaedic medicine, Diagnosis of soft tissue lesions, vol. 1. 8th ed. London: Balliere Tindall; 1983.
30. Langevin HM. Potential role of fascia in chronic musculoskeletal pain. Integrative pain medicine. Contemp Pain Med. 2008;11:123–32.
31. Langevin HM, Churchill DL, Wu J, Badger GJ, Yandow JA, Fox JR, Krag MH. Evidence of connective tissue involvement in acupuncture. FASEB J. 2002;16:872–4.
32. Rees JD, Wilson AM, Wolman RL. Current concepts in the management of tendon disorders. Rheumatology. 2006;45:508–21.
33. Young M, Ranson C. The role of targeted exercises in the management of Achilles and patellar tendinopathy in sport. Eur Musculoskeletal Rev. 2011;6:1331–36.
34. Mafi N, Lorentzon R, Alfredson H. Superior short-term results with eccentric calf muscle training compared to concentric training in a randomised prospective multicentre on patients with chronic Achilles tendinosis. Knee Surg Sports Traumatol Arthrosc. 2001;9:42–7.
35. Langevin HM, Storch KN, Snapp RR, Bouffard NA, Badger GJ, Howe AK, Taatjes DJ. Tissue stretch induces nuclear remodelling in connective tissue fibroblasts. Histochem Cell Biol. 2010;133:405–15.
36. Osterhues DJ. The use of kinesio taping® in the management of traumatic patella dislocation. A case study. Physiother Theory Pract. 2004;20:267–70.
37. Kellett J. Acute soft tissue injuries – a review of the literature. Med Sci Sports Exerc. 1986;18:489–500.
38. Niemuth PE, Johnson RJ, Myers MJ, Thieman TJ. Hip muscle weakness and overuse injuries in recreational runners. Clin J Sports Med. 2005;15:14–21.
39. Ramelet AA. Exercise-induced vasculitis. J Acad Dermatol Venereol. 2006;20:423–7.
40. Bringard A, Perrey S, Belluye N. Aerobic energy cost and sensation responses during submaximal running exercise – positive effects of wearing compression tights. Int J Sports Med. 2006;27:373–8.

41. Ali A, Caine MP, Snow BG. Graduated compression stockings: physiological and perceptual responses during and after exercise. J Sports Sci. 2007;25:413–9.
42. Herbert RD, Gabriel M. Effect of stretching before and after exercising on muscle soreness and risk of injury: systematic review. BMJ. 2002;325:468–73.
43. Bennell K, Matheson G, Meeuwise W, Brukner P. Risk factors for stress fractures. Sports Med. 1999;28:91–122.
44. Larson-Meyer DE, Willis KS. Vitamin D and athletes. Curr Sports Med Rep. 2010;9:220–6.
45. Nieman DC. Exercise effects on systemic immunity. Immunol Cell Biol. 2000;78:496–501.
46. Ivy JL. Role of carbohydrate in physical activity. Clin Sports Med. 1999;18:469–84.
47. Nybo L. CNS fatigue and prolonged exercise: effect of glucose supplementation. Med Sci Sports Exerc. 2003;35:589–94.
48. Williams D, Brewer J, Walker M. The effect of a high carbohydrate diet on running performance during a 30 km treadmill time trial. Eur J Appl Physiol Occup Physiol. 1985;65:18–24.
49. Sherman WM, Costill DL, Miller JM. Effect of exercise-diet manipulation on muscle glycogen and its subsequent utilization during performance. Int J Sports Med. 1981;2:114–8.
50. Noakes TD, Lambert EV, et al. Carbohydrate ingestion and muscle glycogen depletion during marathon and ultramarathon training. Eur J Appl Physiol Occup Physiol. 1988;57:482–9.
51. Emmett J. The physiology of marathon running. Marathon and beyond. 2007. www.marathonandbeyond.com/choices/emmett.htm. Accessed on 15 Sep 2012.
52. Cheuvront SN, Haymes EM. Thermoregulation and marathon running: biological and environmental influences. Sports Med. 1997;31:743–62.
53. Noakes TD. Fluid replacement during marathon running. Clin J Sport Med. 2003;13:309–18.
54. Murray R, Selfert JG, Eddy DE, Paul GL, Halaby GA. Carbohydrate feeding and exercise: effect of beverage carbohydrate content. Eur J Appl Physiol Occup Physiol. 1989;59:152–8.
55. Davis DP, Videen JS, Marino A, Vilke GM, Dunford JV, Van Camp SP, Maharam LG. Exercise associated hyponatremia in marathon runners: a two year experience. J Emerg Med. 2001;21:47–57.
56. Frizzel RT, Lang GH, Lowance DC, Lathan SR. Hyponatremia and ultramarathon running. JAMA. 1986;255:772–4.
57. Roi GS, Giacometti M, Banfi G, Zaccaria M, Gritti I, Von Duvillard SP. Competitive running at high altitude: is it safe? Med Sci Sports Exerc. 1999;31:191.
58. Talbot TS, Townes DA, Wedmore IS. To air is human: altitude illness during an expedition length adventure race. Wilderness Environ Med. 2004;15:90–4.

Chapter 14
Personality Characteristics in Extreme Sports Athletes: Morbidity and Mortality in Mountaineering and BASE Jumping

Erik Monasterio

Contents

Introduction	303
Cloninger's Temperament and Character Inventory (TCI)	305
TCI Findings in Mountaineers and BASE Jumpers	306
Implication of Research Findings	308
Summary	312
References	313

Introduction

"Extreme" risk-taking sports such as mountaineering, kayaking, rock climbing, downhill mountain biking, and BASE jumping have increased in popularity in recent years and capture increasing public interest [1]. These activities court significant dangers and attract individuals who are prepared to put their personal safety, and at times their life, in search of a rush of excitement or an unusual accomplishment.

Mountaineering is the sport of climbing mountains, which incorporates the skills of rock and ice climbing: It has long been regarded as a high-risk sport associated with frequent and often severe, physical injuries and fatalities [2–4]; in mountaineering, climbing falls tend to be longer than those experienced in rock and ice climbing, and since climbing to altitudes over 2,500 m is not uncommon among mountaineers, altitude-related problems (such as cerebral and pulmonary edema) increase the chances of potential morbidity and mortality [3, 5]. Paradoxically, despite these risks, the popularity of mountaineering has continued to increase in

E. Monasterio
Department of Psychological Medicine,
University of Otago, Christchurch School of Medicine,
2 Riccarton Avenue, 4345,
Christchurch 8140, New Zealand
e-mail: erik.monasterio@cdhb.govt.nz

the last 15–20 years, and it is now one of the fastest growing outdoor sporting activities. Media and scientific articles of accidents and tragedies are published as frequently as accounts of successful ascents, leading to ongoing debate on the ethics of the sport, particularly as it has become a commercial venture. Dramatically publicized disasters, such as the 1996 Everest tragedy in which a total of eight climbers died (five from two commercial expeditions) appear to have done little to dissuade climbers from the sport. The number of commercial guiding companies continues to grow, and the list of paying clients increases with many adventure climbing companies offering novices guided ascents of the world's highest peaks, such as Mount Everest, for a fee of US$40,000 to US$50,000 [6]. Two hundred and twenty mountaineers have died in their quest to climb Everest/Sagamartha, 245 to climb New Zealand's highest mountain, Aoraki/Mt Cook, and more than 1,000 in their quest for Europe's highest peak, Mt Blanc.

BASE jumping is arguably the most dangerous of the "extreme" sports: it developed out of skydiving and uses specially adapted parachutes to jump from fixed objects. "BASE" is an acronym that stands for the four categories of fixed objects that one can jump off. These are *B*uilding, *A*ntenna, *S*pan (a bridge, arch, or dome), and *E*arth (a cliff or other natural formation). Although the popularity of the sport is rapidly increasing, the total number of participants worldwide in 2002 was estimated at approximately 700 [7]. Recent studies have calculated the annual fatality risk as one death per 60 participants and the serious injury rate (requiring hospital care) as 0.2–0.4 % per jump; BASE jumping is therefore associated with a 5–16-fold risk for death or injury when compared with skydiving [8–10]. Our experience is that 72 % of experienced BASE jumpers had witnessed the death or serious injury of other participants in the sport, and that 76 % had at least one "near miss" incident and only 6 % had not sustained an injury, near miss, or witnessed a fatality from BASE jumping [11].

Taking into consideration the considerable risks and morbidity and mortality reported in extreme sports, it is not surprising that there exists a widespread belief that extreme sports participants are in some way "unusual." A number of studies have investigated the relationship between personality traits and participation in high-risk physical sports such as mountaineering, surfing, and skydiving, but hitherto there have been no published studies examining the personality characteristics of BASE jumpers; sensation seeking is by far the most consistently studied personality factor in the literature. Most studies have found that high-risk sport participants tend to score higher on Zuckerman's Sensation Seeking (SS) Scale compared to low-risk sports participants and control groups [12–18]. Zuckerman defines sensation seeking as "the need for varied, novel and complex sensations and experiences and the willingness to take physical and social risks for the sake of such experience" [19].

Jack and Ronan investigated sensation seeking tendencies of a diverse group of 166 athletes and found that high-risk sports participants (hang gliding, mountaineering, skydiving, and automobile racers) scored significantly higher in total SS than low-risk sports participants (swimming, marathon running, aerobics, and golf), although there was no difference on the impulsiveness dimension between groups [13]. Cronin and Fowler et al. in separate studies found that male and female climbers scored higher in measures of total SS and the Thrill and Adventure Seeking (TAS) and Experience Seeking (ES) subscales than control populations of students [15, 16]. Diehm and Armatas compared a population of 44 high-risk, surfing sports participants with 41 low-risk, golf participants and found that surfers scored higher on total SS and TAS, Experience Seeking (ES) and Disinhition (Dis) subscales, openness to experience, and intrinsic motivation. The authors commented that surfing could be promoted as a positive risk-taking pursuit [17]. In a cross-sectional study, Franques et al. examined three groups of 34 individuals (opioid-dependent subjects, paragliders, and college staff), in the same geographical environment, and matched for age and sex. They found that opioid-dependent subjects and paragliders scored significantly higher in total SS and the SS subscales of TAS and Dis. In addition, paragliders scored higher than controls in the boredom susceptibility subscale and higher than opioid-dependent subject in the TAS subscale. Higher total scores in SS suggested to the authors that opioid-dependent subjects and paragliders could express different forms of a general tendency to seek intense and abrupt sensations through various behaviors [18].

In addition, a smaller number of studies have also considered other personality variables such as neuroticism, extraversion, and conscientiousness [14, 20]. Freixanet who investigated the personality profiles of mountaineers and alpinists found a positive relationship between extraversion – and an inverse relationship between neuroticism – and engagement in high-risk climbing [14]. Castanier et al. who investigated 302 men involved in high-risk sports (downhill skiing, mountaineering, rock climbing, paragliding, and skydiving) found that personality types with a configuration of low conscientiousness combined with high extraversion and/or high neuroticism were greater risk takers [20].

The author and colleagues have extended on the extant research field, which has tended to focus almost exclusively on the relationship between a particular personality trait, sensation seeking, and participation in extreme sports, by utilizing a more comprehensive assessment of personality functioning. The purpose of this chapter is to summarize the results of this research, applied to a population of mountaineers and BASE jumpers, and discuss the implications of the findings. We have explored the possible psychobiological contribution to mountaineering and BASE jumping, attempting to determine whether particular personality variables are associated with engagement in risk-taking sports, a higher risk of accidents, and psychological resilience in the face of trauma. The personality model we have employed is the Temperament and Character Inventory (TCI) [21].

Cloninger's Temperament and Character Inventory (TCI)

The TCI is a self-report personality questionnaire, which accounts for both normal and abnormal variation in the two major components of personality: temperament and character. The TCI-235 is a 235-item self-reported questionnaire designed to assess differences between people in seven basic dimensions of temperament and character. Temperament refers to the automatic emotional responses that are thought to be moderately heritable, independent, genetically homogenous, and stable over time. Each temperament dimension is hypothesized to be regulated neurochemically by a complex distributed network of brain connections.

There are four temperament dimensions, which are:

1. *Novelty Seeking, NS* – a tendency to activate or initiate new behaviors with a propensity to seek out new or novel experiences, impulsive decision making, extravagance, quick loss of temper, and active avoidance of frustration.
2. *Harm Avoidance, HA* – a tendency to inhibit behaviors with a propensity to worry in anticipation of future problems, fear of uncertainty, rapid fatigability, and shyness in the company of strangers.
3. *Reward Dependence, RD* – a tendency to maintain behaviors manifested by dependency on the approval of others, social attachments, and sentimentality.
4. *Persistence, P* – a tendency to be hardworking, industrious, and persistent despite frustration and fatigue. Character refers to self-concepts and individual differences in goals and values that can be influenced by social factors, learning, and the process of maturation.

The character dimensions are:

1. *Self-directedness, SD* – which refers to self-determination, personal integrity, self-integrity, and willpower.
2. *Cooperativeness, C* – which refers to individual differences in identification with and acceptance of other people.
3. *Self-transcendence, ST* – which refers to feelings of religious faith or viewing oneself as an integral part of the universe in other ways [21].

The benefit of using this model is that it provides broad information on temperament and character, and there is a large volume of research and findings in different clinical, nonclinical, and control populations across a number of different countries.

TCI Findings in Mountaineers and BASE Jumpers

We compared 49 experienced mountaineers [22] and 68 experienced BASE jumpers [23] with a previously collected age-matched control sample utilizing the TCI-235 [24].

Ninety-six percent of mountaineers estimated that (on at least two occasions) they had climbed in situations of high risk. High risk was defined as climbing in dangerous terrain (under unstable ice cliffs, over avalanche-prone terrain, and in crevassed glaciers), in dangerous weather conditions, or in situations where the climber did not feel fully confident in their abilities and where a climbing mistake would lead to significant risk of serious injury or death. This level of risk is inherent

Table 14.1 Climbers' demographic and injury findings

	Minimum	Maximum	Mean
Age (years)	21	56	33
Years climbing	1	>20	>7
Climbing grades – rock	12	29	23
Climbing grades – alpine	2	6+	5
Professional vs. amateur	8 professional	41 amateur	
Injured climbers	47 %	?	
Gender	10 % (female)	90 % (male)	
Marital status	51 % single	49 % married	

[a]Rock climbing grades were rated according to the Australasian Ewbank system (5–34). Above grade 10, ropes and security devices are recommended. Grades above 18 require a significant degree of technical skill. Generally, the higher the grade, the greater the technical challenges and risk of accident

[b]Alpine climbing grades were rated according to the New Zealand and Australian system (1–7). From grade 3 on, technical climbing equipment such as ice axes, crampons, security equipment, and a rope are required. Grade 5 involves sustained technical climbing which may have vertical sections of ice climbing; grade 6 involves vertical sections of ice with poor protection and grade 7 is possible but as yet unaccomplished

Table 14.2 BASE jumpers' demographic and injury findings

	Minimum	Maximum	Mean
Age	21	68	34
Gender	59 males (87 %)	9 females (13 %)	
Martial status	39 single (58 %)	29 married (42 %)	
Time BASE jumping (years)	0.5	17	5.8
Total no. of jumps	12	2,300	286
Injured jumpers	28 injured (42 %)	40 not injured (58 %)	
Severity (AIS)	2	5	3.1

AIS Abbreviated Injury Scale

to high-performance mountaineering. BASE jump volunteers were included if they had been involved in the sport for at least 6 months and had made at least ten jumps; of those, 76 % had at least one "near miss" incident and 72 % had witnessed a serious or fatal accident from the sport.

Demographic and injury data in these populations is summarized in Tables 14.1 and 14.2. Mountaineers and BASE jumpers in the study were predominantly single, male, and in their mid-30s. At baseline, 47 % of mountaineers had been involved in

Table 14.3 Climber ($n=49$) and BASE jumpers ($n=68$) compared with normative population ($n=181$) TCI-235 score means (and SD)

	NS***	HA***	RD	P	SD**	C	ST***
Climbers	21.6 (5.2)	9.1 (4.7)	14.1 (4.4)	5.0 (1.5)	35.5 (5.0)	34.1 (4.6)	11.0 (6.7)
Base jumpers	22.8 (5.7)	7.9 (6.3)	13.8 (4.8)**	5.5 (1.4)	33.4 (6.7)	33.7 (5.6)	12.7 (7.0)
Controls	19.0 (5.8)	12.4 (6.9)	15.6 (4.3)	5.7 (2.1)	32.0 (7.0)	33.6 (6.7)	18.7 (6.3)

NS novelty seeking, *HA* harm avoidance, *RD* reward dependence, *P* persistence, *SD* self-directedness, *C* cooperativeness, *ST* self-transcendence
**$p<0.05$, ***$p<0.001$

a total of 33 accidents: 10 severe, 16 moderate, and 7 mild. Four-year follow-up date was only available in mountaineers, and there were 4 (8.2 %) deaths from climbing misadventure. At baseline, 42 % of BASE jumpers had suffered serious injury (mean AIS score = 3.1) [4, 9].

TCI scores are summarized in Table 14.3. Mountaineers and BASE jumper personality measures differed significantly from age-matched controls; they had higher NS and SD scores, and lower HA and ST scores. In addition, BASE jumpers had lower scores on RD. Overall there was no difference between male and female scores in the BASE jumper population, and there were insufficient females in the mountaineer population to determine whether there were any gender differences. There was no difference in personality variables between mountaineers and BASE jumpers. Interestingly, all TCI scores, except for HA, were distributed relatively normally. As Figs. 14.1 and 14.2 show, HA scores had a markedly skewed distribution. In particular, a significant proportion of BASE jumpers had extremely low HA scores; 40 % have a score of 4 or less.

In mountaineers, the Spearman correlation coefficients noted a significant inverse relationship between cooperativeness and the total number of accidents (−0.313, $p<0.05$) and severity of accidents (−0.475, $p<0.05$); in this group, there was no significant correlation between other personality traits and number or severity of accidents. Interestingly, there was no association between personality traits and injury measures in the BASE jump group, with the strongest Spearman's $r=-0.09$.

Implication of Research Findings

Overall, when compared to age-matched control populations, mountaineers and BASE jumpers scored higher on the temperament measure of NS and the character measure of SD and lower on the temperament measure of HA and the character measure of ST, with only BASE jumpers scoring lower on the temperamental measure of RD. However, the relatively large variation evident in the standard deviations across the measures of temperament and character suggests that there is not a tightly defined personality profile among mountaineers and BASE jumpers, and that factors other than personality are also likely to contribute to engagement in these sports. Such factors may include opportunity and access to the natural climbing

Jumpers HA spread

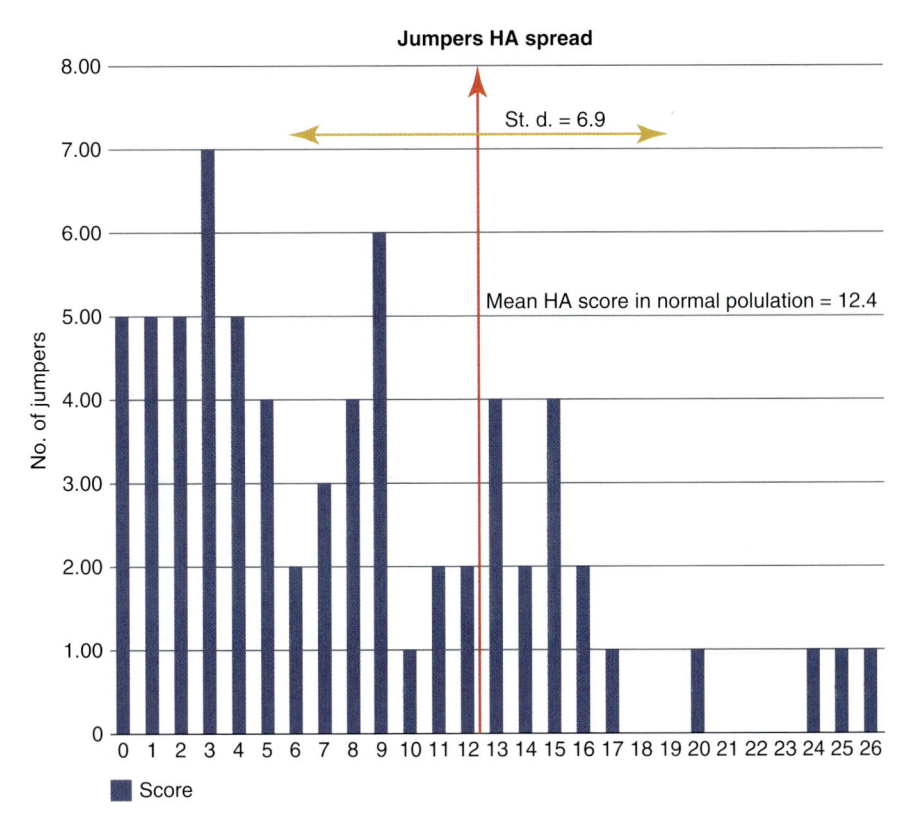

Fig. 14.1 HA scores in BASE jumpers

environment, peer influence, increased popularity, media attention, and commercialization of these activities.

There is a high correlation between Zuckerman's SS and Cloninger's NS scales [25], and, therefore, the finding of high NS in the research population is consistent with the previously demonstrated relationship between SS and participation in risk-taking sports [12–18]. According to Cloninger's model of personality, high novelty seekers enjoy exploring unfamiliar places and situations. They are easily bored; try to avoid monotony and so tend to be quick-tempered, excitable, and impulsive; and enjoy new experiences and seek out thrills and adventures, even if other people think that they are a waste of time. NS is reinforced by a constellation of genetically determined neurotransmitters, particularly those in the dopamine/pleasure system [26, 27]. High NS and SS suggests that mountaineers and BASE jumpers have lower levels of circulating dopamine and therefore may be in a state of under arousal, which may in turn contribute to engagement in risk-taking sports.

There is also a correlation between Eysenck's neuroticism (N) and Cloninger's HA scales [25], and so the findings of low HA in our population are consistent with the finding of Freixanet's study, which found that elite alpinists scored lower on N compared to controls and other mountaineers [14]. Forty percent of BASE jumpers

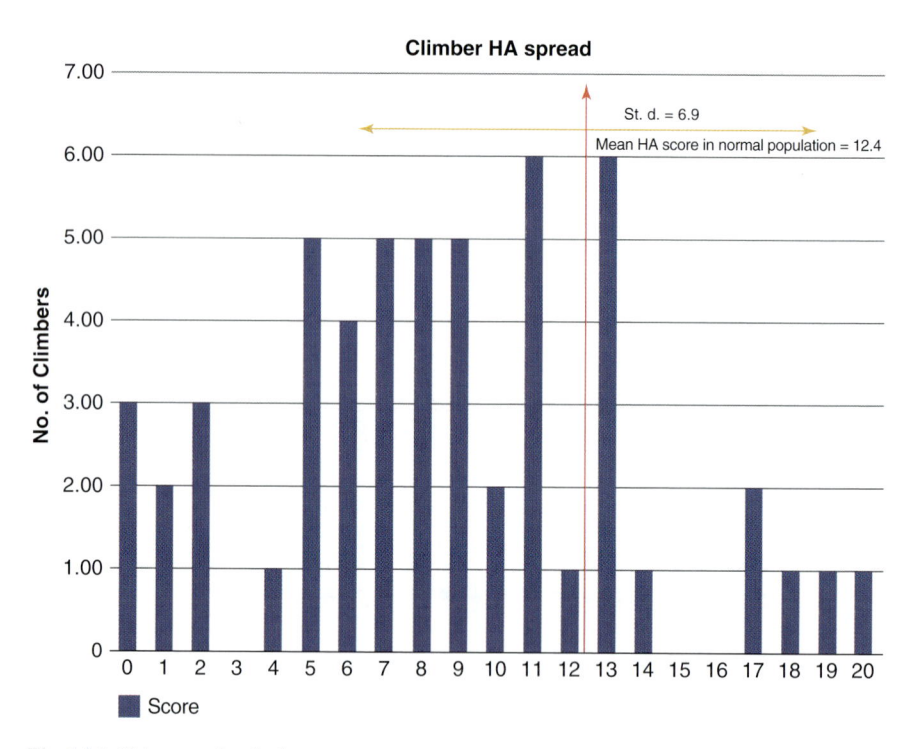

Fig. 14.2 HA scores in climbers

and 17 % of mountaineers had extremely low HA scores. In a normal population, around 5 % have HA scores of 4 or less. The eight- and threefold increase in BASE jumpers and mountaineers, respectively, suggests that a large proportion have a temperament profile characterized by low HA. HA consists of a heritable bias in the inhibition or cessation of behaviors, while high scores are positively correlated with pessimistic worry in anticipation of future problems, passive avoidant behaviors such as fear of uncertainty and shyness of strangers, and rapid fatigability. The findings of low HA are therefore not surprising or counterintuitive, as individuals with low scores on this dimension are described as carefree, relaxed, daring, courageous, composed, and optimistic even in situations which worry most people. These individuals are described as outgoing, bold, and confident. Their energy levels tend to be high, and they impress others as dynamic, lively, and vigorous. The advantages of HA are confidence in the face of danger and uncertainty, leading to optimistic and energetic efforts with little or no distress. The disadvantages are related to unresponsiveness to danger, which can lead to foolhardy optimism [21].

There is a high prevalence of witnessed and experienced serious trauma and near misses among mountaineers and BASE jumpers; despite this, participants persisted in their chosen activity, and this persistence in the face of trauma suggests that they possess considerable psychological resilience to trauma. This observation is consistent with the findings from a study of professional mountain guides ($n = 1,347$) in Switzerland; researchers found that in this study, which has the largest population of mountaineers and guides in the literature, 78 % had experienced at least one potentially traumatic event, yet the prevalence rate for post-traumatic stress disorder (PTSD) was 2.7 % and subsyndromal PTSD was 1.5 %. In interpreting their findings, the researchers reviewed other studies related to PTSD in different types of rescue workers, such as fire and ambulance service workers, of similar age and with comparable duration of professional experience, and found that those workers reported PTSD prevalence rates of more than 18 % [28]. Therefore, mountain guides had only 15–20 % prevalence of PTSD, despite similar exposure to trauma. A number of studies have examined the relationship between Cloninger's temperamental traits and risk of PTSD and other anxiety disorders in general, with a consistent finding of elevated HA [29–31]. Although some patients differed in other aspects of their temperament, this depended on comorbid features besides anxiety [31]. Low HA scores in mountaineers and BASE jumpers may confer some protection against PTSD and anxiety disorders in general and so contribute to psychological resilience in the face of considerable trauma.

Low scores in RD generally suggest that there is less reliance or indifference toward approval from others; therefore, lower RD scores among BASE jumpers may indicate a bias toward engagement in a sport that does not rely on the participation of others.

Interestingly, there was an inverse correlation between C and the frequency and severity of injury ($Rs = -0.313$ and $Rs = -0.475$, respectively) in mountaineers, but no other association between temperament and character measures and accidents (strongest Spearman's $r = 0.148$), in either population. In general, individuals who score low on C are described as self-absorbed, unhelpful and uncooperative, and less likely to engage in teamwork; this in turn is likely to increase the risk of injury in mountaineering where safety and risk management requires a team approach, but not in BASE jumping where participants do not rely on teamwork for safety and participation. To the author's knowledge, this is the first study that has identified an association between a specific personality trait and risk of injury in extreme sports. Replication of this finding could have implications for risk assessment and management in mountaineers and potentially other extreme sports that require team participation. Assessment of C may identify mountaineers who have low C and therefore may serve to alert them to possible increased risk and the need for behavior modification; mountain guides may also identify clients with increased risk potential.

In order to participate in extreme sports such as mountaineering and BASE jumping, participants require highly developed skills that can only be developed by repeated and consistent practice over time, and which are generally acquired after undergoing a fairly rigorous apprenticeship. As SD refers to self-determination and maturity or the ability of an individual to control, regulate, and adapt behavior to fit the situation in accord with individually chosen goals and values, it is understandable that mountaineers and BASE jumpers scored high on this measure. High SD with an emphasis on discipline and skill acquisition helps to explain why these sports people engage in risk-taking behaviors by normative rather than impulsive/

disorganized antisocial means (such as drug use and criminal behavior). Previous research has shown that a combination of high NS and low HA increases the risk of drug use [32, 33].

Self-transcendence (ST) is a character trait that in general denotes a propensity to religious and transpersonal experience and a tendency to self-forgetfulness. The finding of low ST in these populations has not been previously reported and is counterintuitive and difficult to account for. However, as extreme sports are often pursued in unstable environments and require a high level of performance under extreme stress, meticulous attention to detail, and split-second decision making, a capacity for sustained focus over prolonged periods of time and in situations of physical and psychological stress is important. High ST with its attendant propensity for self-forgetfulness and openness to transpersonal experience is likely to be disadvantageous as it may lead to distractibility and diminished focus on a highly specific task. Individuals who score low on ST tend to be proud, impatient, unfulfilled, self-aware, and generally struggle to accept failure [21]; this may also contribute to their drive to achieve in extreme sports despite exposure to risk. The difficulty in accepting failure with equanimity and the inability to achieve extreme sports goals in individuals who score particularly low in ST may lead to adjustment difficulties with advancing years, when individuals are faced with mounting injuries and impaired performance.

Cloninger's model of personality has been applied to the study of non-risk-taking sport populations with mixed results. Seznec et al. utilized the TCI to examine a sample of 18 elite racing cyclists from the French junior racing team and compared them with 26 age- and gender-matched controls of the same nationality. The only significant difference between the populations related to higher RD in cyclists [34]. Han et al. examined a mixed population of 277 high school boys engaged in endurance, combat, power, and team sports and compared them with a population of 152 nonathlete high school boys to determine whether there were any differences in temperament and state and trait anxiety. HA scores of athletes were higher than in nonathletes, and there was no difference in other temperaments between groups. Endurance athletes showed highest NS and lowest P scores among the four different types of sports. Levels of trait and state anxiety were higher in the athletes than nonathletes group [35]. These sport participants did not show the characteristic findings of our study populations, and, therefore, the differences in temperament and character of mountaineers and BASE jumpers cannot be attributed to regular, general participation in sports. It is likely that the risk-taking component in the extreme sports groups to a substantial extent account for the differences.

Summary

The study of risk-taking sports people yields interesting results. Sports such as mountaineering and BASE jumping are associated with significant risk of injury and death. The results of the studied populations indicate that in general mountaineers,

BASE jumpers and other extreme sport participants score differently on measures of temperament and character when compared to normative and low-risk sport populations. In addition, a substantial proportion of the BASE jumpers studied presented extremely low scores in the temperament measure of HA, the extent of which has not been reported in any other population. As temperament traits are thought to be neurochemically regulated and moderately heritable, it is likely that to some extent engagement in these sports is genetically determined and "hardwired." Overall, however, the relatively large variation evident in the standard deviations across the measures of temperament and character suggests that there is not a tightly defined personality profile among mountaineers and BASE jumpers, and that factors other than personality contribute to engagement in these sports. Such factors may include opportunity and access to the natural climbing environment, peer influence, increased popularity, media attention, and commercialization of these activities.

References

1. Pain MTG. Risk taking in sport. Lancet. 2005;366:S33–4.
2. Malcolm M. Mountaineering fatalities in Mt Cook National Park. N Z Med J. 2001;114(1127):78–80.
3. Pollard A, Clarke C. Deaths during mountaineering at extreme altitude. Lancet. 1988;1:1277.
4. Monasterio ME. Accident and fatality characteristics in a population of mountain climbers in New Zealand. N Z Med J. 2005;118(1208):U1249.
5. Schoffl V, Morrison A, Schwarz U, et al. Evaluation of injury and fatality risk in rock and ice climbing. Sports Med. 2010;40(8):657–79.
6. Elmes M, Barry D. Deliverance, denial and the death zone: a study of narcissism and regression in the May 1996 Everest climbing disaster. J Appl Behav Sci. 1999;35:163–87.
7. Maeland S. Basehopping- nasjonale- sublime opplevelser. Norsk Antropologisk tidsskrift. 2004;1:80–101.
8. Westman A, Rosen M, Berggren P, Bjornstig U. Parachuting from fixed objects; descriptive study of 106 fatal events in BASE jumping 1981–2006. Br J Sports Med. 2008;42(6):431–6.
9. Monasterio ME, Mei-Dan O. Risk and severity of injury in a population of BASE jumpers. N Z Med J. 2008;121(1277):70–5.
10. Soreide K, Ellingsen L, Knutson V. How dangerous is BASE jumping? An analysis of adverse events in 20,850 jumps from Kjerag Massif, Norway. J Trauma. 2007;62:1113–7. Abstract at http://www.jtrauma.com/pt/re/jtrauma/abstract.00005373-200705000-00006.htm;jsessionid=LysVWzSWmJfTKBsLRQ6WGZnnyvF88vQDplfcJXCmWNtnpHy1nzf3!851130288!181195628!8091!-1.
11. Zuckerman M. Sensation seeking and sports. Pers Indiv Differ. 1983;4:285–93.
12. Mei-Dan O, Carmont MR, Monasterio EM. The epidemiology of severe and catastrophic injuries in BASE jumping. Clin J Sport Med. 2012;22(3):262–7.
13. Jack SJ, Ronan KR. Sensation seeking among high- and low-risk sports participants. Pers Indiv Differ. 1998;25(6):1063–83.
14. Freixanet MG. Personality profile of subjects engaged in high physical risk sports. Pers Indiv Differ. 1991;12:1087–92.
15. Cronin C. Sensation seeking among mountain climbers. Pers Indiv Differ. 1991;12:653–4.
16. Fowler CJ, von Knorring L, Oreland L. Platelet monoamine oxidase activity in sensation seekers. Psychiatr Res. 1980;3:272–9.

17. Diehm R, Armatas C. Surfing: an avenue for socially acceptable risk-taking, satisfying needs for sensation seeking and experience seeking. Pers Indiv Differ. 2004;36:663–77.
18. Franques P, Auriacombe M, Piquemal E, Verger M, et al. Sensation seeking as a common factor in opioid dependent subjects and high risk sport practicing subjects. A cross sectional study. Drug Alcohol Depend. 2003;69:121–6.
19. Zuckerman M. Sensation seeking: beyond the optimal level of arousal. Hillsdale: Erlbaum; 1979.
20. Castanier C, Le Scanff C, Woodman T. Who takes risks in high-risk sports? A typological personality approach. Res Q Exerc Sport. 2010;81(4):478–84.
21. Chapter 4: Basic description of the personality scales. In: Cloninger CR, Przybeck TR, Svrakic DM, et al., editors. The Temperament and Character Inventory (TCI): a guide to its development and use. St Louis: Center for Psychobiology of Personality, Washington University; 1994. p. 19–29.
22. Monasterio E, Alamri Y, Mei-Dan O. Personality variables in a population of mountain climbers (in press).
23. Monasterio E, Mulder R, Frampton C, Mei-Dan O. Characteristics of BASE Jumpers. Journal of Applied Sports Psychology 2012;24(4): 391–400. doi: 10.1080/10413200.2012.666710.
24. Chapter 9: Norms and demographic correlates of the TCI. In: Clonninger CR, Przybeck TR, Svrakic DM, et al., editors. The Temperament and Character Inventory (TCI): a guide to its development and use. St Louis: Center for Psychobiology of Personality, Washington University; 1994. p. 85–91.
25. Zuckerman M, Cloninger CR. Relationship between Clonninger's, Zuckerman's, and Eysenck's dimensions of personality. Pers Indiv Diff. 1996;21(2):283–5.
26. Golimbet VE, Alfimova MV, Gritsenko IK, Ebstein RP. Relationship between dopamine system genes and extraversion and novelty seeking. Neurosci Behav Physiol. 2007;37:601–6.
27. Schinka JA, Letsch EA, Crawford FC. DRD4 And novelty seeking: results of meta-analyses. Am J Med Genet. 2002;114:643–8.
28. Sommer I, Ehlert U. Prevalence and predictors of posttraumatic stress disorder symptoms in mountain guides. J Psychosom Res. 2004;57(4):329–35.
29. Gil S, Caspi Y. Personality traits, coping style, and perceived threat as predictors of posttraumatic stress disorder: a prospective study. Psychosom Med. 2006;68(6):904–9.
30. Richman H, Frueh BC. Personality and PTSD II: personality assessment of PTSD-diagnosed Vietnam veterans using the Cloninger Tridimensional Personality Questionnaire (TPQ). Depress Anxiety. 1997;6:70–7.
31. Chapter 3: Applications to anxiety disorders. In: Cloninger CR, Przybeck TR, Svrakic DM et al., editors. The Temperament and Character Inventory (TCI): a guide to its development and use. St Louis: Center for Psychobiology of Personality, Washington University; 1994. p. 107–11.
32. Wills TA, Vaccaro D, McNamara G. Novelty seeking, risk taking, and related constructs as predictor of adolescent substance use: an application of Cloninger's theory. J Subst Abuse. 1995;6(1):1–20.
33. Gunnarsdottir ED, Pingitore RA, Spring BJ, Konopka LA, et al. Individual differences among cocaine users. Addict Behav. 2000;25(5):641–52.
34. Seznec JC, Lepine JP, Pelissolo A. Dimensional personality assessment of the members of the French national team of road cycling. Encéphale. 2003;29(1):29–33.
35. Doug HH, Kim JH, Lee YS, Bae SJ, et al. Influence of temperament and anxiety on athletic performance. J Sports Med. 2006;5:381–9.

Chapter 15
Endocrine Aspects and Responses to Extreme Sports

Karen Tordjman, Naama Constantini, and Anthony C. Hackney

Contents

Introduction...	315
Hormonal Response to Physical Activity: Exercise	316
Ultra-endurance Extreme Events..	318
Extreme Sports with Mental Stress...	320
Conclusions..	321
Epilogue	322
References..	323

Introduction

In the last few decades, extreme sports have gained in popularity worldwide. These activities are popular not only with adventurous elite athletes but more and more everyday people are participating in extreme sports activities on a recreational basis. As an illustration of this phenomenon, a 2008 report approximated that the

K. Tordjman (✉)
Institute of Endocrinology, Metabolism, and Hypertension, Tel Aviv-Sourasky Medical Center, Tel Aviv, Israel
Sackler Faculty of Medicine, Tel Aviv University,
Tel Aviv, Israel
e-mail: karent@tlvmc.gov.il

N. Constantini
Department of Orthopedic Surgery, Sport Medicine Center, The Hadassah-Hebrew University Medical Center, Jerusalem, Israel

A.C. Hackney
Endocrine Section-Applied Physiology Laboratory, Department of Exercise & Sport Science, University of North Carolina,
Chapel Hill, NC, USA

O. Mei-Dan, M.R. Carmont (eds.), *Adventure and Extreme Sports Injuries*,
DOI 10.1007/978-1-4471-4363-5_15, © Springer-Verlag London 2013

number of extreme sport participants in the United States alone was nearly 275 million person-events, attempting participation in 14 different types of extreme sports activities [1].

With increasing numbers of persons becoming involved in extreme sports, it becomes exceedingly important to understand the physiological responses to such activities on the human body due to their potentially stressful nature. The hormonal responses of the endocrine system to stresses, either distress or eustress, result in a multitude of subsequent responses in many physiological systems (e.g., cardiovascular, metabolic, and respiratory) affecting the entire body in both a positive, as well as a deleterious manner. Thus, a clear and thorough understanding of the endocrine responses to extreme sports participation is critical to allow health-care researchers and clinicians to develop the necessary guidelines to mitigate risks or contraindications to individuals' participation. That is, this type of knowledge can allow for health-care researchers and clinicians to develop evidence-based guidance as to which activities may create, or have, a greater negative health risk associated with them.

To this end, the intent of this chapter is to provide a brief summary-overview of the endocrine responses to a variety of extreme sports. Regrettably, the number of research studies examining the endocrine responses of participants in such activities is very few and somewhat limited in the nature of their scientific approach and design due to them being field-base studies. Organizationally, this chapter addresses the endocrine response to extreme sports by categorizing the sport activities into two broad classifications: (*a*) ultra-endurance events and (*b*) events with extreme mental stress. It is recognized that these classifications are neither mutually exclusive nor do they completely capture the essence of each sports' individual characteristics, but due to the small number of research investigations available, some sports activities have been combined based upon a marginal degree of similarities within the activities. Additionally, to provide a point of reference for the reader, a brief section on the representative hormonal responses to exercise is presented initially.

Hormonal Response to Physical Activity: Exercise

Many of the extreme sports have elements of adventure, danger of physical harm, and/or undue levels of fatigue associated with them. Such elements can place tremendous physical demands and stress on the physiological systems of the body.

One physiological system that is highly responsive to such demands-stresses is the endocrine system [2, 3]. When properly activated, this complex system is capable of orchestrating an array of physiological responses that, for the most part, ultimately promote the desired level of performance while maintaining homeostasis. In order to appreciate the endocrine changes operating under extreme sports conditions, a general review of some typical responses of the endocrine system to conventional athletic-sporting activities is in order. It is beyond the scope of this chapter to give a detailed account of all the documented alterations that occur with such activities. It should be noted however that marked differences exist between trained and untrained individuals, and that the type of activity (aerobic vs. anaerobic primary energy demands) and its duration (short-term vs. prolonged endurance) are key modulators of these responses [4–6].

By and large, the hormonal responses to physical activity are geared at making energy substrates readily available, enabling the cardiovascular system to maintain adequate tissue oxygenation and cardiac output, preserving fluid and electrolyte homeostasis, optimizing mental functions, and providing a sense of well-being to withstand the physical and emotional challenges.

The sympathetic nervous system responds rapidly to exercise with catecholamine discharge, which is proportional to the type, intensity, and duration of the effort [7]. Both epinephrine and norepinephrine release affect cardiovascular function and respiratory adjustment. The surge in these catecholamines ensures blood diversion to muscles, skin, and other critical organs, as well as energy substrate release through glycogenolysis, lipolysis, and gluconeogenesis.

The major glucocorticoid hormone, cortisol, also has a fundamental role in substrate availability, and it has long been established that exercise elicits the activity of the hypothalamic-pituitary-adrenal axis (HPA) [8]. This response appears to be dependent both on the level of exercise intensity and its duration, but not on neither gender nor age [9]. The additional benefit of plasma cortisol increase with exercise is the suppression of the inflammatory insult due to potential muscle injury or trauma [3].

Exercise is a very potent physiological stimulus for growth hormone secretion. In contrast to cortisol, growth hormone release with exercise is strongly related to age and gender. Women tend to have higher basal growth hormone levels and larger responses to exercise than men, and responses diminish somewhat with age in both gender [10]. Growth hormone secretion in response to exercise serves an immediate energetic purpose by allowing mobilization of fatty acids through lipolysis during exercise, but it also promotes muscle growth through its anabolic action during the recovery from exercise.

Fluid and electrolyte balance is also finely coordinated during exercise by a concerted hormonal mechanism(s) that aims to limit the fluid losses incurred by sweating and heat dissipation. The aforementioned sympathetic activity response to exercise is a major stimulus for renal renin secretion (i.e., the rate-limiting step of the renin-angiotensin-aldosterone [RAA] system controlling fluid balance). Activation of the RAA system results in elevation of angiotensin II, a potent dipsogenic hormone, and aldosterone (also promoted by the activation of the HPA), which in turn promote increased thirst and sodium and water retention to restore fluid homeostasis. Finally, baroreceptors and osmoreceptors, which sense the volume and sodium depletion that tends to occur with exercise, elicit arginine vasopressin (also called antidiuretic hormone) secretion, further contributing to the restoration of euvolemia [11, 12].

Prolactin, a pleiotropic anterior pituitary hormone, mostly known for its role in lactation, is also a typical stress hormone that rises acutely, but transiently, in response to exercise. Although, it has been implicated (in rare circumstances) in the amenorrhea common in female athletes involved in regular high-intensity activity, its rise with exercise appears to have a predominantly immunomodulatory role as it seems to counteract the immunosuppressive effect of cortisol [13].

Acute and chronic physical activity has a major impact on both male and female gonadal function. Short bouts of exercise tend to increase testosterone levels in men. While endurance training can induce some reproductive dysfunction in men, the so-called exercise-hypogonadal male condition [14], it is rarely of major clinical significance (although, oligospermic and osteopenia conditions have been reported). In contrast, the neuroendocrine impact of intense exercise on female reproductive function has been well characterized and extensively documented. The state of hypogonadotropic hypogonadism leading to amenorrhea appears to be linked to an energy drain [15]. Indeed, it has been suggested that low leptin levels associated with negative energy balance are instrumental in these derangements [16]. This suppression of gonadal function combined with low energy availability put the athletes at increased risk for low bone mineral density [17].

Finally, psychological stress and exercise stimulate release of beta (β)-endorphins that foster mood elevation with training. This is postulated to serve as an endogenous reward system, thus promoting further adherence to exercise [18].

Implicit in all the above, it is easy to envision how exaggeration of any of these hormonal responses, such as may happen in extreme sports situations, can act as double-edged sword becoming maladaptive and entailing deleterious effects rather than being beneficial.

Ultra-endurance Extreme Events

One of the classic ultra-endurance events of the extreme sport world is the Hawaiian Ironman. In a unique opportunity, Ginsburg et al. [19] performed a large-scale study of participants ($n = 57$) in this championship. The primary intent of the study was to look at potential gender differences in the degree of exercise-induced oxidative stress. Following the race, the susceptibility of plasma lipids to peroxidation was reduced in males but no so in the females. In men, the race also induced a significant increase in estradiol (i.e., a hormone with antioxidant properties), while a concurrent reduction in testosterone occurred. No significant hormonal changes were noted in the women. The authors concluded that there are marked gender-based differences in aspects of oxidative stress responses to participation in an Ironman triathlon. It was unclear to the authors if the testosterone reduction in the men was due to increased peripheral tissue conversion of testosterone to estradiol or stress-induced gonadal suppression.

South Africa has a rich history of holding ultra-endurance events. For example, the Comrades Marathon is an ultramarathon running event (~90 km) between the cities of Durban and Pietermaritzburg and is the world's largest and oldest ultramarathon race (started in 1921). In 2007, researchers at the University of Cape Town [20] completed a comprehensive study examining the endocrine responses to athletes who performed three different exercise sessions: an ultramarathon race (56 km; "Two Ocean's"), a laboratory-base running maximal (VO_{2max}) test, and a submaximal (60 min) running laboratory test. The intent of this study was primarily to examine fluid balance hormones and compare these across the three bouts of exercise; however, in so doing, these authors studied a variety of hormones. For oxytocin, NT-proBNP, aldosterone, IL-6 (inflammatory cytokine), cortisol, corticosterone, and 11-deoxycortisol, the ultramarathon event results in more substantial postexercise increases than the other two forms of exercise. Interestingly, this was not the case with arginine vasopressin which was more elevated following the VO_{2max} test. Findings suggest the extended duration of the ultramarathon induces more of a hormonal stress response and overall physiological demands on the stress reactivity and fluid balance regulation aspects of the endocrine system. Kraemer et al. [21] also studied the hormonal responses to an ultra-endurance event; specifically, the 160-km "human-powered ultramarathon" event held in the extreme cold of Arctic Alaska. The competitors in this race could complete the marathon using either skiing, running, or cycling as means of locomotion; however, this study only examined runners and cyclists. No differences were found between the hormonal responses of the two types of athletes. Participation in this ultramarathon induced substantial increases in growth hormone, cortisol, and the proinflammatory cytokine IL-6. Conversely, there was a concomitant reduction in the testosterone levels that was suspected to be associated with the elevated adrenal stress response observed for cortisol. In a somewhat related study, Bishop et al. [22] examined the psychological and select hormonal responses of a two-man expedition to ski across Greenland (~350 km, 17 days). Psychological parameters of stress varied throughout the expedition but tended to relate to the physical difficulties inherent to the terrain and participant's fatigue level. The testosterone to cortisol ratio was assessed prior to and at select time during this expedition. The ratio showed a progressive decline during the expedition, which was also thought to be due to reductions in testosterone as induced by elevations in the cortisol levels (i.e., cortisol can inhibit the steroidogenesis process of testosterone production) [2, 14]. While not involving extreme sports activities, Aakvaag and Opstad [23, 24] conducted a series of classic studies with military personnel doing severe, prolonged marching-maneuver activities (3–5 days) with little sleep, food, and typically in cold weather. These studies showed similar suppression of testosterone and elevations of cortisol as well as another stress hormone, prolactin. Additionally, substantial suppression of the thyroid axis was displayed in these soldiers by the end of the marching-maneuver activities which persisted into the recovery days following the activities. Another cold weather-related study was that of Benso and associates [25] who examined the hormonal status of mountain climbers doing a Mt. Everest expedition involving approximately 2 months of ascent and descent trekking at altitudes ranging from 5,200 to 8,852 m. This demanding physical activity at high altitude resulted in an activation of the GH/IGF-I axis as assessed by blood measurements, but a substantial suppression of the hypothalamic-pituitary-thyroid axis–related hormones resulted in the development of a "low T_3 syndrome" condition (i.e., a situation of low serum triiodothyronine [T_3] and elevated reverse T_3 occurring from a nonthyroidal illness or event, without preexisting hypothalamic-pituitary and thyroid gland dysfunction) [2, 25]. This work of Benso supports earlier findings of Hackney et al. [26] who several years earlier demonstrated a low T_3 syndrome condition developed in as little as 2 weeks of sustained trekking at approximately 5,000 m.

Extreme Sports with Mental Stress

One of the most popular extreme sport commercial activities is bungee jumping, perhaps due to lack of a requirement for prior physical training [1] and the fact that no previous experience, personal equipment, or specific skills or talent are needed. Nonetheless, bungee jumping places a great deal of mental and emotional stress on the participant. In 1994, Henning and associates [27] examined novice bungee jumpers to investigate the influence of the psychological stress on endocrine and immune reactivity. As would be expected, the subjective ratings of anxiety were increased prior to the jump and clearly reduced afterward. After the jump, cortisol, β-endorphins, and leukocyte number were increased from pre-jump levels but gradually declined to baseline levels during the recovery time following the jump. The levels of β-endorphins, but not cortisol, after the jump correlated with ratings of euphoric sensation. In later supportive work, Van Westerloo et al. [28] found bungee jumping resulted in significant and substantial increases in blood catecholamine and cortisol concentrations both before and immediately after jumping. Interestingly, the stress associated with preparing for, as well as completing, the jump resulted in cytokine responses invoking a suppression of aspects of the innate immune system.

In a more physically demanding, yet also emotionally stressful activity, Stenner et al. [29] examined the endocrine responses to exploration of a cave, that is, Alpine potholing. Subjects spend nearly 20 h exploring a cave to a depth of 700 m in an environment characterized by darkness, low temperatures, and high humidity. The responses were compared to a control, rest day in normal environmental conditions. Growth hormone, cortisol, and free thyroxine showed slight but significant increases during the caving day. Interestingly, however, cortisol displayed a reduction on the descent portion of the caving (opposite of what was expected). The authors were puzzled by this latter outcome but speculated it was due to the elite nature of their subject pool who might not necessary consider the environmental condition encountered as extremely stressful.

In a somewhat related physical activity, Sherk et al. [30] focused on the hormonal responses to rock climbing. Specifically, these researchers measured growth hormone, testosterone, and cortisol responses before and after a continuous vertical climb on a fixed climbing route (climbing for 30 min or until exhaustion). This type of endurance climbing activity would equally result in more physical and less mental stress demands. On average, the subjects (males) climbed for 24.9 ± 1.9 min. Circulating testosterone and growth hormone concentrations were significantly increased following the climb, but cortisol was unchanged. By 15 min into the recovery from the climb, testosterone returned to baseline, but growth hormone remained elevated significantly. In another study, Hodgson and associates [31] conducted a unique study examining cortisol responses to rock climbing using varying rope safety protocols which were designed to induce low, moderate, and high degrees of physical and mental stress. Results of this study demonstrated cortisol responses and subject anxiety were directly related to perceived subjective anxiety and the increasing difficulty/risk of the rope safety protocol employed.

Finally, aerial activities such as skydiving and paragliding have been popular for many years and are well known to evoke hormonal stress responses [1, 2]. For example, Chatterton et al. [32] examined the relationship between the hormonal and psychological responses of men about to engage in their first skydiving jump. A psychological rating of events indicated significantly increased intensity and sympathetic nervous system activity; the latter, as assessed by the salivary amylase response, was increased over prior control day values. Conversely, salivary cortisol and testosterone levels were significantly lower on the morning of the jump than on the control day. The level of anxiety and subjective stress measures rose to their highest levels just before the jump. With the exception of testosterone, which remained suppressed, cortisol, prolactin, and growth hormone all increased greatly and reached peak values before or shortly after landing from the jump and declined significantly within the next hour. Anxiety and subjective stress measures declined to those of control values within 15 min after landing. In paragliders, Filaire et al. [33] evaluated motivation, anxiety, and cortisol throughout a day of a competition in comparison to a control, rest day. The subjects in this study were all found to be paratelic-dominant (i.e., "playful mind-set," a person who has a fun-loving attitude to a situation, seeks excitement and/or pleasure) in their motivational demeanor and approach. Furthermore, their cortisol was elevated on the competition day, and responses were correlated with the cognitive anxiety of the subjects prior to the paraglide jump. In earlier work, Thatcher et al. [34] found similar findings to that of Filaire et al., with respect to there being a paratelic state and elevated cortisol in their subjects who were skydivers.

Conclusions

Participation in extreme sports is becoming more and more popular worldwide. Individuals of varying physical fitness level, age, health, and gender are attempting to partake in a variety of extreme sports events. Due to this increasing popularity and prevalence of participation, it becomes important for health-care researchers and clinicians to fully understand the physiological implications of such activities. This is especially true in light of the fact that some extreme sports have elements of adventure, increased danger of physical harm, and excessive levels of fatigue associated with them. Such elements are well known to place tremendous physical demands and stress on the endocrine systems of the human body. There is a substantial amount of research literature characterizing the hormonal responses of the endocrine system to regular physical activity, exercise, and typical sports events. To date, however, the research studies examining the hormonal responses to extreme sports are exceptionally few and limited. The available studies would suggest there is a great deal of stress reactivity response within the endocrine system by extreme sport participation (i.e., high circulating levels of stress-reactive hormones – catecholamines, cortisol, prolactin, growth hormone). It is most certain, however, that some of these hormonal changes in response to extreme sports activities, especially those of a prolonged endurance nature (i.e., ultramarathons), are also occurring in an attempt to bring about metabolic, immunological, and cardiovascular adjustments necessary to perform the physical exercise [3]. That is, the aforementioned hormones are implementing key physiological roles and adjustments within the body. Nevertheless, at this time due to the extremely few studies available researching extreme sports, it is difficult and most certainly premature to completely characterize the hormonal responses as being only those as just depicted above. Much further work is necessary in to completely portray the endocrinological responses and implications of extreme sports participation before a conclusive characterization can be conveyed to health-care workers and clinicians.

Epilogue

The immense popularity and high visibility of top-level sporting events and the sizeable roster of world-class athletes with medical conditions, together with improved therapeutic tools, are now setting the stage for a growing number of patients with endocrine diseases to engage in extreme sports events. Relative to endocrine diseases one of the most prevalent is diabetes mellitus [35]. Hossain and colleagues reported in the *New England Journal of Medicine* that the number people in the world with diabetes will to increase from 171 to 366 million by the year 2030 [35]. The immensity of these numbers alone suggests many more diabetic subjects will be participating in all types of sporting events, extreme and otherwise, in the future. Realizing the challenge, and given the growing interest of diabetic patients to participate in sports in general, several professional organizations have issued guidelines for the nutritional and medical management of this condition in recreational and competitive athletes [36]. However, specific recommendations for those diabetic individuals taking part in extreme sports or similarly potentially hazardous stressful events are still lacking. Nonetheless, a body of preliminary literature is emerging that supports diabetics are able to participate in highly demanding and stressful sporting events such as marathons [37–39], mountaineering treks [40, 41], and/or activities involving hyperbaric exposure (i.e., scuba diving) [42–44] without an undue excessive risk of developing life-threatening hypo- or hyperglycemic events. However, the limited available evidence suggests in such situations it is critical that the diabetic subject be in good levels of physical fitness prior to such events and medically monitored in a rigorous fashion throughout and after such participation. This said though, the need exists for specific, careful research work in a sound clinical and scientific fashion on what, if any, limits there would be on diabetic individuals wishing to participate in extreme sports events. Most certainly, this work is warranted and needed in the near future.

References

1. Sporting Goods Manufacturers Association (SGMA) Analysis of the Sports & Fitness Participation Report, 2008 edition. Available at (http://www.sgma.com/press/2_Extreme-Sports%3A-An-Ever-Popular-Attraction). Accessed on 1 Nov 2011.
2. Charmandari E, Tsigo C, Chrousos G. Endocrinology of the stress response. Annu Rev Physiol. 2005;67:259–84.
3. Hackney AC. Stress and the neuroendocrine system: the role of exercise as a stressor and modifier of stress. Expert Rev Endocrinol Metab. 2006;1(6):783–92.
4. Duclos M, Corcuff JB, Pehourcq F, Tabarin A. Decreased pituitary sensitivity to glucocorticoids in endurance-trained men. Eur J Endocrinol. 2001;144(4):363–8.
5. Tremblay MS, Copeland JL, Van Helder W. Influence of exercise duration on post-exercise steroid hormonal responses in trained males. Eur J Appl Physiol. 2005;94(5–6):505–13.
6. Vanhelder WP, Radomski MW, Goode RC, Casey K. Hormonal and metabolic response to three types of exercise of equal duration and external work output. Eur J Appl Physiol Occup Physiol. 1985;54(4):337–42.
7. Mazzeo RS. Catecholamine response to acute and chronic exercise. Med Sci Sports Exerc. 1991;23(7):839–45.
8. Few JD. The effect of exercise on the secretion and metabolism of cortisol. J Endocrinol. 1971;51(2):10–1.
9. Traustadóttir T, Bosch PR, Cantu T, Matt KS. Hypothalamic-pituitary-adrenal axis response and recovery from high-intensity exercise in women: effects of aging and fitness. J Clin Endocrinol Metab. 2004;89(7):3248–54.
10. Wideman L, Weltman JY, Hartman ML, Veldhuis JD, Weltman A. Growth hormone release during acute and chronic aerobic and resistance exercise: recent findings. Sports Med. 2002;32(15):987–1004.
11. Luger A, Deuster PA, Debolt JE, Loriaux DL, Chrousos GP. Acute exercise stimulates the renin-angiotensin-aldosterone axis: adaptive changes in runners. Horm Res. 1988;30(1):5–9.
12. Wade CE. Hormonal regulation of fluid homeostasis during and following exercise. In: Warren MP, Constantini NW, editors. Contemporary endocrinology: sports endocrinology. Totowa: Humana Press; 2000. p. 207–25.
13. Dohi K, Kraemer WJ, Mastro AM. Exercise increases prolactin-receptor expression on human lymphocytes. J Appl Physiol. 2003;94(2):518–24.
14. Hackney AC. Effects of endurance exercise on the reproductive system of men: the "exercise-hypogonadal male condition". J Endocrinol Invest. 2008;31(10):932–8.
15. Warren MP. The effects of exercise on pubertal progression and reproductive function in girls. J Clin Endocrinol Metab. 1980;51(5):1150–7.
16. Loucks AB, Thuma JR. Luteinizing hormone pulsatility is disrupted at a threshold of energy availability in regulatory menstruating women. J Clin Endocrinol Metab. 2003;88:297–311.
17. De Souza MJ, West SL, Jamal SA, Hawker GA, Gundberg CM, Williams NI. The presence of both an energy deficiency and estrogen deficiency exacerbate alterations of bone metabolism in exercising women. Bone. 2008;43(1):140–8.
18. Schwarz L, Kindermann W. Changes in beta-endorphin levels in response to aerobic and anaerobic exercise. Sports Med. 1992;13(1):25–36.
19. Ginsburg GS, et al. Gender differences in exercise-induced changes in sex hormone levels and lipid peroxidation in athletes participating in the Hawaii Ironman triathlon. Clin Chim Acta. 2001;305(1–2):131–9.
20. Hew-Butler T, et al. Acute changes in endocrine and fluid balance markers during high-intensity, steady-state, and prolonged endurance running: unexpected increases in oxytocin and brain natriuretic peptide during exercise. Eur J Endocrinol. 2008;159:729–37.
21. Kraemer WJ, et al. Hormonal response to a 160-km race across frozen Alaska. Br J Sports Med. 2008;42(2):116–20.
22. Bishop SL, et al. Relationship of psychological and physiological parameters during an Arctic ski expedition. Acta Astronaut. 2001;49(3):261–70.

23. Aakvaag A, Sand T, Opstad PK, Fonnum F. Hormonal changes in serum in young men during prolonged physical strain. Eur J Appl Physiol Occup Physiol. 1978;39(4):283–91.
24. Opstad PK, Aakvaag A. The effect of a high calory diet on hormonal changes in young men during prolonged physical strain and sleep deprivation. Eur J Appl Physiol Occup Physiol. 1981;46(1):31–9.
25. Benso A, et al. Endocrine and metabolic responses to extreme altitude and physical exercise in climbers. Eur J Endocrinol. 2007;157:733–40.
26. Hackney AC, Feith S, Pozos R, Seale J. Effects of high altitude and cold exposure on resting thyroid hormone concentrations. Aviat Space Environ Med. 1995;66:325–9.
27. Henning J, et al. Biopsychological changes after bungee jumping: beta-endorphin immunoreactivity as a mediator of euphoria? Neuropsychobiology. 1994;29(1):28–32.
28. Van Westerloo DJ, et al. Acute stress elicited by Bungee Jumping suppresses human innate immunity. Mol Med. 2011;17(3–4):80–8.
29. Stenner E, et al. Hormonal responses to a long duration exploration in a cave of 700 M depth. Eur J Appl Physiol. 2007;100(1):71–8.
30. Sherk VD, et al. Hormone responses to a continuous bout of rock climbing in men. Eur J Appl Physiol. 2011;111(4):687–93.
31. Hodgson CI, et al. Perceived anxiety and plasma cortisol concentrations following rock climbing with differing safety rope protocols. Br J Sports Med. 2009;43(7):531–5.
32. Chatterton RT, Vogelsong KM, Lu Y, Hudgens GA. Hormonal responses to psychological stress in men preparing for skydiving. J Clin Endocrinol Metab. 1997;82(8):2503–9.
33. Filaire E, et al. Motivation, stress, anxiety and cortisol responses in elite paragliders. Percept Mot Skills. 2007;104(3):1271–81.
34. Thatcher J, et al. Motivation, stress, and cortisol responses to skydiving. Percept Mot Skills. 2003;97(3):995–1002.
35. Hossain P, Kawar B, El Nahas M. Obesity and diabetes in the developing world – a growing challenge. N Engl J Med. 2007;356:213–5.
36. Joint Position Statement of the American College of Sports Medicine. The American Dietetic Association and Dietitians of Canada: nutrition and athletic performance. J Am Diet Assoc. 2000;12:1543–56.
37. Meinders AE, Willekens FL, Heere LP. Metabolic and hormonal changes in IDDM during long-distance run. Diabetes Care. 1988;11(1):1–7.
38. Tuominen JA, Ebeling P, Koivisto VA. Exercise increases insulin clearance in healthy man and insulin-dependent diabetes mellitus patients. Clin Physiol. 1997;17(1):19–30.
39. Boehncke S, Poettgen K, Maser-Gluth C, Reusch J, Boehncke WH, Badenhoop K. Endurance capabilities of triathlon competitors with type 1 diabetes mellitus. Dtsch Med Wochenschr. 2009;134(14):677–82.
40. Moore K, Vizzard N, Coleman C, McMahon J, Hayes R, Thompson CJ. Extreme altitude mountaineering and Type 1 diabetes: the Diabetes Federation of Ireland Kilimanjaro Expedition. Diabet Med. 2001;18:749–55.
41. Pavan P, Sarto P, Merlo L, Casara D, Ponchia A, Biasin R, Noventa D, Avogaro A. Metabolic and cardiovascular parameters in type 1 diabetes at extreme altitude. Med Sci Sports Exerc. 2004;36(8):1283–9.
42. Edge CJ, Grieve AP, Gibbons N, O'Sullivan F, Bryson P. Control of blood glucose in a group of diabetic scuba divers. Undersea Hyperb Med. 1997;24(3):201–7.
43. Edge CJ, St Leger Dowse M, Bryson P. Scuba diving with diabetes mellitus – the UK experience 1991–2001. Undersea Hyperb Med. 2005;32(1):27–37.
44. Adolfsson P, Ornhagen H, Jendle J. Accuracy and reliability of continuous glucose monitoring in individuals with type 1 diabetes during recreational diving. Diabetes Technol Ther. 2009;11(8):493–7.

Chapter 16
Preventing Injuries in Extreme Sports Athletes

John Nyland and Yee Han Dave Lee

Contents

Introduction	325
Injury Prevention Must Equal Performance Enhancement	326
Periodization in Training	327
Self- and Skilled Peer Assessments	329
Specific Adaptations to Imposed Demands	329
Example 1: Kayaker	330
Example 2: Downhill Skier	333
Example 3: Climber	333
Summary	334
References	335

Introduction

Designing an injury prevention plan for extreme sports participation is a multifaceted task. Essential to any plan is for the participant to possess or otherwise develop the capacity to objectively assess themselves on a number of key physiological, psychological, and behavioral factors as they relate to unique features of the specific extreme sport that they perform. For example, in addition to having endurant grip strength for rock or mountain climbing [1–5], the climber needs to possess a high strength/mass ratio and have sufficient joint flexibility to enable their whole-body center of mass to be positioned close to the climbing surface as forces are applied (Fig. 16.1). This simple characteristic decreases the resistance moment arms developed through their upper and lower extremities, thereby reducing neuromuscular activation demands. Having a sufficient power/weight ratio is similarly important in mountain biking [6]. In addition

J. Nyland, DPT, SCS, EdD, ATC, CSCS, FACSM (✉) • Y.H.D. Lee, M.D.
Division of Sports Medicine, Department of Orthopaedic Surgery, University of Louisville,
550 South Jackson St., First Floor ACB, Louisville, KY 40202, USA
e-mail: john.nyland@louisville.edu

Fig. 16.1 Lateral plank with hip abduction, front plank, "C"-roll progression to develop endurant upper and lower extremity strength integrating the trunk and core regions

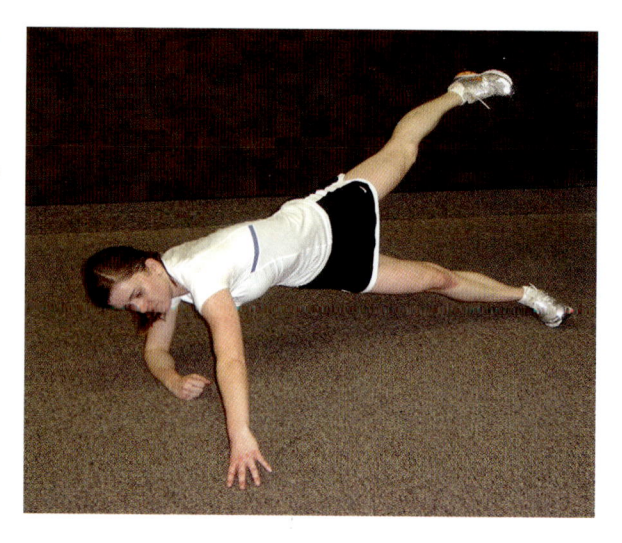

to evaluating their inherent physical characteristics (including the influence of current and past medical or injury histories), the extreme sports athlete needs to be able to honestly appraise their actual versus perceived skill level and risk-taking tendencies, the influence of central and peripheral fatigue on activity performance and cognitive decision-making capability [7], and have a thorough understanding of the most likely injury risk factors associated with their sport [8]. For example hang gliding, base jumping, and paragliding are associated with a high frequency of back and lower extremity injuries (often resulting in vertebral fracture and/or spinal cord injury) due to improper landing techniques [9–12]. In contrast, whitewater kayaking is more likely to predispose the extreme sports athlete to glenohumeral joint injuries, particularly anterior-inferior labral and rotator cuff injuries, both from chronic and acute injury mechanisms. Downhill skiing on the other hand often results in knee injuries through sudden improper postural alignment when landing on one lower extremity, peripheral and/or central fatigue that compromises lower extremity neuromuscular shock absorption system function, poor decision-making, or any combination of these factors. Because of the influence of anxiety [13–15], fatigue, and other stressors on performance capability, the extreme sports athlete is advised to always underestimate their skill and expertise levels prior to participation. All too often, the spur-of-the-moment "thrill factor" which can occur at anytime during extreme sports participation supersedes sound judgment resulting in serious injury or death [16–18]. The extreme sports athlete is challenged with avoiding the seduction or rapture of the event, never letting it override sound judgment.

Injury Prevention Must Equal Performance Enhancement

In designing an injury prevention plan, the extreme sports athlete should remember that any appropriately designed strategy also represents a performance enhancement plan. Establishing this simple link in the athlete's mind may be the ultimate key to program compliance. As the plan is developed, the extreme sports athlete should be committed to the fact that for any conditioning step that is undertaken, there should be a sound rationale. The extreme sports athlete is advised to have a better understanding of their own intrinsic strengths (S) and weaknesses (W) in addition to the opportunities (O) for improvement available to them and potential threats (T) to safely returning from a sports outing. This type of S-W-O-T analysis as is commonly performed in business is a good idea, particularly if more skilled peers are encouraged to provide their perceptions regarding an extreme sports athlete's capabilities.

What are the physiological requirements of the extreme sport [19]? What factors unique to the selected extreme sport have the greatest influence on physiological energy system (short-term or long-term anaerobic or aerobic) regulation and nutrition or hydration requirements? For the selected extreme sport, where, what, and when are injuries or system failures most likely to occur? For example, forward falling when mountain biking on a steep downhill run may increase in likelihood when decision-making is compromised either due to central fatigue or the thrill associated with excessive speed [20–22]. The ocean kayaker is generally more likely to drown if they decide to swim toward shore after capsizing rather than staying with their boat [23]. For sports with a high fall risk, it is essential that the extreme sports athlete understand the scenarios where falls are most likely to occur, the likely circumstances, biomechanical alignment, and pathomechanics associated with the fall, and how to effectively dissipate the energy associated with the fall into a safe rollout rather than relying on an outstretched arm or leg or failing to tuck the head-neck and upper back [24]. Do the fall risks involve potential high-speed one leg landings, forward or side rolling, or do they involve slow-speed balance loss events? On what surface are they likely to occur? What is the fall prevention strategy? Incorporating fall training, similar to judo and wrestling, into extreme sports training is essential. With purposeful practice, safe falling techniques become more second nature, reflexive, and subconsciously driven [25, 26]. Therefore, the extreme sports athlete will be more likely to automatically perform an appropriate reaction when the potentially injurious situation arises. As with neuromuscular training programs designed to prevent knee injury, the extreme sports athlete needs to eventually direct performance program focus more toward honing neuromuscular responsiveness to sudden, unexpected perturbations during injury mechanism simulations that are safe, yet somewhat similar to potentially injurious events [8].

Periodization in Training

Just as periodized training (preparatory phase, competitive event phase, and transition phase) contributes to improved performance among track-and-field athletes and weight lifters, similar principles can be applied to extreme sports preparation [27]. Early preparatory periods of strength-power development can be gradually and strategically translated into sport-specific functional need capabilities over the course of a year. Although early preparatory periods focus primarily on improving "raw"

Fig. 16.2 Forward walk out using Woggler™ (Elrey Enterprises, Inc., Corydon, IN) and stability ball performing a one arm reach at terminal position. An excellent way to train coordinated upper extremity and trunk-core region endurant strength

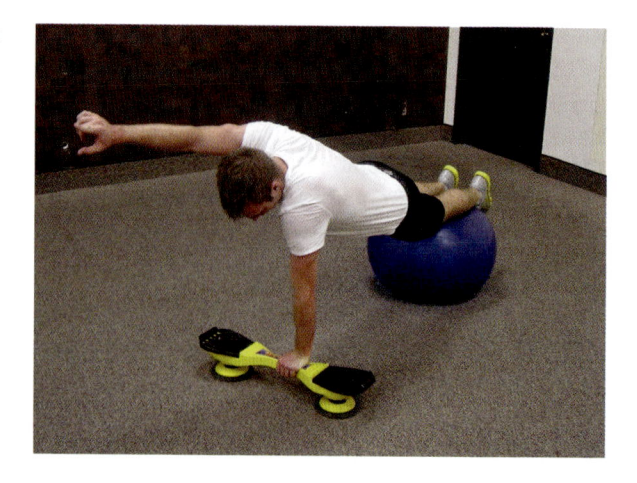

strength, power, endurance, and joint flexibility-tissue extensibility capabilities, during the later part of the preparatory phase, as the extreme sports athlete nears the time for their event, they should focus almost exclusively on refined movements involving coordinated trunk-core and upper-lower extremity function in a manner that simulates extreme sports performance (Fig. 16.2) [28]. During the later part of the preparatory phase, there is a strong overlay of neuromuscular responsiveness training given possible extreme sports scenarios where injury would be most likely to occur. These scenarios are not always limited to intrinsic extreme sports athlete or equipment issues, but also should consider extrinsic environmental factors such as low oxygen levels, limited freshwater supplies, extreme temperature or humidity conditions, wind, conditions that reduce vision (such as glare or fog), and conditions that reduce hearing. Additionally, the surface and surface-foot or surface-hand interface [29, 30] possibilities that are likely to be associated with an extreme sports injury warrant particular attention. Concerns related to this may affect both energy expenditure and safety. Performance training should incorporate possible injury scenarios and appropriate contingency strategies into the plan. The classic phrase "for want of a nail, all was lost," may be analogous to lack of proper contingency planning. Lack of simple preparation such as how to adequately protect the skin on the hand, foot, face, or bony prominences of the pelvic region may have dire consequences [31].

In addition to use of a periodization conditioning model to prepare for their extreme sport, athletes are advised to include adequate, rehydration, and nutrition [32] between work-out sessions to enhance system recovery tissue remodeling, and avoid overtraining. These days do not necessarily have to consist of complete rest but should include active rest working on perceived weak points such as balance [33, 34] via Tai Chi training or more dynamic perturbation response training, stretching, and cognitive mental planning practice through "chalk talks" (if-then scenarios) and other event planning strategies. Addressing perceived (and peer-validated performance) weaknesses enables the extreme sports athlete to both improve their injury prevention readiness and allow for connective tissue healing, remodeling, and strengthening through the application of the specific adaptations to imposed demands principle of training. As with many other sports that are loved by their participants, overtraining is a problem with extreme sports athletes, and insufficient tissue healing recovery periods can compromise future performance and safety. A significant difference with the extreme sports athlete however is that overtraining combined with underpractice, underplanning, poor skill development or inaccurate skill appraisal in combination with the instantaneous thrill of the event, and added stressors such as central fatigue are more likely to result in serious injury or death.

Self- and Skilled Peer Assessments

In addition to physiological system preparation and development of a conditioning training log that provides a record of their preparation, the extreme sports athlete is advised to similarly improve their capacity for honest contemplation or reflection, self-assessment of their risk-taking tendencies, how the "thrill factor" of their extreme sport may override sound decision-making, and overall appraisal of their personal skill level. Just as soccer, basketball, and football athletes tend to overrate their perceived return to play readiness following reconstructive knee surgery, we believe that many extreme sports athletes also tend to overrate their true skill level and underrate their risk-taking behavior. Men are generally more likely to overrate their skill levels than women [35]. Young and novice males are the most likely group to inaccurately assess their skill level and take greater risks. These extreme sports athletes are reminded to learn the old axiom: "There are old cowboys and there are bold cowboys, but there are no old, bold cowboys." Acquiring an objective skill appraisal from a peer or higher skilled extreme sports athlete may be especially important to decrease the injury risk among this group of extreme sports athlete.

Specific Adaptations to Imposed Demands

Specificity of training (perfect preparation prevents poor performance) refers to having a comprehensive understanding of physiological and psychological extreme sports demands, the primary movements involved with differing performance techniques, the equipment-athlete interface, their influence on joints and muscle group recruitment, neuromuscular activation characteristics (concentric, isometric, eccentric), the velocity of joint movements, and potential pathomechanics that are most likely to result in acute-sudden injuries such as a poorly controlled single-leg landing or fall during skiing [36], or more chronic, overuse-type injuries such as the potential influence of distance kayak paddling on rotator cuff muscle health. For both injury prevention and extreme sports performance, the athlete should focus on developing efficient trunk-core neuromuscular integration for force-momentum transfer to the upper and lower extremities and endurant low back strength with neutral lumbopel-

Fig. 16.3 Alternating upper-lower extremity raise from a quadruped position. Cup with tennis or agility balls is placed on low back to encourage smooth movements and neutral lumbopelvic alignment

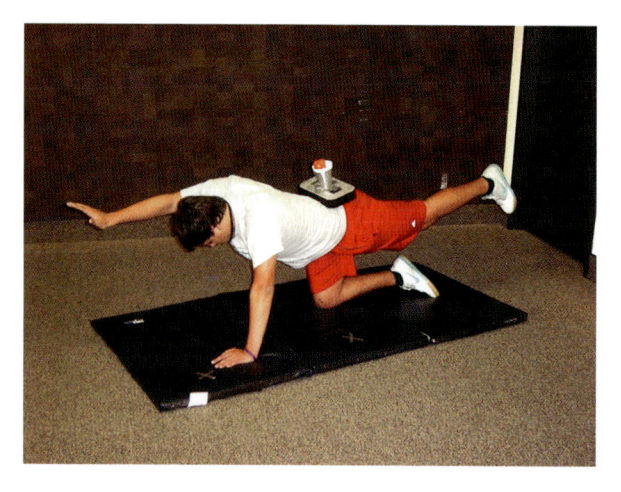

vic alignment (avoiding excessive lordosis or kyphosis) (Fig. 16.3). The extreme sports athlete should determine if they possess inherently loose or hyperelastic joint connective tissues that enable excessive range of motions (particularly at the hands, wrists, elbows, hips, knees, and ankles) [37]. They may need to adjust their training to focus more on improving dynamic joint stability and midrange neuromuscular strength and control while being cognizant of maintaining the athletic position (slight hip, knee, and ankle flexion) during weightbearing to avoid breaking down capsuloligamentous joint "bumpers or excessive joint range restrictors" from repetitious conditioning practices and potentially overused dependence on postures that rely predominantly on noncontractile tissues. Although seemingly paradoxical, the extreme sports athlete with intrinsically hyper-lax joint connective tissues at the knee, for example, may also need to increase musculotendinous extensibility throughout the back and lower extremities, particularly at biarticular muscles (such as the hamstrings, rectus femoris, gastrocnemius, biceps brachii) or any other muscle with pelvic attachments to enable functionally safe positions to be assumed and maintained during extreme sports like rock or mountain climbing, kayaking, and distance running. Although it is essential for the extreme sports athlete to check, verify, familiarize, and practice with the equipment of their sport (including both primary and secondary technique and/or equipment adjustments), greater focus should be placed on the human decision-making side of the equation. As Paul McCartney wrote in the song Hey Jude, "…The movement you need is on your shoulders."

Example 1: Kayaker

Extreme sports whitewater kayaking places intense demands on the glenohumeral joints and rotator cuff muscles as the kayaker executes sudden turns, quick acceleration or deceleration, and rolls [38]. As with anyone who repetitively reaches or

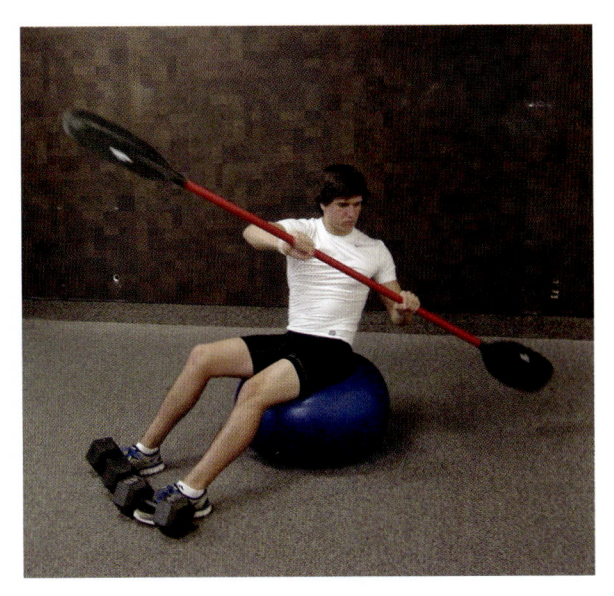

Fig. 16.4 Long-sitting paddling simulation on a stability ball with feet braced by dumbbells

throws overhead, the glenohumeral joint and rotator cuff muscle group health of the extreme sport kayaker is directly influenced by scapulothoracic and lumbopelvic alignment, active mobility, coordination, and endurant strength-power. In addition to the repetitive demands placed on the upper extremities through repetitive paddling over long distances or the sudden bursts of maneuvering, the extreme sports kayaker needs to consider the accumulative effects of portaging, overhead carrying, or dragging their boats, as well as the likelihood of falling on an outstretched upper or lower extremity. Each of these mechanisms may further contribute to glenohumeral joint and rotator cuff muscle group injury. Foundational to any injury prevention-performance enhancement program but particularly important to the shoulder complex (glenohumeral joint and scapulothoracic articulation) is achieving and maintaining complete pain-free active range of motion in positions of function [39]. A position of function refers to evaluating and stretching the muscle or muscle group of interest into the length at which it must function during extreme sports performance, including slight exaggeration during training. Since during paddling and boat maneuvering the shoulder complex functions from a long-sitting position, it is essential to evaluate and train the system from this position (Fig. 16.4). Since portaging the boat likely involves use of the shoulder complex in a standing position, it is likewise essential also to evaluate and train the system from this position (Fig. 16.5a, b). In the first scenario, the kinetic chain functions from a base on the ischial tuberosities of the pelvis [40] with the lower extremities attempting to provide additional stabilization by bracing within the boat. In the second scenario, the kinetic chain functions from one or both lower extremities during weightbearing, transferring forces and momentum proximally through the lumbopelvic region and trunk to the upper extremities. As with one who repetitively performs overhead reaching or throwing, the rotator cuff of the glenohumeral joint is vulnerable to

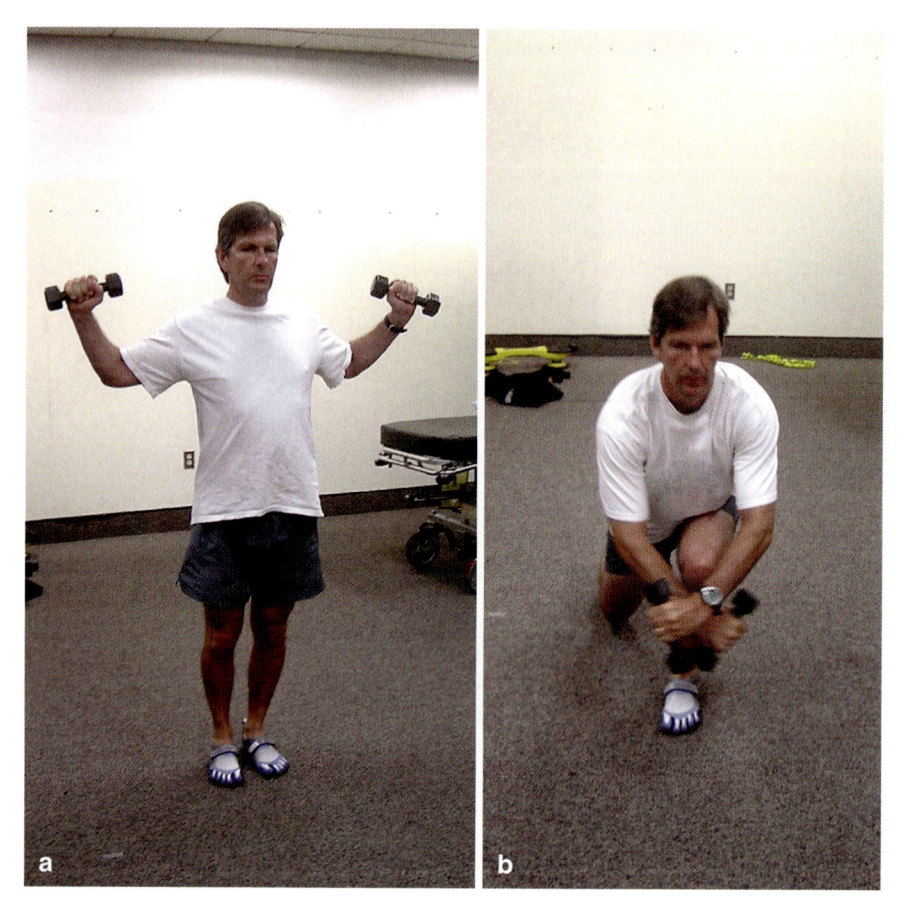

Fig. 16.5 Forward lunge with resisted rotator cuff and scapular retractor muscle strengthening. (**a**) Start position in standing with glenohumeral joints abducted and externally rotated and scapulae retracted. (**b**) Moving into a full lunge position with the glenohumeral joints adducted, internally rotated, and scapulae protracted before returning to the start position. Weighted vest can be added to provide additional training load

impingement through the loss of balanced function anywhere along the entire kinetic chain resulting in superior humeral head migration at the glenoid process of the scapula impinging the rotator cuff muscle group. Additionally, boat maneuvering may also place the whitewater kayaker at risk for glenohumeral joint instability associated with activity-related neuromuscular strength imbalances from repetitive shoulder extension-internal rotation, tending to inhibit and weaken rotator cuff muscle function. This loss of intrinsic rotator cuff muscle function in combination with the range of motion demands of paddling can combine to increase the likelihood of increasing capsulolabral laxity at the glenohumeral joints and dysfunction at the rotator cuff and scapulothoracic muscle groups [39, 41].

A program designed to prevent the occurrence of either rotator cuff injury or acquired glenohumeral joint laxity should begin with an assessment of the extreme sports athlete's own tissue type. Using Beighton Scale test movements [37], the kayaker, for example, can determine if they have characteristics that reflect a genetic predisposition to laxity-related shoulder complex injury. Although maintaining nonimpaired shoulder complex mobility is essential to any neuromuscular strength or power training program, extreme sports athletes with these inherent capsuloligamentous characteristics should focus more on achieving midrange dynamic joint stability during training and avoid repetitively assuming extreme joint range of motion positions that stretch out or grind down the noncontractile bumpers provided by capsuloligamentous and osseous joint structures such as the glenohumeral ligaments, the glenoid labrum, and the glenoid fossa of the scapula.

Example 2: Downhill Skier

During downhill skiing, the kinetic chain of the extreme sports athlete functions during upright weightbearing through the entire body. The knee joints are at particular injury risk. The extensors of the hip, knee, and ankle joints provide primary dynamic shock absorption [42]. Knee injury likelihood increases when it moves from its preferred predominately neuromuscularly balanced sagittal plane (flexion-extension) alignment to poorly controlled, sudden single-leg weightbearing where frontal plane genu valgus (hip adduction, knee abduction) and transverse plane (internal or external rotation) forces place the entire lower extremity in alignments where noncontractile tissues must absorb a greater percentage of the composite knee joint loading forces. While knee injuries predominant during extreme sport downhill skiing, snowboarders are more prone to ankle injuries [43, 44]. Noncontractile capsuloligamentous tissues were not designed to repetitively withstand these demands. This condition is exacerbated if the downhill skier has a genetic predisposition to have hyperelastic knee capsuloligamentous tissues, is female, or if they have otherwise acquired increased knee joint laxity (through previous injury or monthly menstrual cycle), if their technique is poor, if the course is too difficult, poorly groomed, impacted by severe weather, or if they have poor neuromuscular conditioning for the demands of the extreme sports event. Developing increased resistance to both peripheral and central fatigue is essential for the extreme sports downhill skier (Fig. 16.6) both in terms of lower extremity and whole-body neuromuscular control but also in terms of the decision-making associated with knowing when to stop or otherwise reduce activity intensity.

Example 3: Climber

As mentioned earlier, during climbing, the extreme sports athlete must have a high strength/mass ratio, adequate joint flexibility and musculotendinous tissue extensibility to enable positioning of the body's center of mass near the climbing surface.

Fig. 16.6 Single-leg stance on Bosu Ball™ with "ski poles" and with blindfold to deny vision contributions to postural awareness. Athlete attempts to maintain balanced upright stance and safe lower extremity alignment while touching cones with the foot of the non-weightbearing lower extremity upon verbal cue

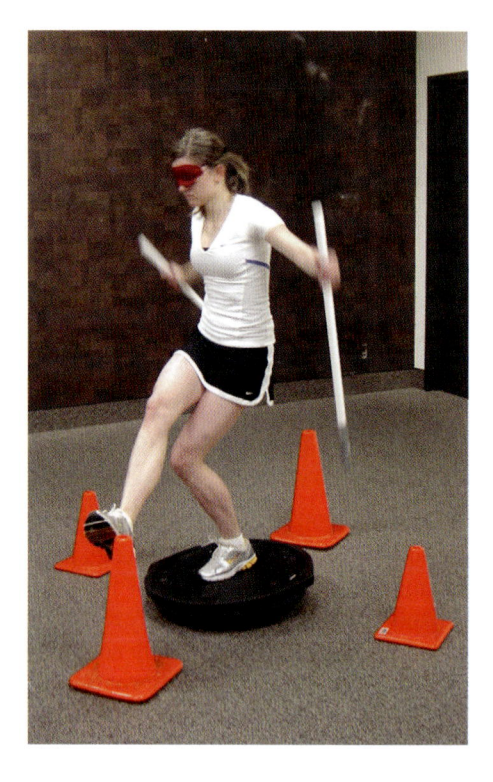

These simple but vital characteristics greatly reduce the work required to maintain position on the climbing surface and to traverse it as needed. For obvious reasons, having sufficient endurant grip strength [1–5], ankle plantar flexor, and subtalar joint invertor-evertor strength are important to both initiate and complete a climbing movement. The climber has to be adept at transferring forces between contralateral and ipsilateral upper and lower extremities through the lumbopelvic and scapulothoracic regions [38, 39]. Innovative devices like the Ground Force 360 device™ (Center of Rotational Exercise, Clearwater, FL) provide adjustable exercise environments that enable trunk-core-lower extremity region coordination and endurant strength-power training using a wide variety of foot placements, trunk-lower extremity flexion angles, resistance modes, and ranges of motion (Fig. 16.7) [45, 46].

Summary

To prevent injury, extreme sports athletes need to consider both the key physiological requirements of their sport and the unique psychobehavioral characteristics of their participation in that sport. Self-assessment of their risk-taking tendencies and the likelihood of letting the thrill of the activity override sound decision-making is essential. Performing a S-W-O-T analysis in addition to self- and skilled-peer appraisals of the extreme sports athlete's skill level is highly recommended.

Fig. 16.7 Long-axis rotational training on the Ground Force 360 device™ (Center of Rotational Exercise, Clearwater, FL), an excellent method for improving lower extremity, trunk, and lumbopelvic region functional integration using concentric, eccentric, and combined eccentric-concentric resistance modes

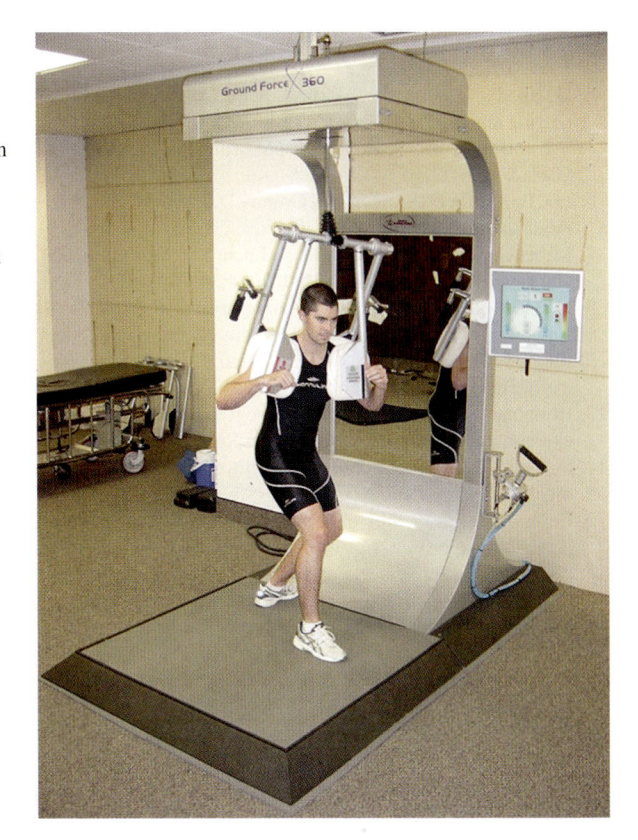

Developing a periodized performance training approach is highly recommended in addition to maintaining a training log as a progressive program attempts to optimize endurant strength-power, joint flexibility, musculotendinous extensibility, strength/mass ratio, and fall risk prevention as needed while also allowing for specific tissue remodeling and psychophysiological system adaptations to imposed exercise demands to take place while avoiding overtraining (active rest, hydration, nutrition). Optimized upper and lower extremity coordination of the trunk and core regions is essential as the athlete learns to respond appropriately to sudden perturbations which mimic potential injury producing pathomechanics by displaying subconsciously mediated dynamic joint stability, neuromuscular postural control, and effective fall prevention response strategies.

References

1. Cutts A, Bollen SR. Grip strength and endurance in rock climbers. Proc Inst Mech Eng H. 1993;207:87–92.
2. Mallo GC, Sless Y, Hurst LC, Wilson K. A2 and A4 flexor pulley biomechanical analysis: comparison among gender and digit. Hand (NY). 2008;3:13–6.

3. Quaine F, Martin L. A biomechanical study of equilibrium in sport rock climbing. Gait Posture. 1999;10:233–9.
4. Quaine F, Vigouroux L, Martin L. Effect of simulated rock climbing finger postures on force sharing among the fingers. Clin Biomech (Bristol, Avon). 2003;18:385–8.
5. Schweizer A, Hudek R. Kinetics of crimp and slope grip in rock climbing. J Appl Biomech. 2011;27:116–21.
6. Lee H, Martin DT, Anson JM, Grundy D, Hahn AG. Physiological characteristics of successful mountain bikers and professional road cyclists. J Sports Sci. 2002;20:1001–8.
7. Millet GY, Lepers R. Alterations of neuromuscular function after prolonged running, cycling, and skiing exercises. Sports Med. 2004;34:105–16.
8. Noe F. Modifications of anticipatory postural adjustments in a rock climbing task: the effect of supporting wall inclination. J Electromyogr Kinesiol. 2006;16:336–41.
9. Filaire E, Alix D, Rouveix M, Le Scanff C. Motivation, stress, anxiety, and cortisol responses in elite paragliders. Percept Mot Skills. 2007;104(3 Pt 2):1271–81.
10. Brummer V, Schneider S, Abel T, Vogt T, Struder HK. Brain cortisol activity is influenced by exercise mode and intensity. Med Sci Sports Exerc. 2011;43:1863–72.
11. Schulze W, Richter J, Schulze B, Esenwein SA, Butner-Janz K. Injury prophylaxis in paragliding. Br J Sports Med. 2002;36:365–9.
12. Castanier C, Le Scanff C, Woodman T. Who takes risks in high-risk sports? A typological personality approach. Res Q Exerc Sport. 2010;81:478–84.
13. Chamarro A, Fernandez-Castro J. The perception of causes of accidents in mountain sports: a study based on the experiences of victims. Accid Anal Prev. 2009;41:197–201.
14. Pimentel GG. Socio-cultural aspects regarding the perception of quality of life amongst people engaging in extreme (high-risk) sports. Rev Salud Publica (Bogota). 2008;10:561–70.
15. Exadaktylos AK, Sclabas G, Eggli S, Schonfeld H, Gygax E, Zimmermann H. Paragliding accidents – the spine is at risk. A study from a Swiss Trauma Centre. Eur J Emerg Med. 2003;10:27–9.
16. Monasterio E, Mei-Dan O. Risk and severity of injury in a population of BASE jumpers. N Z Med J. 2008;121:70–5.
17. Rekand T, Schaanning EE, Varga V, Schattel U, Gronning M. Spinal cord injuries among paragliders in Norway. Spinal Cord. 2008;46:412–6.
18. Soreide K, Ellingsen CL, Knutson V. How dangerous is BASE jumping? An analysis of adverse events in 20,850 jumps from Kjerag Massif, Norway. J Trauma. 2007;62:1113–7.
19. van Somersen KA, Palmer GS. Prediction of 200-m sprint kayaking performance. Can J Appl Physiol. 2003;28:505–17.
20. Chow TK, Kronisch RL. Mechanisms of injury in competitive off-road bicycling. Wilderness Environ Med. 2002;13:27–30.
21. Dodwell ER, Kwon BK, Hughes B, Koo D, Townson A, Aludino A, Simons RK, Fisher CG, Dvorak MF, Noonan VK. Spinal column and spinal cord injuries in mountain bikers: a 13-year review. Am J Sports Med. 2010;38:1647–52.
22. Gaulrapp H, Weber A, Rosemeyer B. Injuries in mountain biking. Knee Surg Sports Traumatol Arthrosc. 2001;9:48–53.
23. Bailey I. An analysis of sea kayaking incidents in New Zealand 1992–2005. Wilderness Environ Med. 2010;21:208–18.
24. Aleman KB, Meyers MC. Mountain biking injuries in children and adolescents. Sports Med. 2010;40:77–90.
25. Coyle D. The talent code. New York: Bantam Books, A Division of Random House; 2009.
26. Powers CM, Fisher B. Mechanisms underlying ACL injury-prevention training: the brain-behavior relationship. J Athl Train. 2010;45:513–5.
27. Garcia-Pallares J, Garcia-Fernandez M, Sanchez-Medina L, Izquierdo M. Performance changes in world-class kayakers following two different training periodization models. Eur J Appl Physiol. 2010;110:99–107.
28. Liow DK, Hopkins WG. Velocity specificity of weight training for kayak sprint performance. Med Sci Sports Exerc. 2003;35:1232–7.

29. Holtzhausen LM, Noakes TD. Elbow, forearm, wrist, and hand injuries among sport rock climbers. Clin J Sport Med. 1996;6:196–203.
30. Killian RB, Nishimoto GS, Page JC. Foot and ankle injuries related to rock climbing. The role of footwear. J Am Podiatr Med Assoc. 1998;88:365–74.
31. Polliack AA, Scheinberg S. A new technology for reducing shear and friction forces on the skin: implications for blister care in the wilderness setting. Wilderness Environ Med. 2006;17: 109–19.
32. Enqvist JK, Mattsson CM, Johansson PH, Brink-Elfegoun T, Bakkman L, Ekblom BT. Energy turnover during 24 hours and 6 days of adventure racing. J Sports Sci. 2010;28:947–55.
33. Chapman DW, Needham KJ, Allison GT, Lay B, Edwards DJ. Effects of experience in a dynamic environment on postural control. Br J Sports Med. 2008;42:16–21.
34. Hrysomallis C. Balance ability and athletic performance. Sports Med. 2011;41:221–32.
35. Demirhan G. Mountaineers' risk perception in outdoor-adventure sports: a study of sex and sports experience. Percept Mot Skills. 2005;100(3 Pt 2):1155–60.
36. Bere T, Florenes TW, Krosshaug T, Koga H, Nordsletten L, Irving C, Muller E, Reid RC, Senner V, Bahr R. Mechanisms of anterior cruciate ligament injury in World Cup alpine skiing: a systematic video analysis of 20 cases. Am J Sports Med. 2011;39(7):1421–9.
37. Beighton P, Solomon L, Soskolne CL. Articular mobility in an African population. Ann Rheum Dis. 1973;32:413–8.
38. McKean MR, Burkett B. The relationship between joint range of motion, muscular strength, and race time for sub-elite flat water kayakers. J Sci Med Sport. 2010;13:537–42.
39. Roseborrough A, Lebec M. Differences in static scapular position between rock climbers and a non-rock climber population. N Am J Sports Phys Ther. 2007;2:44–50.
40. Flodgren G, Hedelin R, Henriksson-Larsen K. Bone mineral density in flatwater sprint kayakers. Calcif Tissue Int. 1999;64:374–9.
41. Hagemann G, Rijke AM, Mars M. Shoulder pathoanatomy in marathon kayakers. Br J Sports Med. 2004;38:413–7.
42. Hame SL, Oakes DA, Markolf KL. Injury to the anterior cruciate ligament during alpine skiing: a biomechanical analysis of tibial torque and knee flexion angle. Am J Sports Med. 2002; 30:537–40.
43. Delorme S, Tavoularis S, Lamontagne M. Kinematics of the ankle joint complex in snowboarding. J Appl Biomech. 2005;21:394–403.
44. Funk JR, Srinivasan SC, Crandall JR. Snowboarder's talus fractures experimentally produced by eversion and dorsiflexion. Am J Sports Med. 2003;31:921–8.
45. Nyland J, Burden R, Krupp R, Caborn DN. Single leg jumping neuromuscular control is improved following whole body, long-axis rotational training. J Electromyogr Kinesiol. 2011;21:348–55.
46. Nyland J, Burden R, Krupp R, Caborn DN. Whole body, long-axis rotational training improves lower extremity neuromuscular control during single leg lateral drop landing and stabilization. Clin Biomech (Bristol, Avon). 2011;26:363–70.

Chapter 17
Rehabilitation of Extreme Sports Injuries

Peter Malliaras, Dylan Morrissey, and Nick Antoniou

Contents

Acute Injuries	340
Traumatic Anterior Shoulder Dislocation	340
A2 Pulley Rupture	344
Anterior Cruciate Ligament Rupture	346
Overuse Injuries	349
Wrist Extensor Tenosynovitis and Intersection Syndrome	349
Ulnar Nerve Neuropathy	350
Extension-Related Low Back Pain	351
Long Head of Biceps Tendinopathy	354
Common Aspects of Rehabilitation	355
Psychological Aspects	355
References	356

Rehabilitation of injury in extreme sports athletes involves consideration of injury etiology, pathology, tissue healing, pain mechanisms, and reconciling athlete-specific functional deficits with sport-specific requirements. In this chapter, rehabilitation of common acute and chronic extreme sports injuries will be outlined with an emphasis on progressive exercise, sport-specific rehabilitation, and return to sport considerations.

Acute soft tissue injury is characterized by pain and healing via a tri-phasic inflammatory response that includes inflammatory, proliferative, and remodeling phases that have been described in detail elsewhere [1]. Inflammation is an

P. Malliaras (✉) • D. Morrissey
Centre for Sports and Exercise, Queen Mary,
University of London, Mile End Hospital, London E1 4DG, UK
e-mail: p.malliaras@qmul.ac.uk

N. Antoniou
Melbourne Hand Therapy,
Elgar Hill Medical Suites, Suite 7, 28 Arnold Street, Box Hill 3128,
Melbourne, VIC, Australia

important prerequisite for healing in acute injury and is supported rather than blunted [2]. Although peaking at 2–3 weeks, the proliferative phase has an early onset at about 1–2 days post injury, and, therefore, active movement and protected loading are often commenced in the first week to maximize this response. Overuse injury may be characterized by inflammatory pathology (e.g., wrist extensor tenosynovitis) or a failed healing response, as in chronic tendinopathy (e.g., long head of biceps tendinopathy). Early reactive and later degenerative phases of tendon overuse injury have recently been described in detail elsewhere [3].

Acute Injuries

Traumatic Anterior Shoulder Dislocation

Traumatic anterior shoulder dislocation is common in many extreme sports, including surfing, snowboarding, skiing, and kayaking. The mechanism of injury usually involves end range glenohumeral abduction and external rotation. In kayaking, it commonly occurs during a high brace or roll, often associated with poor technique or rough water (e.g., white water kayaking) where the hand–shoulder alignment is compromised. An example would be a kayaker descending in white water and bracing with the near side paddle in the wall of water, but instead of the body weight being maintained above the hand position, the water forces the hand up, and hence the arm is forced into abduction/external rotation. Surfers commonly dislocate their shoulders while paddling with wide arms (poor technique) or in rough water [4]. The most common mechanism for shoulder dislocation among skiers and snowboarders is a fall onto the outstretched hand with an element of rotation. This is more common among snowboarders [5, 6], probably because both legs are bound in the same direction, so the lower limb dissipates less rotator force than in skiing (where ACL injury is more common, see section "Anterior Cruciate Ligament Rupture" below) [6]. The common features of the injury are high force and speed, poor technique or trauma, and forced external rotation in abduction.

Men below the age of 25 are most commonly affected [7], and recurrence rates may be above 70 % among athletes [8–10]. The threshold for surgical reconstruction is relatively low in these athletes, especially if there is significant capsular or labral injury, such as a Bankart lesion [11], especially among young and active athletes [12–14].

Treatment Modalities and Rehabilitation

Rehabilitation following traumatic anterior shoulder dislocation has been described in detail elsewhere [15–17] and is outlined in this section (Table 17.1) with reference to extreme sports. The initial 3 weeks following traumatic shoulder dislocation the

Table 17.1 Rehabilitation following traumatic anterior dislocation with reference to kayaking and surfing

	Modalities and exercise	Time commenced
Early rehabilitation	Immobilization in ER	Immediate
	NSAID	
	Scapular isometric setting exercises, addressing excessive rotation in any of the three cardinal planes	
	Wrist, hand, and elbow supported active range of motion to maintain function	
	Remote trunk and lower limb kinetic chain exercise to address individual functional deficits (e.g., leg extension)	
	Cardiovascular maintenance exercise (e.g., stationary cycling) – after third day to ensure no further bleeding is caused	
Optimizing scapulohumeral and kinetic chain integrated function	(A) Gradually restore full range of pain-free movement	3 weeks
	Active and active assisted exercises, manual therapy	
	(B) Scapulohumeral function	
	Rotary glenohumeral joint control in increasing elevation and under load (e.g., isometric progressing to isotonic ER and IR) ensuring minimal displacement of axis of GH rotation	
	Weight-bearing exercises (e.g., four point kneeling, push-up plus)	
	Glenohumeral joint elevation under load	
	Global shoulder function – pushing and pulling (e.g., chest press, rowing)	
	(C) Kinetic chain function	
	Strengthening of the elbow, wrist, and hand	
	Integrated kinetic chain exercises (e.g., PNF D2 pattern, plank exercises)	
	Sports specific kinetic chain	
	Surfing examples	
	Trunk extensor strength (paddling position)	
	Prone trunk extension and glenohumeral ER on fitball (Fig. 17.1a)	
	Kayaking examples	
	Unstable sitting with glenohumeral rotation (Fig. 17.1c)	
Power and sport-specific function	*Surfing examples*	12+ weeks
	Paddling with resistance and increasing speed (Fig. 17.1b)	
	Pop-ups	
	Kayaking examples	
	Swiss ball cable chop (Fig. 17.1d, e)	
	Isometric holds in abduction, in rotation with repeated body drop to mimic injury mechanism	

IR internal rotation, *ER* external rotation, *PNF* peripheral neuromuscular facilitation

focus is on pain management and reduction of inflammation. Current practice is to immobilize the shoulder in external rotation [18, 19] but only for a restricted period of 2–4 weeks to limit secondary stiffness, muscle wasting, and loss of neuromuscular control. Cryotherapy and interferential current are useful if there is pain.

Scapulothoracic exercise emphasizing mid-inner range upward scapular rotation, external rotation, and posterior tilt; wrist, hand, and elbow range of motion; trunk and lower limb kinetic chain exercise; and cardiovascular exercise can commence at an early stage.

From approximately 3 weeks, the goal of rehabilitation is to restore full range of motion and coordinated and sport-specific function of scapular and glenohumeral muscles with the entire kinetic chain (Table 17.1). The shoulder is inherently unstable, so aside from the passive stabilizing structures (e.g., glenohumeral capsule, ligaments, labrum), active stabilizers, primarily the rotator cuff, are essential for joint stability during function [20, 21]. Rehabilitation is tailored to the individual athlete, for example, addressing underlying glenohumeral internal rotation deficit (Table 17.1, A). It is important to reestablish rotator and elevation function under load while maintaining a stable glenohumeral joint and with minimal or no symptoms (Table 17.1, B). The scapula provides a stable base for shoulder function and is a key link in transfer of power from the lower limbs and trunk to the arm during sporting function. Weight-bearing exercises stimulate proprioception and encourage co-contraction of scapular and rotator cuff muscles [22, 23] (Table 17.1, B). Activation of subscapularis is important, but overactivity in pectoralis major should be avoided [17]. Muscular balance in pushing and pulling is important in kayaking [24], and global muscle exercises including rowing and chest and shoulder press should be incorporated, although machine pectoralis major exercises in shoulder abduction and external rotation (e.g., "pec deck") should be avoided.

Sport-specific kinetic chain function exercises are designed to replicate the strength and endurance demands of the trunk, shoulder girdle, and glenohumeral joint during sport (Table 17.1, C and Fig. 17.1). The final rehabilitation phase involves introduction of power (force times velocity) and replicating sport-specific challenges to the glenohumeral joint (Table 17.1 and Fig. 17.1). Speed should not be commenced until single-arm loaded shoulder rotation and elevation strength is a minimum of 80 % of the unaffected side and can be performed with minimal or no pain.

Return to Sport

The most important principle of safe return to extreme sport following shoulder dislocation is reducing the risk of recurrence by modifying sporting activity in the short term. This includes avoiding kayaking and surfing in rough water and avoiding challenging and wet snow slopes that increase the risk of falling. Returning to kayaking is particularly challenging as the lower limbs and trunk are fixed and contribute less to absorption of rotator forces, and abduction and external rotation of the shoulder under load are characteristic of common kayaking maneuvers, including the brace and roll. This highlights the necessity for tailored sport-specific rehabilitation replicating the demands placed upon the shoulder in kayaking prior to full return to sport. Athletes may return to sport with accelerated rehabilitation program by 4 months [25], although this may be longer depending on the intensity of sports

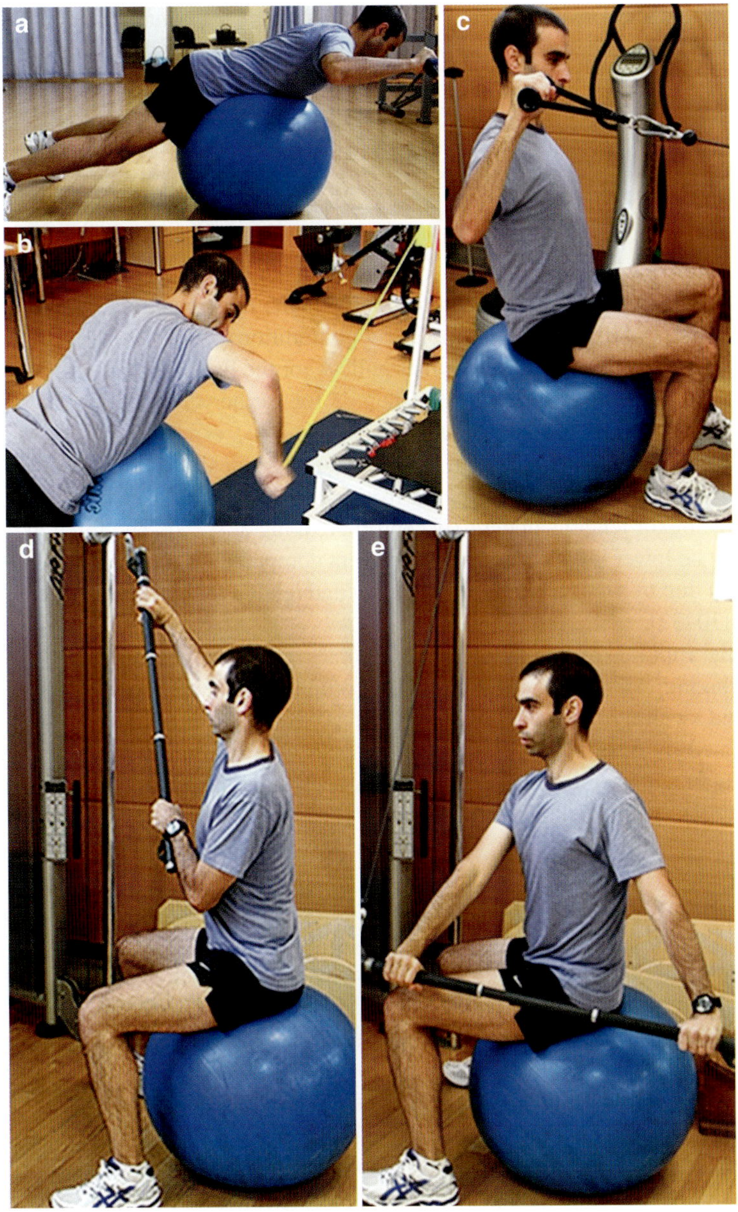

17 Rehabilitation of Extreme Sports Injuries

Fig. 17.1 Sport-specific surfing exercises: (**a**) glenohumeral external rotation in trunk extension on fitball, (**b**) simulated paddling with glenohumeral control with increasing speed. Sport-specific kayaking exercises: (**c**) glenohumeral external rotation during unstable sitting on fitball, (**d**, **e**) cable chop on fitball – right glenohumeral relative abduction and external rotation in initial position (e.g., white water kayaking). Prior to return to sport, any technique faults need to be identified and addressed by developing strength and flexibility or modifying high-risk positions.

A2 Pulley Rupture

Finger injuries are the most common upper limb region injured in climbers, and A2 and A4 finger pulley injuries (climber's finger) the most common climbing injury [26, 27], particularly in sports compared with traditional climbers [27]. Briefly, several retinacular thickenings function as pulleys for the flexor digitorum superficialis and profundus tendons. Please see Chap. 2 for further description of A2 pulley injury (Figs. 2.7, 2.8 and 2.10, pages 22–23).

The most common mechanism involves moving quickly from a crimp to a more open grip, often due the foot slipping from a foot hold [28, 29]. During this movement, the flexor tendons undergo eccentric breaking at speed. The force in the tendon may be lower in this eccentric movement compared to a concentric movement, probably due to friction between the pulley and tendon that increases risk of pulley injury [30–32].

Partial ruptures of the A2 or A4 pulley may not present with clinically obvious bowstringing, whereas this is a feature of complete A2 and A4 pulley rupture [33]. Pain and swelling is usually localized to the base of the proximal phalanx and is aggravated by flexion, especially when resisted. There is often a loss of power in gripping functions, most likely related to reduced moment arm of the flexor tendons, but may also be related to pain inhibition in the acute phase.

Treatment Modalities and Rehabilitation

The treatment of pulley injuries depends on the extent of pathology (assessed accurately with ultrasound or MRI), and this has been fully described by Schoffl et al. [28]. A strain or partial rupture may not require any immobilization, although the fingers are taped for pulley protection. Complete pulley ruptures are immobilized for up to 2 weeks with a hand-based resting splint in a functional position (Fig. 17.2a) that minimizes forces at the A2 pulley by preventing metacarpophalangeal (MCP) flexion. Activities involving MCP joint flexion increase A2 pulley load and should be avoided. In the acute phase, nonsteroidal anti-inflammatory drugs (NSAID) are recommended, although this depends on the extent of swelling and pain. Soft tissue therapy and ultrasound to reduce swelling and encourage healing are indicated.

At between 2 (partial rupture) and 2–4 weeks (complete rupture), functional therapy including range of motion exercise is commenced, followed by progressive loading of the flexor tendons. An MCP joint block ring splint (Fig. 17.2b) can be used for ongoing protection of the A2 pulley. Active (unloaded) exercise is progressively replaced with resistance (loaded) exercise (Fig. 17.2c). Gradual increase of

17 Rehabilitation of Extreme Sports Injuries

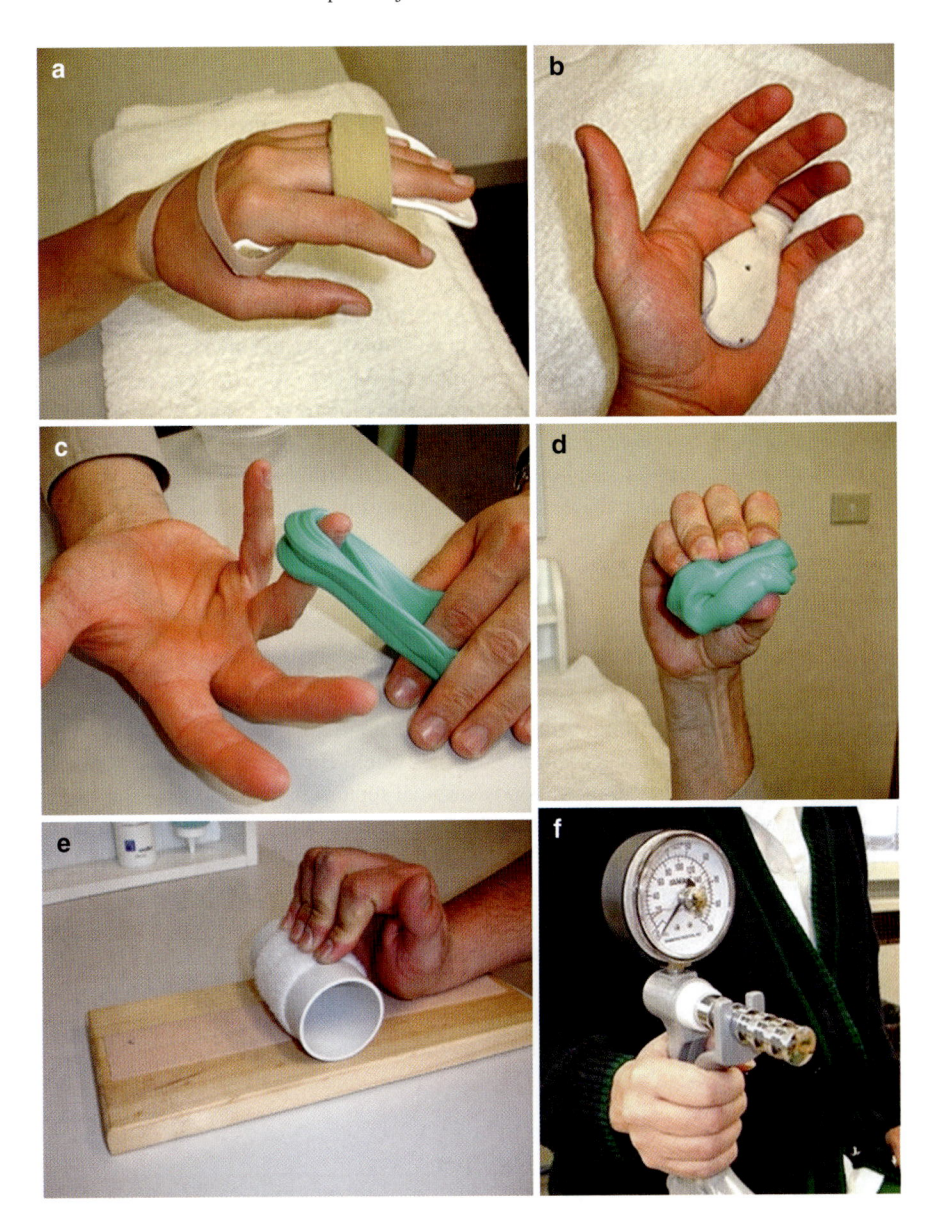

Fig. 17.2 Rehabilitation of A2 pulley injuries: (**a**) immobilization in resting splint, (**b**) MCP joint block ring splint, (**c**) resisted isolated fourth MCP flexion, (**d**) simulated crimp grip with putty resistance, (**e**) resisted MCP and PIP flexion with DIP extension, (**f**) grip strength measurement with handheld dynamometer

forces acting at the A2 pulley during the rehabilitation phase is paramount to facilitate pseudo-pulley formation. Consequently, loaded MCP joint flexed positions and "crimp" positions are introduced in the later stages of recovery (Fig. 17.2d, e). As exercises are progressed, finger pulleys can be protected during rehabilitation with circular tape or a thermoplastic ring. Schweizer [34] demonstrated a biomechanical advantage in reducing the extent of flexor tendon bowstringing by taping the distal aspect of the proximal phalanx instead of over the A2 pulley.

Finger pulley injuries often occur at the end of a climb [35] and are more common in sports climbers who perform more challenging ballistic movements; this highlights the importance of adequate muscular strength rehabilitation in both the upper and lower limb kinetic chains. General grip strength can be measured with dynamometer (Fig. 17.2f). Using the first rung position of the Jamar dynamometer will enable measurement of grip in an intrinsic (lumbricals and interossei) dominant position of MCP flexion – the adopted posture for the "crimp" climbing position. In this way, response to treatment can be objectively monitored as can readiness for a return to climbing activities.

Multiple pulley rupture and bowstringing are indications for surgical repair [28, 36]. Postoperative treatment involves immobilization for 2–4 weeks (ring splint) followed by a similar functional therapy and rehabilitation program to a complete pulley rupture from 4 weeks.

Return to Sport

Once grip strength is a minimum of 80 % of the unaffected side, climbing activity can commence. This is usually a minimum of 4 weeks for a partial rupture, 6 weeks for complete rupture, and 4 months postsurgical repair [28]. Crimp grip should be avoided for a further 6–8 weeks following complete A2 pulley ruptures and surgical repair [36], given the much larger A2 pulley forces with this grip [37]. Strength criteria and careful symptom monitoring as progressing too quickly are common and are often associated with overconfidence of the climber in attempting difficult climbs too early. Circular tape as described above is commonly used by climbers, but cadaver evidence suggests it may not increase the maximum load at failure that the pulley can sustain [38], whereas other studies have found that taping is minimally effective in absorbing flexor tendon bowstringing forces [34].

Anterior Cruciate Ligament Rupture

Anterior cruciate ligament rupture is common in skiing and less so in snowboarding [5]. The mechanism of injury often involves external knee rotation and valgus (lateral to medial) loading while turning and catching the inside edge of the downhill ski or an unbalanced landing from a jump in higher level skiers [39]. Regardless of the level of the athlete, they can expect to return to sport after management, usually involving surgical repair (ACLr) followed by prolonged rehabilitation for higher level skiers. Nonsurgical management may be suitable for skiers at all levels [40, 41], and conservative management success is predicted by a lack of concomitant ligament or meniscal injury, reasonable function (e.g., performance on hopping tests), and minimal or no giving way [42]. There is an emphasis on criteria-based progression through a structured rehabilitation program with both nonsurgical and surgical management, and this facilitates a timely and safe return to sport.

Treatment Modalities and Rehabilitation

Generic post-ACLr rehabilitation has been described in detail elsewhere [43, 44]. In this section, a suitable rehabilitation program for skiers and snowboarders will be outlined with reference to sport-specific exercises and progression criteria. The early rehabilitation phase (0–4 weeks) focuses on managing surgical pain and swelling with ice, compression, elevation, relative immobilization, soft tissue therapy and muscle recruitment strategies, and critically, reestablishing pre-injury level of knee extension and flexion. Core and trunk strength exercise and rehabilitation of specific kinetic chain deficits can commence. Bracing post ACLr is a common practice; however, a recent review concluded that it may not influence re-injury rate and function at long-term follow-up [45]. Decisions regarding duration of brace use are based on athlete confidence, adequacy of muscle control during activities of daily living, and the stability of secondary knee restraints.

In the second phase (5–16 weeks), the focus is on muscle strength, hypertrophy, and power, as well as neuromuscular control flexibility. The emphasis is on single-leg exercise to address lower limb kinetic chain asymmetry and should focus on quadriceps and hamstring strength and hypertrophy as well as strength in the distal (calf) and proximal (gluteal, hip flexors) kinetic chain. There is an ongoing debate about the relative efficacy of closed- versus open-chain exercises. Tagesson et al. [46] built on the work of Morrissey et al. [47] showing no difference in laxity, pain, hamstring strength, jump performance, and functional outcome (Knee Injury and Osteoarthritis Outcome Score) between open- and closed-chain rehabilitation. The only difference was greater quadriceps strength in the open-chain group, suggesting that open-chain exercise should be considered in ACLr rehabilitation programs. It is therefore an athlete-specific decision regarding how to balance open- and closed-chain exercise depending on sport-specific requirements. Depending on the graft, there needs to be a focus on restoring quadriceps strength (patellar tendon graft) or hamstring strength (hamstring graft) [48].

Afferent proprioceptive input moderates neuromuscular control in both feedforward and feedback mechanisms to allow efficient and coordinated athletic function. In the second rehabilitation phase, this involves balance, nonimpact ski-specific exercises (e.g., Fig. 17.3), and unexpected support surface perturbation exercises. In the third phase of rehabilitation (17–22 weeks), the emphasis is on advanced neuromuscular exercise involving impact. This includes agility, plyometric, running, and sport-specific training. The addition of neuromuscular training to conventional resistance training may improve pain and functional scores [49, 50]. There is an emphasis on reproducing sport-specific lateral knee movements under increasingly challenging conditions.

Fig. 17.3 Ski-specific neuromuscular rehabilitation on a "fitter"

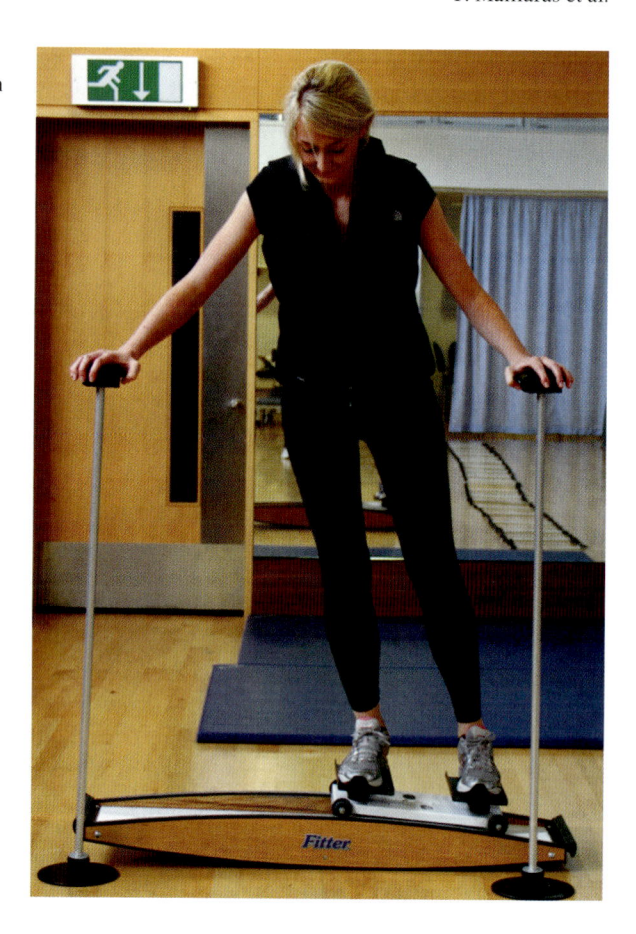

Return to Sport

The fourth and final phase of ACLr rehabilitation involves return to play. Important return to sport criteria include a lack of functional instability or giving way, strength, power, functional outcome score within 10 % of opposite side, and successful completion of agility, plyometric (e.g., crossover triple hop), and sport-specific drills and training [44, 51]. Skiers who wore a functional knee brace when returning to sport were found to have a 2.74 times lower risk of knee injury [52]. Adequate warm-up is the keystone of ACL prevention and should involve a neuromuscular warm-up addressing trunk and lower limb control and coordination in functional tasks [53]. Several warm-up programs (e.g., "the PEP," "the 11+") including balance, strength, plyometric, and agility exercises have been shown to reduce the risk of first-time ACL injury [54–56]. Factors that increase the propensity for the knee to move into a valgus pattern in single-leg squatting and landing should be addressed, particularly in females among whom this pattern is recognized [57].

Fig. 17.4 Intersection syndrome symptoms are localized to the crossover between the first and second extensor compartment tendons, 4–6 cm proximal to Lister's tubercle

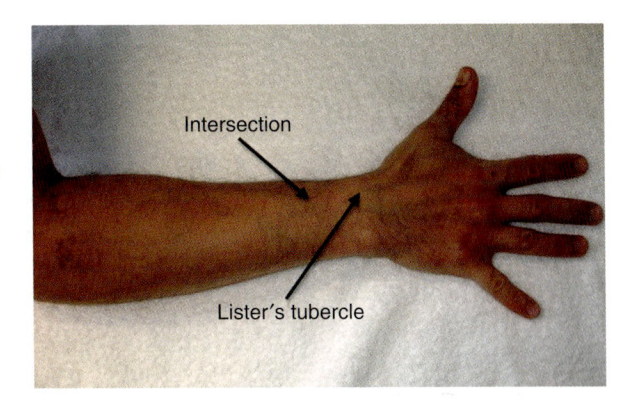

Overuse Injuries

Wrist Extensor Tenosynovitis and Intersection Syndrome

Tenosynovitis of the distal extensor tendons of the wrist is common in kayakers/canoeists as well as other sports (rowing, racquet sports). In long distance kayaking, the incidence of overuse injuries to the wrist is between 21 and 50 % [58, 59]. Intersection syndrome is commonly reported in kayakers and alpine skiers and occurs where the tendons of the first extensor compartment cross over the tendons of the second extensor compartment 4–5 cm proximal to Lister's tubercle (Fig. 17.4). Palmer et al. [60] reported a 12 % prevalence of intersection syndrome among alpine skiers. The etiology of intersection syndrome may involve friction between the first and second compartment extensors [61] and hypertrophy of the APL and EPB tendons [62].

The mechanism of both injuries is repetitive excessive wrist extension, for example, during the pull phase in kayaking. Among kayakers, injury is more common in longer stages (>38 km), rougher water, or kayaking on multiple consecutive days, and greater training prior to events is preventative [59]. Weakness and inefficient use of the proximal upper limb kinetic chain and trunk may also increase wrist overuse and lead to injury. The underlying pathology is inflammatory, with swelling and crepitus often evident in the distal and radial aspect of the dorsal forearm.

Treatment Modalities and Rehabilitation

The key element of management is reducing repetitive loads and correcting technique faults predisposing to injury. This includes addressing functional deficits in the entire upper limb kinetic chain and trunk, for example, reduced trunk strength that may increase wrist extension when the kayaker is pulling. Complete rest from kayaking and skiing is often required initially, although partial rest may be sufficient in less severe cases. If symptoms do not settle, immobilization in a static wrist splint (prefabricated thermoplastic wrist splint in 15° extension) for 2 weeks is indicated [63]. Conservative treatment includes ice, distal to proximal massage (fingers to elbow), stretching the wrist extensors, crepe bandage to encourage reduction in swelling worn at night or times of activity [64]. Wrist extensor stretching should not be performed if painful as this may indicate further compression and injury to the tendon sheath [3]. Ultrasound-guided cortisone injection into the extensor tendon common sheath is indicated if symptoms do not settle within 1–2 weeks following immobilization/load modification [65]. There are currently no outcome studies comparing the influence of platelet-rich plasma in tenosynovitis; however, this is an area which may benefit from this new modality.

Return to Sport

The risk of tenosynovitis may increase during multiple day events [59]; therefore, it is important when returning to kayaking to allow sufficient rest time between endurance training sessions (48–72 h initially). Modification of equipment may help to relieve symptoms, such as changing the diameter of ski poles among skiers [66] that may improve the length-tension relationship of the wrist extensors.

Ulnar Nerve Neuropathy

Compression of the ulnar nerve in Guyon's canal (cyclists palsy) is common in long distance cycling, including mountain biking [67]. Guyon's canal is formed by the pisiform medially and hook of hamate laterally. The motor branch of the ulnar nerve to the hypothenar muscles is given off before Guyon's canal, and compression at this site leads to weakness of all ulnar-innervated hand muscles (hypothenar, interossei, third and fourth lumbricals) and skin sensation. Compression at Guyon's canal or distally is associated with only sensory loss and/or intrinsic muscle weakness (interossei, third and fourth lumbricals and adductor pollicis), depending on whether the superficial sensory or deep motor branches are compressed [68]. Differential diagnosis includes stress fracture of the hook of hamate.

Patterson et al. [69] assessed ulnar nerve sensory function among 18 mountain bike and 32 road bike riders before and after a 600-km ride. Thirty-nine percent had signs of ulnar nerve motor deficit and 33 % and had sensory loss; mountain bikers were more likely to report sensory loss than road bikers. Risk factors include long distance cycling, asymmetrical weight bearing on the handlebars, poor core stability, poor seat or handle bar position encouraging wrist hyperextension, and inadequate handlebar and glove padding [69–71].

Management

The most important aspect of management is to minimize compression of the ulnar nerve during cycling. This can often be achieved by adjusting the mountain bike riders grip and hand position on the handlebars, padded handlebars, and gloves and frequently changing hand position while mountain biking [72]. Padded gloves have been shown to reduce hypothenar pressure in cycling by between 10 and 28 % [73]. If symptoms persist, it is important to progressively reduce the volume of mountain bike riding until there is adequate resolution of symptoms. This is particularly important if the mountain bike rider is experiencing pain or weakness with daily activities such as gripping.

Management should include assessment and treatment of cervical and upper limb neurodynamic dysfunction, seeking evidence of subtle "double crush" nerve compromise. Smith et al. [74] found that cyclists with ulnar nerve compression symptoms at the wrist were more likely to have positive thoracic outlet provocative tests and concurrent neck and shoulder pain compared with matched controls. Neurodynamic dysfunction is initially addressed by working on neural interfaces such as mobilization of the shoulder and first rib, while trying to reduce nerve irritation by avoiding end of range positions, followed by more direct nerve gliding techniques (e.g., upside down goggles stretch) in progressively more provocative positions [75]. Surgical release of Guyon's canal is uncommon but indicated in recalcitrant cases.

Extension-Related Low Back Pain

Low back pain (LBP) is common among sailors, surfers, and windsurfers, often related to prolonged maintenance of end range postures or repetitive movement. This often happens in "pumping" the sails to accelerate the boat and "hiking," which involves positioning (usually in lumbar extension) the body to prevent the boat leaning away from the wind. During surfing, hyperextension of the lumbar spine occurs during paddling out into the surf. Twelve percent of injuries in big boat sailing [76] and 22 % in windsurfing [77] may involve the lumbar spine. Extension-related LBP is also common in cross-country skiing and has been linked with increased thoracic kyphosis and lumbar lordosis [78]. The most common underlying pathology is facetal and disc spondylosis in older and pars defects in younger sailors and windsurfers, probably related to repetitive extension movement [79, 80]. Symptoms can be localized unilateral or bilateral low back pain aggravated by prolonged extension postures and standing.

Treatment Modalities and Rehabilitation

The principles of treating extension-related LBP in sailors and windsurfers are outlined in Table 17.2. Initial management involves avoidance of aggravating activities or postures, while rehabilitating motor patterns demonstrate segmental

Table 17.2 Rehabilitation for extension-related LBP among sailors and windsurfers

	Exercises	Time commenced
Early rehabilitation	Load management (e.g., sailing, excessive standing/walking)	Immediate
	Ice, NSAID	
	Remote upper and lower limb kinetic chain exercises to address individual deficits (e.g., calf raises)	
	Cardiovascular maintenance exercise (e.g., upper limb ergometer)	
	Dissociation of extension from distal (hip) and proximal (shoulders) kinetic chain	
Optimising lumbopelvic muscle function	Lumbopelvic muscle-tendon compliance and strength	2 weeks
	Hip flexor flexibility (tensor fascia lata, rectus femoris, sartorius) (e.g., split squats into end of range)	
	Abdominals (e.g., crunches)	
	Gluteals (e.g., bridging)	
	Hip flexor strength (e.g., standing hip flexion with pulleys)	
	Avoid back extension exercise into end of range in favour of exercises loading the back extensors isometrically (e.g., McGill birddog exercise, ref)	
	Local and global muscle activation	
	Kinetic chain function	
	Integrated kinetic chain exercises (e.g., squats)	
	Sports specific kinetic chain	
	Front plank progressions for abdominals, hip flexors Fig. 17.5	
Sport-specific exercise and graded return to sport	Simulated 'pumping' – pulleys	6+ weeks
	Increasing volume and speed	
	Graded return to windsurfing and sailing	

NSAID non-steroidal anti-inflammatory drugs

or region-specific extension /rotation overstrain and sport-specific strength. This period may be between 7 days and 3 months, depending on the severity of symptoms, underlying pathology, athlete engagement, and motor learning skill. For example, a pars defect may require 2–3 months rest from end of range extension postures (e.g., pumping, hiking) [81–83]. NSAID, ice, and kinetic chain exercises remote from the painful site are indicated in this phase. Efficient transfer of load from the lower limbs to the spine is critical in windsurfing and sailing, for example, in hiking. Quadriceps strength is an important determinant of average hiking moment produced by sailors, and this in turn predicts race scores among Laser sailors [84].

The second phase focuses on optimizing lumbopelvic function while maintaining movement patterns that reduce end range extension stress on previously painful structures. Improving the flexibility of pelvic muscles that maintain lumbar lordosis [85–87], including the tensor fascia lata (Table 17.2), may reduce lumbar extension moment and load on damaged spinal structures. Strong abdominal and hip flexor muscles are necessary to control lumbar spine posture in pumping [88]. They can be strengthened with progressive front plank exercises (Fig. 17.5). Compliant hip flexors allow greater combined hip and lumbar extension that may relatively off-load the spine. End range functional eccentric exercise for the hip flexors such as lunging can increase hip flexor musculotendinous compliance [89, 90]. Lumbar extensor muscle weakness is associated with low back pain in sports involving repetitive extension [91] and should be addressed with isometric loading exercises that avoid end of range. Recruitment of deep stabilizing muscles [92] has been shown to improve function and pain in spondylosis [93] but need to be progressed to include challenge to both local and global muscles systems [94]. A functional core strengthening exercises may be best suited to younger athletes with lumbar hypermobility [95, 96].

The final phase of rehabilitation involves graded return to sport-specific functional and provocative activities (Table 17.2). This can commence when extension-related symptoms settle, abdominal strength has improved (e.g., timed prone bridge), and there has been sufficient time for healing of any underlying pars defect. Successful return to sport is dependent on restoration of function equivalent to the demands of the level of sailing/windsurfing that the injured athlete is returning to. Athletes can start by introducing simulated pumping, for example, using Thera-Band or pulleys, and progressively increasing the volume and load as symptoms permit.

Return to Sport and Prevention

Harnesses that include rigid padding, support from the shoulder to buttock, and leg strap support [97] may allow easier maintenance of neutral spine postured and reduce low back pain risk during hiking. For first onset overuse back pain, technique in

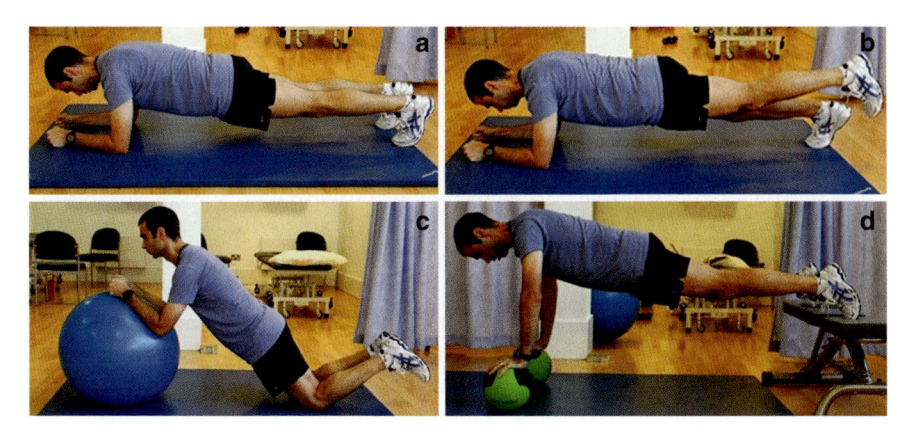

Fig. 17.5 Front plank progressions: (**a**) double leg, (**b**) single leg, (**c**) on knees with fitball, (**d**) on bench with medicine balls

repetitive (e.g., pulley ropes) and sustained tasks (e.g., grinding) needs to be examined and corrected [77]. Pars injuries are most likely seen in adolescent athletes highlighting the need to allow sufficient recovery from sailing/windsurfing in this demographic group.

Long Head of Biceps Tendinopathy

Long head of biceps (LHB) tendinopathy is common among sailors, with the shoulder and upper arm estimated to account for 15 % of injuries in big boat sailing, 38 % of which involve the LHB [76]. Windsurfers are also commonly affected. The mechanism is repetitive loading of the shoulder in flexion, as in pumping. The long head of biceps is thought to be an important anterior glenohumeral stabilizer [98, 99], and this role may be more important in sailors/windsurfers with rotator cuff weakness or loss of integrity [100]. The biceps show increased activity [101], and the LHB tendon is thickened among people with a chronic rotator cuff tear [102]. In younger athletes, there may be associated glenohumeral instability or a SLAP lesion [22].

Predisposing factors include weakness and poor endurance of scapular, trunk, and lower limb muscles, poor technique (e.g., increased glenohumeral internal rotation in sailing postures), and sharp increases in training volume or intensity. The scapula is an important kinetic chain link between the trunk and upper limb, providing a stable base for glenohumeral function. Scapular dyskinesis or movement faults have been linked with biceps tendon problems [23, 103]. Clinical features are tenderness and occasionally palpable thickening or subluxation of the LHB tendon in the biceps groove, pain with flexion, horizontal flexion, and end range internal rotation in shoulder elevation, as well as positive biceps provocation tests (e.g., Speed's, Yergason's test) [104–106]. Ultrasound and MRI imaging can confirm biceps tendon and sheath pathology and associated tissue pathology that may also need to be considered (i.e., rotator cuff tendons, subacromial bursa) [107].

Management

Conservative management of LHB tendinopathy can be divided into three phases. Phase one focuses on rest from provocative sailing postures for 2–8 weeks and restoring full pain-free range of motion in flexion. NSAIDs are useful for pain at rest and image-guided corticosteroid injection indicated in recalcitrant cases [106]. Isometric load in nonprovocative midrange positions may be helpful to maintain tendon tensile load without provoking symptoms [3]. Active-assisted and active-movement exercises are used to restore mobility. Soft tissue restriction (e.g., posterior capsule and pectoralis minor in particular) that may contribute to poor scapular mechanics and associated impingement [104] can be addressed with muscle energy techniques, soft tissue release, stretching, and trigger point therapy. Therapeutic ultrasound may have limited value; a systematic review showed no evidence for the use of ultrasound in managing shoulder pain [108].

The second phase involves restoring scapulothoracic biomechanics and glenohumeral muscle strength, endurance, and power. Rotator cuff muscle weakness should be addressed, especially in older athletes that may be more likely to have degenerative change or loss of integrity [109]. Optimizing rotator cuff strength to control an anteriorly displacing axis of rotation will potentially reduce the stabilizing demand on the LHB tendon. Serratus anterior and trapezius (especially lower fibers) need to be considered as they have an important role in scapular lateral rotation in flexion [23], ensuring optimal scapulohumeral function for repetitive flexion elevation activities in windsurfing and sailing. Inefficiency in these muscles can lead to inefficient load transfer and overload of the LHB tendon. Examples of exercises that demonstrate high EMG for serratus anterior and lower trapezius are detailed elsewhere [110–112]. Proprioceptive and sensorimotor function can be developed among younger athletes who may have an element of instability by using an unstable base proximally or distally (e.g., Fig. 17.5c).

The third phase involves developing kinetic chain strength and power and graded return to sport. Power generated in the lower limbs needs to be transferred effectively to the upper limbs via the trunk [113]. Sport-specific rehabilitation can commence utilizing movement patterns in hiking, pumping, and other aspects of windsurfing and sailing and progressively increasing the volume and intensity. Technique faults such as excessive glenohumeral internal rotation during flexion should be addressed prior to sailing and windsurfing activity.

Common Aspects of Rehabilitation

Rehabilitation of many of the extreme sports injuries discussed in this chapter involves some common principles. Returning to kayaking after glenohumeral joint dislocation, skiing after ACL rupture, and sailing after extension-related back pain are dependent upon functional stability or optimal neuromotor system function [114]. Aside from muscular strength, endurance, and power, it is essential that the proprioceptive component of rehabilitation is integrated and progressed from an early stage. This can involve co-contraction exercises, rhythmic stabilization, balance training, core stability, and plyometric exercise. Proprioceptive challenge is increased by performing exercises with reduced base of support (e.g., Fig. 17.1c) and introducing destabilizing equipment (e.g., physioball, duradisc, Bosu ball, trampette, e.g., Fig. 17.5c, d). Rehabilitation should also include repetition of sport-specific exercises that reproduce the functional positions, strength, and power demands of their sport (e.g., Fig. 17.2d). This will enable specific motor learning for the athletes sporting demands.

Psychological Aspects

Injury rehabilitation will be a stressful period for an athlete who is eager to return to sporting activity. Overtly recognizing this fact with the athlete is a useful tactic. It is critically important for the clinician and athlete to work together in setting goals that are challenging yet realistic and specific to functional sporting demands. Involving the athlete and other stakeholders such as the coach enables the athlete to have a greater sense of control and may also increase reinforcement [115]. It may be important to involve coaching staff with elite athletes in order to reach agreement about realistic timeframes for return to activity, although this needs to be balanced with the primary duty of care to the athlete. Some extreme sports athletes may be obsessive about their sporting activities and display overadherence to rehabilitation or return to sport prior to achieving the necessary goals. Empowering athletes with knowledge of their deficits, the rehabilitation process, and necessary milestones prior to safe return to sport is likely to improve appropriate adherence to rehabilitation [116]. Use of a rehabilitation diary may help to focus the athlete on their goals and improve adherence [117]. Another technique that may be useful is imagery, or recreating the experience of sporting activity or competition [118], which helps athletes make the link between rehabilitation, of movement patterns for example, and later incorporation into sporting technique.

Given the risk factors associated with extreme and adventure sports, athletes must ensure that they are fully rehabilitated before returning to their sport. This requires specific sports rehabilitation programs.

References

1. Peterson L, Renström P, Grana WA. Sports injuries: their prevention and treatment. London: Martin Dunitz; 2001.
2. Hardy MA. The biology of scar formation. Phys Ther. 1989;69:1014–24.
3. Cook J, Purdam CR. Is tendon pathology a continuum? A pathology model to explain the clinical presentation of load-induced tendinopathy. Br J Sports Med. 2009;43:409–16.
4. Nathanson A, Bird S, Dao L, Tam-Sing K. Competitive surfing injuries. Am J Sports Med. 2007;35:113–7.
5. Sutherland A, Holmes J, Myers S. Differing injury patterns in snowboarding and alpine skiing. Injury. 1996;27:423–5.
6. Ogawa H, Sumi H, Sumi Y, Shimizu K. Glenohumeral dislocations in snowboarding and skiing. Injury. 2011;42(11):1241–7.
7. Hovelius L. The natural history of primary anterior dislocation of the shoulder in the young. J Orthop Sci. 1999;4:307–17.
8. Simonet WT, Cofield RH. Prognosis in anterior shoulder dislocation. Am J Sports Med. 1984;12:19–24.
9. Lewis A, Kitamura T, Bayley J. (ii) The classification of shoulder instability: new light through old windows! Curr Orthop. 2004;18:97–108.
10. Robinson CM, Howes J, Murdoch H, Will E, Graham C. Functional outcome and risk of recurrent instability after primary traumatic anterior shoulder dislocation in young patients. J Bone Joint Surg Am. 2006;88:2326–36.
11. Handoll H, Al-Maiyah M. Surgical versus non-surgical treatment for acute anterior shoulder dislocation. Cochrane Database Syst Rev. 2004;(1):CD004325. DOI: 10.1002/14651858.
12. Jakobsen BW, Johannsen HV, Suder P, Sojbjerg JO. Primary repair versus conservative treatment of first-time traumatic anterior dislocation of the shoulder: a randomized study with 10-year follow-up. Arthroscopy. 2007;23:118–23.
13. Kirkley A, Griffin S, Richards C, Miniaci A, Mohtadi N. Prospective randomized clinical trial comparing the effectiveness of immediate arthroscopic stabilization versus immobilization and rehabilitation in first traumatic anterior dislocations of the shoulder. Arthroscopy. 1999;15:507–14.

14. Yanmis I, Tunay S, Komurcu M, Yildiz C. Outcomes of acute arthroscopic repair and conservative treatment following first traumatic dislocation of the shoulder joint in young patients. Ann Acad Med Singapore. 2003;32:824–7.
15. Hayes K, Callanan M, Walton J, Paxinos A, Murrell G. Shoulder instability: management and rehabilitation. J Orthop Sports Phys Ther. 2002;32:497–509.
16. Burkhead Jr W, Rockwood Jr C. Treatment of instability of the shoulder with an exercise program. J Bone Joint Surg Am. 1992;74:890–6.
17. Jaggi A, Lambert S. Rehabilitation for shoulder instability. Br J Sports Med. 2010;44:333–40.
18. Itoi E, Hatakeyama Y, Sato T, et al. Immobilization in external rotation after shoulder dislocation reduces the risk of recurrence. J Bone Joint Surg Am. 2007;89:2124–31.
19. Miller BS, Sonnabend DH, Hatrick C, et al. Should acute anterior shoulder dislocations of the shoulder be immobilised in external rotation? A cadaveric study. J Shoulder Elbow Surg. 2004;13:589–92.
20. Magarey ME, Jones MA. Dynamic evaluation and early management of altered motor control around the shoulder complex. Man Ther. 2003;8:195–206.
21. Labriola JE, Lee TQ, Debski RE, McMahon PJ. Stability and instability of the glenohumeral joint: the role of shoulder muscles. J Shoulder Elbow Surg. 2005;14:S32–8.
22. Wilk KE, Meister K, Andrews JR. Current concepts in the rehabilitation of the overhead throwing athlete. Am J Sports Med. 2002;30:136.
23. Kibler B. Current concepts: scapular dyskinesis. Br J Sports Med. 2010;44:300–5.
24. McKean MR, Burkett B. The relationship between joint range of motion, muscular strength, and race time for sub-elite flat water kayakers. J Sci Med Sport. 2010;13:537–42.
25. Kim SH, Ha KI, Jung MW, et al. Accelerated rehabilitation after arthroscopic Bankart repair for selected cases: a prospective randomized clinical study. Arthroscopy. 2003;19:722–31.
26. Peters P. Orthopedic problems in sport climbing. Wilderness Environ Med. 2001;12:100–10.
27. Paige TE, Fiore DC, Houston JD. Injury in traditional and sport rock climbing. Wilderness Environ Med. 1998;9:2–7.
28. Schöffl V, Hochholzer T, Winkelmann HP, Strecker W. Pulley injuries in rock climbers. Wilderness Environ Med. 2003;14:94–100.
29. Gabl M, Rangger C, Lutz M, et al. Disruption of the finger flexor pulley system in elite rock climbers. Am J Sports Med. 1998;26:651–5.
30. Schöffl I, Oppelt K, Jüngert J, et al. The influence of concentric and eccentric loading on the finger pulley system. J Biomech. 2009;42:2124–8.
31. Schweizer A, Frank O, Ochsner P, Jacob H. Friction between human finger flexor tendons and pulleys at high loads. J Biomech. 2003;36:63–71.
32. Schweizer A, Moor BK, Nagy L, Snedecker JG. Static and dynamic human flexor tendon-pulley interaction. J Biomech. 2009;42:1856–61.
33. Klauser A, Frauscher F, Bodner G, et al. Finger pulley injuries in extreme rock climbers: depiction with dynamic US1. Radiology. 2002;222:755–61.
34. Schweizer A. Biomechanical effectiveness of taping the A2 pulley in rock climbers. J Hand Ther. 2000;25:102–7.
35. Schöffl VR, Kuepper T. Injuries at the 2005 World Championships in rock climbing. Wilderness Environ Med. 2006;17:187–90.
36. Kubiak EN, Klugman JA, Bosco J. Hand injuries in rock climbers. Bull Hosp Jt Dis. 2006;64:172–7.
37. Vigouroux L, Quaine F, Labarre-Vila A, Moutet F. Estimation of finger muscle tendon tensions and pulley forces during specific sport-climbing grip techniques. J Biomech. 2006;39: 2583–92.
38. Warme WJ, Brooks D. The effect of circumferential taping on flexor tendon pulley failure in rock climbers. Am J Sports Med. 2000;28:674–8.
39. Bere T, Flørenes TW, Krosshaug T, et al. Mechanisms of anterior cruciate ligament injury in World Cup alpine skiing. Am J Sports Med. 2011;39:1421–9.
40. Frobell RB, Roos EM, Roos HP, Ranstam J, Lohmander LS. A randomized trial of treatment for acute anterior cruciate ligament tears. N Engl J Med. 2010;363:331–42.

41. Fitzgerald G, Axe MJ, Snyder-Mackler L. Proposed practice guidelines for nonoperative anterior cruciate ligament rehabilitation of physically active individuals. J Orthop Sports Phys Ther. 2000;30:194–203.
42. Hurd WJ, Axe MJ, Snyder-Mackler L. A 10-Year prospective trial of a patient management algorithm and screening examination for highly active individuals with anterior cruciate ligament injury. Am J Sports Med. 2008;36:4856.
43. Nyland J, Brand E, Fisher B. Update on rehabilitation following ACL reconstruction. Open Access J Sports Med. 2010;1:151–66.
44. Myer GD, Paterno MV, Ford KR, Quatman CE, Hewett TE. Rehabilitation after anterior cruciate ligament reconstruction: criteria-based progression through the return-to-sport phase. J Orthop Sports Phys Ther. 2006;36:385–402.
45. Wright RW, Preston E, Fleming BC, et al. A systematic review of anterior cruciate ligament reconstruction rehabilitation. J Knee Surg. 2008;21:225–34.
46. Tagesson S, Öberg B, Good L, Kvist J. A comprehensive rehabilitation program with quadriceps strengthening in closed versus open kinetic chain exercise in patients with anterior cruciate ligament deficiency. Am J Sports Med. 2008;36:298–307.
47. Morrissey MC, Drechsler WI, Morrissey D, et al. Effects of distally fixated versus nondistally fixated leg extensor resistance training on knee pain in the early period after anterior cruciate ligament reconstruction. Phys Ther. 2002;82:35–43.
48. Lautamies R, Harilainen A, Kettunen J, Sandelin J, Kujala UM. Isokinetic quadriceps and hamstring muscle strength and knee function 5 years after anterior cruciate ligament reconstruction: comparison between bone-patellar tendon-bone and hamstring tendon autografts. Knee Surg Sports Traumatol Arthrosc. 2008;16:1009–16.
49. Risberg MA, Holm I, Myklebust G, Engebretsen L. Neuromuscular training versus strength training during first 6 months after anterior cruciate ligament reconstruction: a randomized clinical trial. Phys Ther. 2007;87:737–50.
50. Fitzgerald GK, Axe MJ, Snyder-Mackler L. The efficacy of perturbation training in nonoperative anterior cruciate ligament rehabilitation programs for physically active individuals. Phys Ther. 2000;80:128–40.
51. Myer GD, Paterno MV, Ford KR, Hewett TE. Neuromuscular training techniques to target deficits before return to sport after anterior cruciate ligament reconstruction. J Strength Cond Res. 2008;22:987–1014.
52. Sterett WI, Briggs KK, Farley T, Steadman JR. Effect of functional bracing on knee injury in skiers with anterior cruciate ligament reconstruction. Am J Sports Med. 2006;34:1581–5.
53. Myklebust G, Steffen K. Prevention of ACL injuries: how, when and who? Knee Surg Sports Traumatol Arthrosc. 2009;17:857–8.
54. Soligard T, Myklebust G, Steffen K, et al. Comprehensive warm-up programme to prevent injuries in young female footballers: cluster randomised controlled trial. Br Med J. 2008;337:a2469.
55. Gilchrist J, Mandelbaum BR, Melancon H, et al. A randomized controlled trial to prevent noncontact anterior cruciate ligament injury in female collegiate soccer players. Am J Sports Med. 2008;36:1476–83.
56. Mandelbaum BR, Silvers HJ, Watanabe DS, et al. Effectiveness of a neuromuscular and proprioceptive training program in preventing anterior cruciate ligament injuries in female athletes. Am J Sports Med. 2005;33:1003–10.
57. Hewett TE, Myer GD, Ford KR, et al. Biomechanical measures of neuromuscular control and valgus loading of the knee predict anterior cruciate ligament injury risk in female athletes. Am J Sports Med. 2005;33:492–501.
58. Carmont M, Baruch M, Burnett C, Cairns P, Harrison J. Injuries sustained during marathon kayak competition: the devizes to Westminster race. Br J Sports Med. 2004;38:650–3.
59. du Toit P, Sole G, Bowerbank P, Noakes TD. Incidence and causes of tenosynovitis of the wrist extensors in long distance paddle canoeists. Br J Sports Med. 1999;33:105–9.
60. Palmer DH, Lane-Larsen CL. Helicopter skiing wrist injuries. A case report of "bugaboo forearm". Am J Sports Med. 1994;22:148–9.

61. Howard NJ. Peritendinitis crepitans: a muscle-effort syndrome. J Bone Joint Surg Am. 1937;19:447–59.
62. Grundberg A, Reagan D. Pathologic anatomy of the forearm: intersection syndrome. J Hand Surg. 1985;10:299–302.
63. Ankarath S. Chronic wrist pain: diagnosis and management. Curr Orthop. 2006;20:141–51.
64. May JJ, Lovell G, Hopkins WG. Effectiveness of 1 % diclofenac gel in the treatment of wrist extensor tenosynovitis in long distance kayakers. J Sci Med Sport. 2007;10:59–65.
65. Hanlon DP, Luellen JR. Intersection syndrome: a case report and review of the literature. J Emerg Med. 1999;17:969–71.
66. Servi JT. Wrist pain from overuse: detecting and relieving intersection syndrome. Physician Sports Med. 1997;25:41–4.
67. Cherington M. Hazards of bicycling: from handlebars to lightning. Semin Neurol. 2000;20:247–54.
68. Hankey GJ, Gubbay SS. Compressive mononeuropathy of the deep palmar branch of the ulnar nerve in cyclists. J Neurol Neurosurg Psychiatry. 1988;51:1588–90.
69. Patterson JMM, Jaggars MM, Boyer MI. Ulnar and median nerve palsy in long-distance cyclists. Am J Sports Med. 2003;31:585–9.
70. Richmond D. Handlebar problems in bicycling. Clin J Sports Med. 1994;13:165–73.
71. Maimaris C, Zadeh H. Ulnar nerve compression in the cyclist's hand: two case reports and review of the literature. Br J Sports Med. 1990;24:245–6.
72. Ruchelsman DE, Lee SK. Neurovascular injuries of the hand in athletes. Curr Orthop Prac. 2009;20:409–15.
73. Slane J, Timmerman M, Ploeg HL, Thelen DG. The influence of glove and hand position on pressure over the ulnar nerve during cycling. Clin Biomech. 2011;26:42–8.
74. Smith TM, Sawyer SF, Sizer PS, Brismée JM. The double crush syndrome: a common occurrence in cyclists with ulnar nerve neuropathy-a case–control study. Clin J Sports Med. 2008;18:55–61.
75. Butler DS, Matheson J, Boyaci A. The sensitive nervous system. Unley: NOIgroup Publications; 2000.
76. Neville V, Molloy J, Brooks J, Speedy D, Atkinson G. Epidemiology of injuries and illnesses in America's Cup yacht racing. Br J Sports Med. 2006;40:304–11.
77. Dyson R, Buchanan M, Hale T. Incidence of sports injuries in elite competitive and recreational windsurfers. Br J Sports Med. 2006;40:346–50.
78. Alricsson M, Werner S. Young elite cross-country skiers and low back pain – a 5-year study. Phys Ther Sport. 2006;7:181–4.
79. Debnath UK, Harshavardhana N, Scammell BE, Freeman BJC. Lumbar pars injury or spondylolysis-diagnosis and management. Orthop Trauma. 2009;23:109–16.
80. Allen J, De Jong MR. Sailing and sports medicine: a literature review. Br J Sports Med. 2006;40:587–93.
81. Standaert C, Herring S. Spondylolysis: a critical review. Br J Sports Med. 2000;34:415–22.
82. Standaert CJ, Herring SA. Expert opinion and controversies in sports and musculoskeletal medicine: the diagnosis and treatment of spondylolysis in adolescent athletes. Arch Phys Med Rehabil. 2007;88:537–40.
83. Iwamoto J, Sato Y, Takeda T, Matsumoto H. Return to sports activity by athletes after treatment of spondylolysis. World J Orthop. 2010;1:26–30.
84. Tan B, Aziz AR, Spurway NC, et al. Indicators of maximal hiking performance in Laser sailors. Eur J Appl Physiol. 2006;98:169–76.
85. Carlson C. Axial back pain in the athlete: pathophysiology and approach to rehabilitation. Curr Rev Musculoskelet Med. 2009;2:88–93.
86. Kujala UM, Taimela S, Oksanen A, Salminen JJ. Lumbar mobility and low back pain during adolescence. Am J Sports Med. 1997;25:363–8.
87. Krabak B, Kennedy DJ. Functional rehabilitation of lumbar spine injuries in the athlete. Sports Med Arthrosc Rev. 2008;16:47–54.
88. Neville V, Folland JP. The epidemiology and aetiology of injuries in sailing. Sports Med. 2009;39:129–45.

89. Brughelli M, Mendiguchia J, Nosaka K, et al. Effects of eccentric exercise on optimum length of the knee flexors and extensors during the preseason in professional soccer players. Phys Ther Sport. 2010;11:50–5.
90. Brockett CL, Morgan DL, Proske U. Human hamstring muscles adapt to eccentric exercise by changing optimum length. Med Sci Sports Exerc. 2001;33:783–90.
91. Iwai K, Nakazato K, Irie K, Fujimoto H, Nakajima H. Trunk muscle strength and disability level of low back pain in collegiate wrestlers. Med Sci Sports Exerc. 2004;36:1296–300.
92. Bergmark A. Stability of the lumbar spine. A study in mechanical engineering. Acta Orthop Scand Suppl. 1989;230:1–54.
93. O'Sullivan PB, Phyty DM, Twomey LT, Allison GT. Evaluation of specific stabilizing exercise in the treatment of chronic low back pain with radiologic diagnosis of spondylolysis or spondylolisthesis. Spine. 1997;22:2959–65.
94. McGill SM, Karpowicz A. Exercises for spine stabilization: motion/motor patterns, stability progressions, and clinical technique. Arch Phys Med Rehabil. 2009;90:118–26.
95. Hicks GE, Fritz JM, Delitto A, McGill SM. Preliminary development of a clinical prediction rule for determining which patients with low back pain will respond to a stabilization exercise program. Arch Phys Med Rehabil. 2005;86:1753–62.
96. Fritz JM, Whitman JM, Childs JD. Lumbar spine segmental mobility assessment: an examination of validity for determining intervention strategies in patients with low back pain. Arch Phys Med Rehabil. 2005;86:1745–52.
97. Hall SJ, Kent JA, Dickinson VR. Original research comparative assessment of novel sailing trapeze harness designs. J App Biomech. 1989;5:289–96.
98. Paxinos A, Walton J, Tzannes A, et al. Advances in the management of traumatic anterior and atraumatic multidirectional shoulder instability. Sports Med. 2001;31:819–28.
99. Landin D, Myers J, Thompson M, Castle R, Porter J. The role of the biceps brachii in shoulder elevation. J Electromyogr Kinesiol. 2008;18:270–5.
100. Bigliani LU, Kelkar R, Flatow EL, Pollock RG, Mow VC. Glenohumeral stability: biomechanical properties of passive and active stabilizers. Clin Orthop Rel Res. 1996;330:13–30.
101. Sakurai G, Tomita Y, Nakagaki K, Tamai S. Role of long head of biceps brachii in rotator cuff tendon failure: an EMG study. J Shoulder Elbow Surg. 1996;5:S135.
102. Toshiaki A, Itoi E, Minagawa H, et al. Cross-sectional area of the tendon and the muscle of the biceps brachii in shoulders with rotator cuff tears. Acta Orthop. 2005;76:509–12.
103. Ludewig PM, Cook TM. Alterations in shoulder kinematics and associated muscle activity in people with symptoms of shoulder impingement. Phys Ther. 2000;80:276–91.
104. Cools AM, Cambier D, Witvrouw EE. Screening the athlete's shoulder for impingement symptoms: a clinical reasoning algorithm for early detection of shoulder pathology. Br J Sports Med. 2008;42:628–35.
105. Ejnisman B, Monteiro GC, Andreoli CV, de Castro Pochini A. Disorder of the long head of the biceps tendon. Br J Sports Med. 2010;44:347.
106. Ryu JHJ, Pedowitz RA. Rehabilitation of biceps tendon disorders in athletes. Clin J Sports Med. 2010;29:229–46.
107. Ardic F, Kahraman Y, Kacar M, et al. Shoulder impingement syndrome: relationships between clinical, functional, and radiologic findings. Am J Phys Med Rehabil. 2006;85:53–60.
108. Green S, Buchbinder R, Hetrick S. Physiotherapy interventions for shoulder pain. Cochrane Database Syst Rev. 2003;CD004258.
109. Tempelhof S, Rupp S, Seil R. Age-related prevalence of rotator cuff tears in asymptomatic shoulders. J Shoulder Elbow Surg. 1999;8:296–9.
110. Cools AM, Dewitte V, Lanszweert F, et al. Rehabilitation of scapular muscle balance. Am J Sports Med. 2007;35:1744–51.
111. Kibler WB, Sciascia AD, Uhl TL, Tambay N, Cunningham T. Electromyographic analysis of specific exercises for scapular control in early phases of shoulder rehabilitation. Am J Sports Med. 2008;36:1789–98.

112. Escamilla RF, Yamashiro K, Paulos L, Andrews JR. Shoulder muscle activity and function in common shoulder rehabilitation exercises. Sports Med. 2009;39:663–85.
113. Kibler WB. The role of the scapula in athletic shoulder function. Am J Sports Med. 1998;26:325–37.
114. Panjabi MM. Clinical spinal instability and low back pain. J Electromyogr Kinesiol. 2003;13:371–9.
115. Taylor J, Taylor S. Psychological approaches to sports injury rehabilitation. Gaithersburg: Lippincott Williams & Wilkins; 1997.
116. Lind E, Ekkekakis P, Vazou S. The affective impact of exercise intensity that slightly exceeds the preferred level. J Health Psych. 2008;13:464–8.
117. Pizzari T, Taylor NF, McBurney H, Feller JA. Adherence to rehabilitation after anterior cruciate ligament reconstructive surgery: implications for outcome. J Sports Rehabil. 2005;14:201–5.
118. White A, Hardy L. An in-depth analysis of the uses of imagery by high-level slalom canoeists and artistic gymnasts. Sports Psych. 1998;12:377–403.

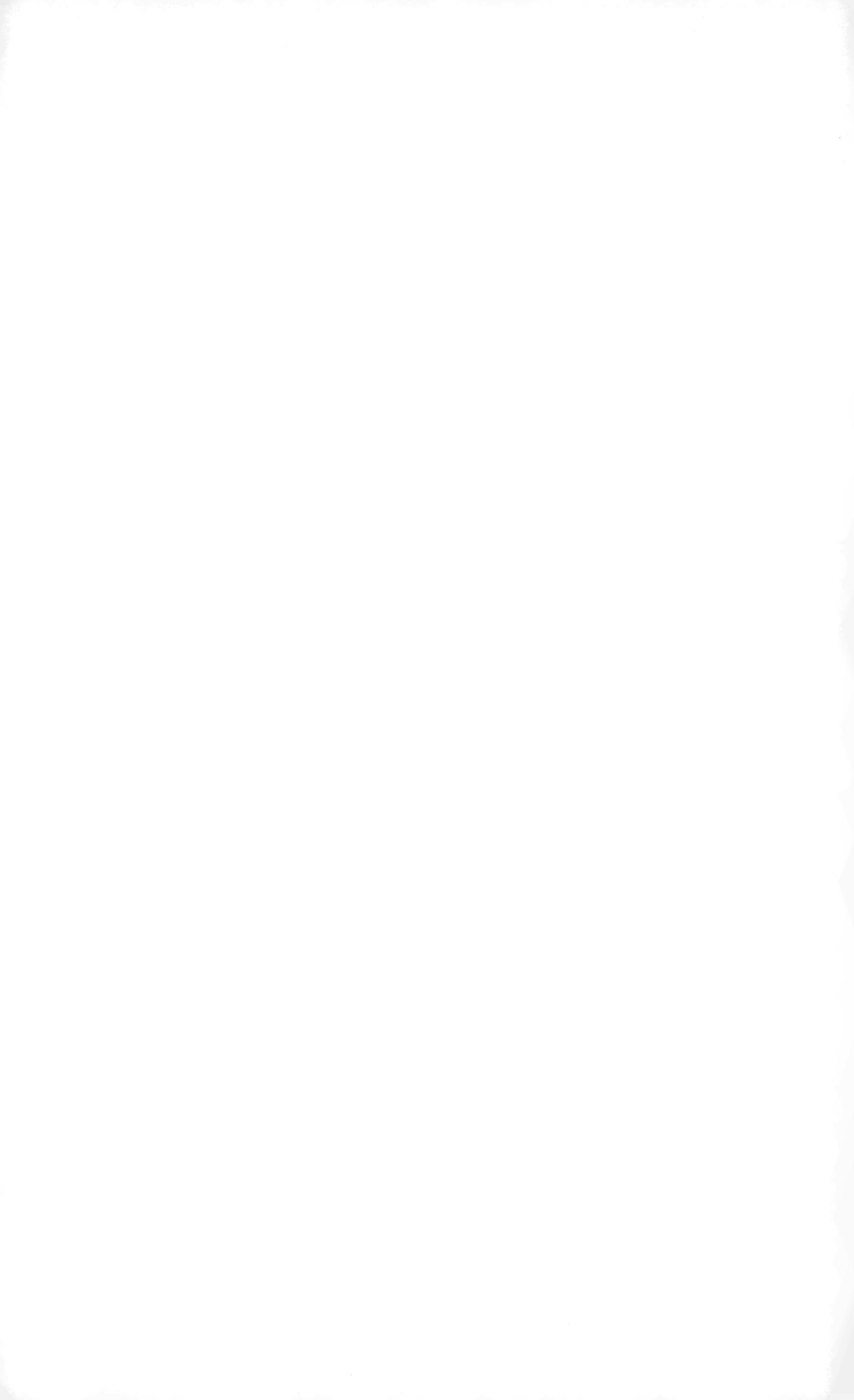

Index

A
Abdominal viscera, mountain biking injuries, 240
ACL. *See* Anterior cruciate ligament (ACL)
Acute mountain sickness (AMS), 299
Alpine skiing
  axial injuries, 57–58
  backcountry injuries, 50
  equipment
    carving skis, 41
    helmets, 42–43
    off-piste (backcountry) equipment, 44–46
    outer clothing layers, 42
    ski binding, 39
    sunglasses and goggles, 43
  helicopter trauma service, 59–61
  injury classification, 47
  injury risk, 44–45, 47
  lower limb injuries
    ankle injuries, 52–53
    femur, 54
    knee injuries, 51–52
    lower leg injuries, 52, 53
  origin and development, 37–38
  prevention measures
    boots and bindings, 62
    equipment options, 58
    instructors, 61, 62
    self-test for ski bindings, 63
    ski patrols, 61
  professional snowboarders, injuries, 50
  risk of death on slopes, 46
  treatment and rehabilitation, 58
  upper limb injuries
    shoulder, 54–55
    thumb, 55–56

Altitude, 280–281, 298
America's Cup yacht racing, 209, 214, 216–217
AMS. *See* Acute mountain sickness (AMS)
Ankle injuries, alpine skiing and snowboarding, 52, 53
Anorexia athletica, climbing, 29
Anterior cruciate ligament (ACL)
  injury, in skiing, 51, 52
  rupture, rehabilitation, 346
    return to sport, 348
    ski-specific neuromuscular rehabilitation on fitter, 348
    treatment modalities, 347
Aortic rupture, paragliding, 262
Arthritis, climbing, 24–25
Association of Surfing Professionals (ASP), 145
Automatic reserve activation devices (AAD), 75
Axial injuries, alpine skiing and snowboarding, 57–58

B
Back injuries, whitewater paddling, 129
Back pain
  sailing, 218
  surfing, 162–164
  windsurfing, 198–199
BASE jumping, 304
  danger of, 103–104
  equipment
    canopy system, 97
    parachuting systems, 97–99
    protective gear and assisting equipment, 99–100

BASE jumping (*cont.*)
  fatalities, 102–103
  injuries, 100–102
  medical aspects
    emergency/prehospital care, 107–108
    hospital care, 108
  object strike and bad landing, 101
  origins of sport and development
    BASE number, 95
    concept, 94–96
    events and records, 96–97
    fixed object jumps, 92–94
    legality of, 96
    parachute, 92
  personality characteristics, of jumpers
    research findings implication, 308–312
    Temperament and Character Inventory (TCI), 306–310
  prevention measures
    courses, 109
    environment issues, 109–110
    mental aspects, temperament score, 110–111
    weather conditions, 110
  rehabilitation, 108–109
  vs. skydiving, 95, 104–105
  wingsuits and proximity flying, 105–107
Blisters, whitewater paddlers, 130, 134
Bodyboarding and bodysurfing, 147–148
Bosu Ball™, 334
Bouldering, 9, 10, 30
Building, Antenna, Span and Earth (BASE) jumping. *See* BASE jumping
Bungee jumping, 320

C
Canopy formation, 71, 72
Cercarial dermatitis/swimmer's itch, 199–200
Climbing
  anorexia athletica, 29
  A2 pulley rupture, rehabilitation
    grip strength measurement, dynamometer, 345, 346
    MCP joint, 344, 345
    return to sport, 346
    treatment modalities, 344–346
  bouldering, 9, 10
  equipment, 13–14
  grading systems, 10, 11

  ice climbing, 10, 11, 31–32
  injuries and overuse syndromes
    arthritis and osteoarthrosis, 24–25
    chronic exertional compartment syndrome of forearms, 28
    crimp and hanging grip technique, 17
    diagnoses, frequent localization, 18
    Dupuytren contracture, 28
    feet, 28–29
    finger injuries, clinical examination and diagnostics of, 16–18
    fingers of rock climbers, 18
    fractures, epiphyseal fractures, 25–26
    joint capsular damage and collateral ligament injury, 24
    lumbrical shift syndrome, 26–27
    normal musculoskeletal adaptations, 19, 20
    pulley injuries, 19, 21–23
    tendon strains and ruptures, 25
    tenosynovitis, 22–24
  injury and fatality risk
    ice climbing, 12
    indoor climbing, 12
    mountaineering, 13
    traditional climbing, sport climbing, and bouldering, 12
  injury prevention, 333–335
    bolts, 30
    bouldering, 30
    preventive measures, 31
  mountaineering, 32–33
  sport climbing/free climbing, with bolts, 9
  training in rock climbing, 14–16
Cold/heat illness, whitewater paddlers, 131
Collateral ligament injury, 24

D
Dehydration/overhydration avoidance, mountain running, 297
Dinghy sailing
  catamarans, 207, 208
  crew, 205, 207
  injuries
    causalgia, 212–213
    cramped conditions, 213
    incidence, 210–211
    region, 211
    type, 211–212
  Olympic triangle, 207, 208
  trapeze, 205, 207

Index

Downhill skier, injury prevention, 333, 334
Dupuytren contracture, 28

E
Elbow injuries
    snowboarding, 56
    whitewater paddling, 128
Elbow pain, sailing, 218
Endocrine aspects and responses
    diabetes, 322
    mental stress
        bungee jumping, 320
        caving, 320
        rock climbing, 320–321
        skydiving and paragliding, 321
    to physical activity, exercise, 316
        catecholamines, 317
        cortisol, 317
        fluid and electrolyte balance, 317
        gonadal function, 318
        growth hormone, 317
        prolactin, 317–318
    research, 316
    ultra-endurance extreme events
        Hawaiian Ironman, 318
        marathon, 318–319
        mountain climbers, 319–320
        testosterone to cortisol ratio, 319
Endurance running, 277, 278
Epicondylitis, whitewater paddling, 128
Epiphyseal fractures, climbing, 26
Exercise, hormonal response, 316–318
Exertional compartment syndrome of forearms, 28
Extension-related low back pain
    front plank progressions, 353
    lumbopelvic muscle function, optimizing, 352–353
    return to sport and prevention, 353–354
    sailors and windsurfers, 351, 352
    treatment modalities and rehabilitation, 351–353
External auditory canal exostosis (EAE), 166

F
Facial injuries, mountain biking, 237–238
Finger injuries, climbing, 16–18
Forearm exertional compartment syndrome, 28, 127–128

Fractures
    climbing, 25–26
    surfing, distribution of, 151
    whitewater injuries, 124, 134
Front plank progressions, low back pain, 353

G
Gastrointestinal illness, whitewater paddlers, 131, 138
Glenohumeral joints, 330–332
    external rotation, 342, 343
Global Positioning System (GPS), paragliding, 251
Ground Force 360 device™, 335
Guyon's canal, 350

H
Harm avoidance (HA) scores, 309–310
Hazardous marine animals, surfing, 166, 167
Head injuries
    mountain biking, 237–238
    paragliding, 261
Hormonal response. *See* Endocrine aspects and responses

I
Ice climbing, 10–12
    equipment, 14
    injuries, 31, 32
    overuse syndromes, 32
Infectious diseases, windsurfing, 200
Injury prevention
    climbing, 30–31
    forward walk out using Woggler™, 328
    injury risk factors, 326
    performance enhancement, 326–327
    periodization in training, 327–329
    self-and skilled peer assessments, 329
    specific adaptations to imposed demands
        climber, 333–335
        downhill skier, 333, 334
        kayaker, 330–333
        upper-lower extremity raise from quadruped position, 330
    S-W-O-T analysis, 327
    upper and lower extremity strength, trunk and core regions, 325, 326
    windsurfing, 200–201
International Canoe Federation (ICF), 114

International Parachuting Commission (IPC), 77, 78
Intersection syndrome, 349–350

J
Jellyfish stings, windsurfing, 199
Joint capsular damage, 24
Joint strains, whitewater injuries, 124

K
Kayaker, injury prevention
    athlete's tissue type, assessment, 333
    forward lunge with resisted rotator cuff and scapular retractor muscle strengthening, 331, 332
    glenohumeral joints and rotator cuff muscles, 330–332
    long-sitting paddling simulation on stability ball, 331
Kayaking, 114, 115, 117, 119, 122–124, 127
    traumatic anterior shoulder dislocation, rehabilitation, 340, 341, 343
Kite surfing
    equipment
        board, 177
        harness, 179
        helmet and board leash, 179
        lines and bar, 178, 179
        quick-release system, 178
        types of kite, 177–178
        wetsuit, 179
        wind conditions, 180
    fractures, 184
    injury and fatality rates
        body sites, 181
        mechanism, 182
        types of, 182
    origin and development, 173–175
    prevention measures, 185–187
    treatments and rehabilitation, 183–185
Knee injuries, 282
    skiing, 51–52

L
Lacerations
    surfing, distribution of, 151
    treatment, whitewater injuries, 133
Leading edge inflatable (LEI) kites, 177, 178
Leashes, surfing, 147, 158, 170
Leg injuries, Alpine skiing, 52, 53
Leptospirosis, whitewater paddlers, 131

Lisfranc dislocation/fracture, windsurfing, 195, 196
Long head of biceps (LHB) tendinopathy, rehabilitation, 354–355
Low back pain (LBP), extension-related, 351–354
Lower extremity injuries
    paragliding, 260–261
    windsurfing
        chronic injuries, foot straps, 195, 197
        knee and leg injuries, 195
        Lisfranc dislocation/fracture, 195, 196
Lower limb injuries
    alpine skiing and snowboarding, 51–54
    mountain biking, 240–241
Lumbrical shift syndrome, 26–27

M
Management of injured extreme sports athlete
    epidemiology, 2–3
    rehabilitation, 4–5
    resuscitation and initial management, 3
    temperament of, 2
    treatment decisions, 3–4
Marathon, endocrine responses, 318–319
Medial collateral ligament (MCL) injury, in skiing, 51
Metacarpophalangeal (MCP) joint, 344, 345
Mountain biking injuries
    adventure racing, 241
    cross-country races, 226, 241
    downhill riding, 226
    injury patterns
        abdominal viscera, 240
        head and face, 237–238
        lower limbs, 240–241
        perineum, 240
        spinal injuries, 239
        upper limbs, 239
    injury prevention, 242–243
    injury rates and demographics
        Canada, 236
        disc brakes, 236
        falling over handlebars, 235
        literature, 228–233
        Mammoth Mountain Ski Area in United States, 234
        NORBA, 228, 235
        questionnaire survey, 228, 235, 236
        recreational mountain biking, 237
    origins of, 225–226
    suspension systems, 227, 228

Index

Mountaineering, 13, 32–33, 303–304
Mountaineers, personality characteristics
   research findings implication, 308–312
   Temperament and Character Inventory (TCI), 306–310
Mountain running
   acute injury, 292–293
   causes of injury
      fatigue, 290
      footwear, 290
      orthotics, 291
      trauma, 289
   chronic injury, 293
   conservative physiotherapy treatment
      connective tissue network, 293, 294
      progressive resistance exercises, 294
   equipment
      altitude, 280–281
      climate, 280
      clothing, 278–279
      food and drink, 280
      footwear, 279–280
      safety requirements, 281
   fatalities, 283
   injury rates, 281–284
   marathon kit list, 279
   origin and development, 274–276
   preventative measures, injury and illness
      acute mountain sickness (AMS), 299
      carbohydrate, 297
      compression garments, 295–296
      core stability and pelvic muscles strengthening, 295
      dangers of training and racing at altitude, 298
      dehydration/overhydration, avoidance, 297
      fat, 298
      immune system, effects on, 296
      protein, 297–298
      running footwear, monitoring of, 295
      stress fractures, factors, 296
      vitamins and minerals, 298
      warm-up, 295
   runner's knee
      cardiac damage, 289
      clinical examination, 285–286
      minor lesions, 286, 288
      pelvic tilt in uphill running, 286
      stress fractures, 288
      superior hamstring lesion and associated structures, 287
      symptoms and signs, 285, 286
      tendon injuries, 288
      ultramarathon, tenosynovitis, 288
      treatment, 291–292
Mount Kinabalu International Climbathon, 277
Muscle strains, whitewater injuries, 124, 136–137
Myelopathy, surfing, 164

N

National Off-Road Bicycling Association (NORBA), 228, 235
Neck pain, surfing, 162–164
Nerve injuries, windsurfing, 197–198
Non-avalanche-related snow immersion death (NARSID), 46

O

Osteoarthrosis, climbing, 25
Otitis externa, surfing, 166
Overuse injuries, rehabilitation
   extension-related low back pain, 351–354
   long head of biceps tendinopathy, 354–355
   ulnar nerve neuropathy, 350–351
   wrist extensor tenosynovitis and intersection syndrome, 349–350

P

Parachute
   BASE jumping, 92, 97–99
   history of, 70
   skydiving, 73, 74, 85–86
Paragliding
   aero-acrobatic maneuver and stunt flying, 256
   cause of accidents, 267–269
   collapse (in-flight deflation), 254–255
   competitive flying disciplines, 255, 256
   cross-country flying, 254
   definition, 248
   development of, 248–249
   endocrine responses, 321
   equipment
      glide ratio, 250
      GPS, 251
      harnesses, 249, 250
      inflatable parafoils, 249
      paraglider, 249–251
      radio, 251
      tethered launches, 251
      variometer, 251

Paragliding (*cont.*)
  injuries, 255
    distribution, 257, 258
    fatality, 262–263
    head injuries, 261
    lower extremities injuries, 260–261
    pelvic injuries, 262
    soft tissue injuries, 262
    spinal injuries and related mechanism, 257, 259–260
    thoracic and abdominal injuries, 262
    upper extremity injuries, 261
  injury patterns and causes
    accidents distribution, during flight phases, 265
    in-flight accidents, 266
    landing accidents, 266–268
    mechanisms, 264, 265
    takeoff/launching accidents, 263, 266
  landing, 253–254
  launching
    forward, 252, 253
    reverse, 252
    towed launch, 252–253
  pilot error, 267
  ram-air design paraglider, 248, 249
  safety requirements and prevention, 269–270
  slope soaring, 254
  speed bar, 252
  spiral dive, 252
  steering, 252
  thermal flying, 254
  training level, 270
Pelvic injuries, paragliding, 262
Perineum, mountain biking injuries, 240
Personality characteristics
  opioid-dependent subjects and paragliders, 305
  research findings implication, mountaineers and BASE jumpers
    cooperativeness, 311
    harm avoidance (HA), 309–310
    nonathletes group, 312
    novelty seeking (NS), 309
    reward dependence (RD), 311
    self-directedness, 311
    self-transcendence (ST), 312
    trauma, 310–311
  sensation seeking (SS), 304–305, 309
  surfing, 305
  Temperament and Character Inventory (TCI)
    dimensions, 306
    mountaineers and BASE jumpers, 306–308
Personal watercraft (PWC), 144, 145
Pilot chute, BASE jumping, 97–99
Post-traumatic stress disorder (PTSD), 311
Proximity flying, BASE jumping, 105–107
Pulley injuries, climbing, 19
  annular, therapy guidelines for, 21
  cadaver image in biomechanic strength test, 23
  diagnostic-therapeutic algorithm, 23
  normal and ruptured, ultrasound image of, 22
Pulley rupture
  A2, 22, 23, 344–346
  rehabilitation, 344–346

R

Rafting. *See* Whitewater canoeing and rafting
Ram-air design paraglider, 248, 249
Ram-air parachute, 73
Rehabilitation, 4–5
  acute injuries, 339
    anterior cruciate ligament rupture, 346–348
    A2 pulley rupture, 344–346
    traumatic anterior shoulder dislocation, 340–344
  BASE jumping, 108–109
  common aspects of, 355
  overuse injuries
    extension-related low back pain, 351–354
    long head of biceps tendinopathy, 354–355
    ulnar nerve neuropathy, 350–351
    wrist extensor tenosynovitis and intersection syndrome, 349–350
  psychological aspects, 355–356
  whitewater paddling, 135
Reserve parachute, 73, 75
Resuscitation and initial management, of injured athlete, 3
Rib fractures, whitewater paddling, 129–130
Rock climbing, 8–12. *See also* Climbing
  campus board training, 14,Z15
  endocrine responses, 320–321
  injuries and overuse syndromes in fingers, 18

Index

Rotator cuff tendinopathy, 128, 137
Roy-Camille classification of sacral fractures, 260
Runner's knee, 285–289

S
Safe Sea™, 200
Sailing. *See also* Yacht sailing
   back pain, 218
   definition, 203
   dinghy sailing (*see* Dinghy sailing)
   elbow pain, 218
   fitness training, 218–220
   hiking, 219
   injury incidence and mechanisms, 210–217
   injury prevention and rehabilitation, 220–221
   knee pain, 218
   origin of, 203–205
   racing, categories and subclasses, 205
   speed records, 205, 206
Seabather's eruption/sea lice, 199
Seafloor, acute injuries, 157–159
Sea ulcers, 168, 169
Sensation seeking (SS), 304–305, 309
Shoulder dislocation
   traumatic anterior, rehabilitation, 340–344
   whitewater injuries, 125, 126, 134, 136
   windsurfing, 197
Shoulder injuries
   alpine skiing and snowboarding, 54–55
   whitewater paddling, 128–129, 137
Shoulder rehabilitation, surfing, 165
Skiing. *See* Alpine skiing
Skin
   infections, whitewater paddlers, 130, 133–134
   problems, windsurfing, 199–200
   surfing, 165, 166
Skydiving
   vs. BASE jumping, 95, 104–105
   endocrine responses, 321
   equipment
      automatic reserve activation devices (AAD), 75
      parachute, 73, 74
      reserve parachute, 73, 75
      supplemental oxygen, 76–77
      wing loading, 75, 76
   fatalities
      IPC, 77, 78
      jump plane crashes, 78–79
      off drop zone landings, 78
   history, 70–71
   injuries
      distribution of, 80
      fracture by miscalculated landing, 82
      mechanisms in reported nonfatal injury, 79, 81
   prevention measures
      after subaquatic diving, decompression sickness, 87
      aviation school considerations, 85
      human factor, 88
      hypoxia, 86
      impact energy, 87–88
      medical fitness, 86
      parachute flight and landing, 85–86
      water landings, 87
   sporting events
      canopy formation, 71, 72
      free fall formations, 71, 72
      high-altitude jumps, 71
      speed skydiving, 71
   treatments
      golden hour, 83
      immediate care, 83
      initial hospital care, 84
      local emergency services, 80, 82–83
      rehabilitation, 84
Skyrunning, 280, 281
   categories, 275, 277
   origin and development, 277
Snowboarding. *See also* Alpine skiing
   backcountry injuries, 50
   elbow injuries, 56
   equipment, 41–42
      helmets, 42–43
      off-piste (backcountry) equipment, 44
   injury classification, 48–50
   injury risk, 44–45, 47, 49
   knee injuries, 52
   origin and development, 37–38
   prevention measures, 58, 61–62, 64
   professional snowboarders, injuries, 50
   risk of death on slopes, 46
   treatment and rehabilitation, 58
   wrist injuries, 55, 56
Snow kiting
   equipment, 180
   injury and fatality rates, 182–183
   origin and development, 175–177
   prevention measures, 185–187
   treatments and rehabilitation, 183–185
Soft tissue injuries, paragliding, 262

Spinal injuries
  alpine skiing and snowboarding, 57
  mountain biking, 239
  paragliding
    lumbar spine, 260
    thoracolumbar region, 259, 260
    vertebral fracture distribution, 259
  surfing, 157, 158
  windsurfing, 199
Spondylolysis, surfing, 163, 164
Stand-up paddle surfing (SUP), 145, 147
Supraspinatus tendon, whitewater injuries, 129
Surfboard, acute injuries, 151, 155–157
Surfing
  acute injuries
    aerial maneuvers, 160, 161
    anatomic distribution, 149, 151
    cervical immobilization, 158, 159
    fin induced chin and thigh laceration, 156
    hospital-based studies, 152–153
    mechanisms of injury, 151, 154
    outpatient studies, 150
    rip currents, 160
    seafloor, 157–159
    surfboard, 151, 155–157
    tube riding, 157, 158
    tympanic membrane (TM) rupture, 159
    wave-force injuries, 159–160
    wave-riding injuries, 160–162
  ASP, 145
  cut-back maneuver, 146
  demographics, 145–146
  environmental injuries
    hazardous marine life, 166, 167
    skin, eyes, and ears, 165–166
  equipment
    blanks, 147
    bodyboarding and bodysurfing, 147–148
    leashes, 147, 170
    longboards and shortboards, 147
    SUP and tow-in, 147
    wetsuits, 148
  fatalities, 149
  floater, 146
  history, 143–145
  injury prevention
    equipment, 169–170
    personal protective gear, 170
    safety recommendations, 169
  injury rates and risk factors, 148–149
  overuse injuries
    neck and back pain, 162–164
    upper extremity pain, 164–165
  personal watercraft (PWC), 144, 145
  stand-up paddle surfing (SUP), 145
  traumatic anterior shoulder dislocation, rehabilitation, 340, 341, 343
  wound care, 168–169

T
Temperament and Character Inventory (TCI)
  dimensions, 306
  mountaineers and BASE jumpers
    demographic and injury findings, 307
    HA scores, 309, 310
    high risk, 306
    with normative population, comparison, 308
    Spearman correlation coefficients, 308
Temperament traits, 2
Tendinopathy, whitewater injuries, 128, 137–138
Tendon injuries, runner's knee, 288
Tendon strains and ruptures, climbing, 25
Tenosynovitis
  climbing, 22–24
  whitewater injuries, 127
Thumb injuries, alpine skiing, 55–56
Traumatic anterior shoulder dislocation, rehabilitation
  glenohumeral external rotation, 342, 343
  kayaking and surfing, 340, 341, 343
  return to sport, 342, 344
  treatment modalities, 340–342
Tympanic membrane (TM) rupture, surfing, 159

U
Ulnar nerve neuropathy, rehabilitation, 350–351
Ultra-endurance extreme events, endocrine responses, 318–320
Upper extremity
  pain, surfing, 164–165
  windsurfing injuries
    nerve injuries, 197–198
    shoulder dislocation, 197
Upper limb injuries
  alpine skiing and snowboarding, 54–56
  mountain biking, 239

Index

V
Variometer, 251

W
Weil's disease, whitewater paddlers, 131
Wetsuits, surfing, 148
Whitewater canoeing and rafting
    accidents and injuries, overview of, 121–124
    acute injuries
        acute muscle strains and joint sprains, 124
        fractures, lacerations, and abrasions, 124
        major traumatic injuries, 125
        shoulder dislocation, 125, 126
    buoyancy, 119, 120
    chronic injuries
        back injuries, 129
        elbow injuries, 128
        hand, wrist, and forearm injuries, 126–128
        pelvic and lower limb injuries, 130
        recreational open canoeist, grade II rapid, 128
        rib fractures, 129–130
        shoulder injuries, 128–129
        tendinitis, 127
        tenosynovitis, 127
    craft, 117, 119
    environmental injuries and illnesses
        cold/heat illness, 131
        gastrointestinal illness, 131
        leptospirosis, 131
        skin, 130
    equipment, 119–120
    injury incidence, 123
    and kayaks, 117, 119, 122–124, 127
    origins and development of paddle sports
        competitive whitewater disciplines, 115–120
        crossbow stroke, C1 paddler, 116
        freestyle kayak paddlers, spectacular maneuvers, 118
        International Scale of River Difficulty, 114, 115
        kayak paddler, 121
        surf paddlers, top turn high, 120
    paddle design, 119, 122
    prevention
        of accidents, 132
        of illness, 133
        of injury, 132–133
    safety recommendations, 120–122
    submersion accidents, 122, 123
    treatment and rehabilitation
        abrasions, lacerations, and contusions, 133
        chronic shoulder injury, 137
        elbow, wrist, and forearm tendinopathies, 137–138
        fractures, 134, 135
        gastrointestinal illness, 138
        muscular strains, 136–137
        shoulder dislocation, 134, 136
        skin and blisters, 133–134
Windsurfing
    equipment and technique, 192
    formula windsurfing, 190
    infectious diseases, 200
    injuries
        back pain, 198–199
        body area, 194
        brain and spinal cord injury, 199
        incidence, 192–194
        lower extremities, 194–197
        prevention, 200–201
        type, 193
        uphauling, 193, 194
        upper extremities, 197–198
    origins and development, 189–191
    pumping technique, 201
    skin problems, 199–200
    wave jumping and riding, 190, 191
Wing loading, 75
Wingsuits, 75, 76
    and proximity flying, BASE jumping, 105–107
Woggler™, 328
Wound care, surfing, 168–169
Wrist extensor tenosynovitis, 349–350
    whitewater injuries, 127
Wrist injuries, snowboarding, 55, 56

Y
Yacht sailing
    America's Cup yacht racing, 209, 214, 216–217
    injuries
        causalgia, 216–217
        grinders and bowmen, 214, 216
        incidence, 214, 215
        region, 214–215
    origin of, 204–205

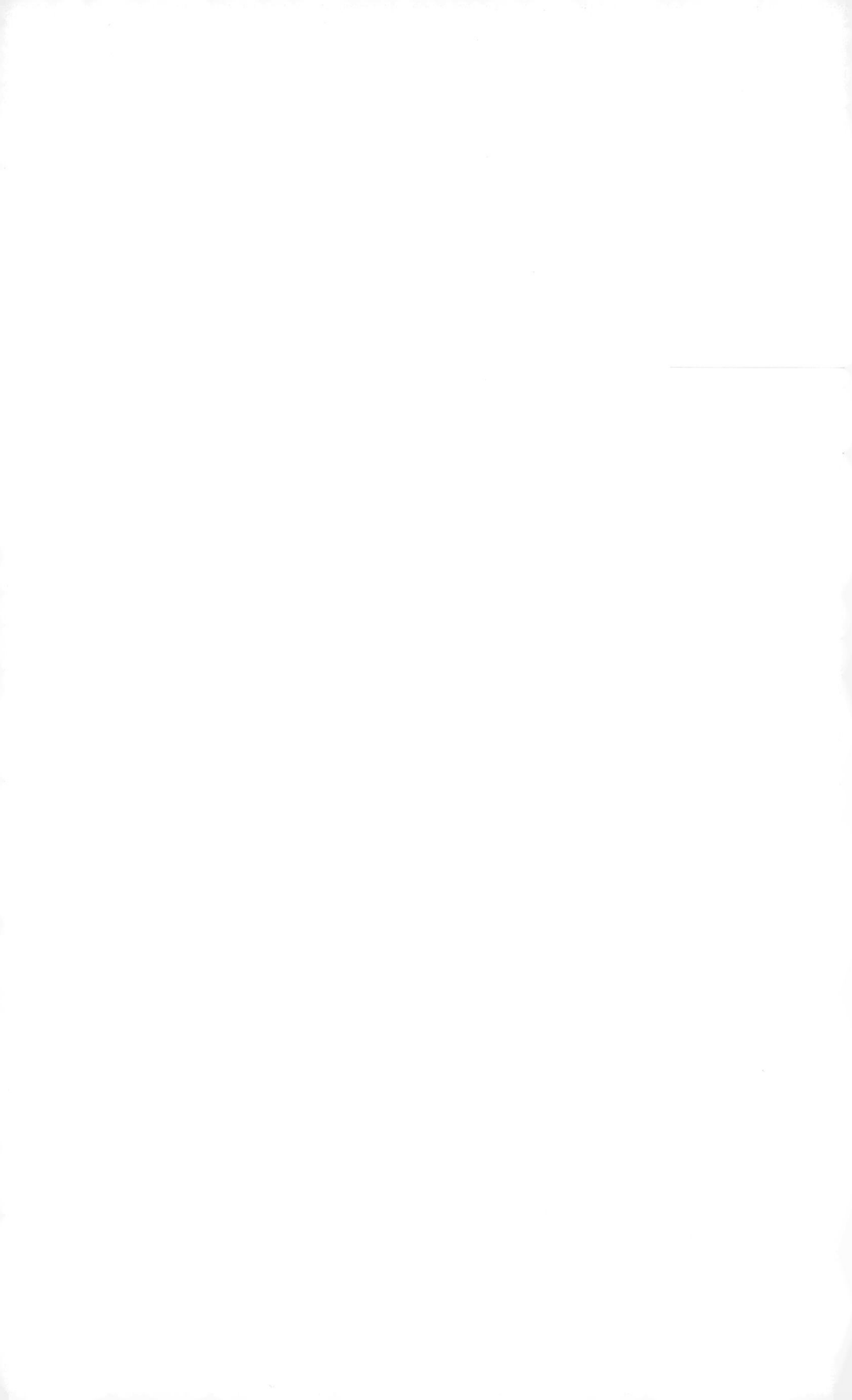